ESSENTIALS OF ANATOMY AND PHYSIOLOGY FOR COMMUNICATION DISORDERS

First Edition

ESSENTIALS OF ANATOMY AND PHYSIOLOGY FOR COMMUNICATION DISORDERS

First Edition

J. Anthony Seikel, PhD
Idaho State University

David G. Drumright, BS

Paula Seikel, PhD
Idaho State University

Illustrations and Photography by Sarah Moore

Essentials of Anatomy and Physiology for Communication Disorders

First Edition

by J. Anthony Seikel, PhD, David G. Drumright, BS, and Paula Seikel, PhD

Vice President, Health Care Business Unit:

William Brottmiller

Editorial Director:

Cathy L. Esperti

Acquisitions Editor:

Kalen Conerly

Developmental Editor:

Juliet Byington

Marketing Director:

Jennifer McAvey

Marketing Coordinator:

Chris Manion

Technology Project Specialist:

Mary Colleen Liburdi

Production Editor:

Anne Sherman

Project Editor:

Daniel Branagh

Art and Design Specialist:

Jay Purcell

Library of Congress Cataloging-in-Publication Data

Seikel, John A.
    Essentials of anatomy and physiology for communication disorders / J. Anthony Seikel, David G. Drumright, Paula Seikel; illustrations and photography by Sarah Moore.—1st ed.
        p. ; cm.
    Includes bibliographical references and index.
    ISBN 0-7668-5946-0

1. Language disorders. 2. Language disorders—Physiological aspects. 3. Anatomy. 4. Physiology.
    [DNLM: 1. Communication Disorders—physiopathology. 2. Hearing—physiology. 3. Nervous System—anatomy & histology. 4. Respiratory Physiology. 5. Respiratory System—anatomy & histology. 6. Speech—physiology. WL 340.2 S459e 2004] I. Drumright, David G. II. Seikel, Paula. III. Title.
RC423.S44 2004
616.85'5—dc22   2003026992

Notice to the Reader

Publisher does not warrant or guarantee any of the products described herein or perform any independent analysis in connection with any of the product information contained herein. Publisher does not assume, and expressly disclaims, any obligation to obtain and include information other than that provided to it by the manufacturer.

The reader is expressly warned to consider and adopt all safety precautions that might be indicated by the activities described herein and to avoid all potential hazards. By following the instructions contained herein, the reader willingly assumes all risks in connection with such instructions.

The publisher makes no representations or warranties of any kind, including but not limited to, the warranties of fitness for particular purpose or merchantability, nor are any such representations implied with respect to the material set forth herein, and the publisher takes no responsibility with respect to such material. The publisher shall not be liable for any special, consequential, or exemplary damages resulting, in whole or part, from the reader's use of, or reliance upon, this material.

Contents

Preface

We are pleased to have the opportunity to take you on a tour of the human speech and hearing mechanisms "from the inside out." You obviously have an interest in the systems of communication. We hope that by giving you an in-depth look at the systems of speech, language, and hearing, we might enhance your appreciation of your chosen profession. Certainly, your knowledge of anatomy and physiology will enhance your work in helping the people you serve in the future.

As you will soon see, the physical systems of communication are extraordinarily complex. We hope that, through reading this text, you will gain the same awe we have for the communicative act.

DEVELOPMENT OF ESSENTIALS OF ANATOMY AND PHYSIOLOGY FOR COMMUNICATION DISORDERS

This text arose from a clear need in the field for a text geared to the needs of the speech-language pathology assistant (SLPA). We recognized that those who have selected this career path need specific, relevant knowledge as they enter the workforce. In choosing material to include in the text, we gained valuable insight from instructors in SLPA programs and we believe that the materials we have provided will meet your needs. We have placed anatomy in a clinical framework with hopes that the person is always kept in mind as more than just the sum of the anatomical parts.

ORGANIZATION OF ESSENTIALS OF ANATOMY AND PHYSIOLOGY FOR COMMUNICATION DISORDERS

This text takes a systemic approach to the study of anatomy and physiology. The first chapter sets the stage, providing you with terminology and background necessary to comprehend the world of anatomy. The succeeding chapters progress through the systems of communication, beginning with the energy source for speech (Chapter 2, Anatomy and Physiology of Respiration), and followed by the sound source for speech (Chapter 3, Anatomy and Physiology of Phonation). We have combined articulation and resonance (Chapter 4, Anatomy and Physiology of Articulation and Resonance) with the philosophy that the resonatory system appropriately fits in the domain of moveable resonance systems (articulation). Chapter 5 (Anatomy and Physiology of Hearing) presents the essentials of hearing, and Chapter 6 (Neuroanatomy and Neurophysiology) focuses on essential components of the nervous system, again with particular attention to the elements most likely to be of use to the SLPA. At the back of the text, you'll find a complete glossary of the terms defined in the margins and an index to make this text an even more valuable resource.

SPECIAL FEATURES OF ESSENTIALS OF ANATOMY AND PHYSIOLOGY FOR COMMUNICATION DISORDERS

We have tried to link the anatomical structures with clinical reality whenever possible. You will notice that we provide frequent "side trips" in the form of clinical notes that illuminate the relevance of the structures under study to your career. We have also included many figures and photographs to help you gain a multidimensional view of anatomy. The figures were chosen to illustrate vital points and areas of discussion, while the photographs provide dimension to the information presented in the drawings.

Anatomy has its own vocabulary, and you will make it yours before the course is through. As new terms are presented in text, they are highlighted in boldface type and defined in the margins as well as in the complete glossary at the back of the book. By inserting key terms in the margins, we hope that you can quickly and easily become familiar with new terms without having to take time to flip to a glossary. However, should you need it, there is a complete glossary for your use. In addition, we are proud to provide ANATESSE, Software for *Essentials of Anatomy and Physiology for Communication Disorders*. We have found that study software is critical to retention of the dense information in anatomy, and we think that this will be very helpful in your studies.

The ANATESSE Software

We have provided a very powerful study tool to use with your computer. The ANATESSE software that accompanies this text gives you one more way to learn the material. It will walk you through the anatomy and physiology, quiz you, and be a virtual laboratory where you can learn at your own pace. This free self-study software reinforces the concepts in the book and makes learning fun and interactive.

How to Use This Instructional Package

We believe that experience is the key to understanding. Needless to say, we can't provide you with a fully equipped cadaver lab, but we can guide you to an understanding of how the various components of anatomy fit together. We offer "guided tours" of your own body's, structures and we hope that these tours will bring your knowledge of anatomy into a cohesive unit.

If you supplement your reading with the relevant computer activities, you will give yourself the best opportunity to gain the knowledge of the anatomy and physiology of communication! We hope that this text and the accompanying software serve you well.

ACKNOWLEDGMENTS

We wish to acknowledge the assistance of Juliet Byington and Chris Manion in their dedicated work on this project at Delmar Learning. We are grateful for the massive accumulated wisdom and knowledge of all the authors referenced in this text. And finally, we thank our students and clients for inspiring us to educate the next generation of speech and hearing professionals.

About the Authors

J. Anthony (Tony) Seikel, PhD

Tony Seikel, PhD, is an Associate Professor in the Department of Communication Sciences and Disorders, and Education of the Deaf at Idaho State University. His background in speech and hearing sciences, oromyofunctional therapy, and neurogenics has drawn him to study the use of speech acoustics for prediction of disease in neurogenic conditions. He has been active in the development of computerized instructional materials for both speech pathology and audiology. His 30-year collaboration with David Drumright has resulted in numerous contributions to instruction in the field, and he has written many papers and given presentations on the topic of instructional pedagogy.

David G. Drumright, BS

David Drumright, BS, has created many nationally distributed software programs for instruction and measurement of speech and hearing, as a result of collaborations at the University of Kansas, Pennsylvania State University, Washington State University, and Idaho State University. He has been coauthor of numerous papers and articles on software and measurement technology in the field. Prior to his work with Washington State University and collaboration with Idaho State University, he worked as a research technician at the Noise Control Laboratory at Pennsylvania State University. He has also taught electronics at a DeVry Branch. His most recent software creation has been distributed for use by audiologists and audiology students who are learning instrumentation.

Paula Seikel, PhD

Paula Seikel, PhD, earned her Doctorate in Clinical Psychology from the University of Kansas and completed her predoctoral internship at the Veterans Administration Hospital in Leavenworth, Kansas. She has worked in community mental health and in university counseling for 17 years. With her husband, Tony, she has coauthored a paper on speech science instruction. Her contribution to this text was writing and editing for clarity and maintaining an awareness of the person, not just the bones.

CHAPTER

1

Basic Elements of Anatomy

OUTLINE

I. Understanding Latin and Greek Terms

A. Plural formation
B. Possessive form of combined terms
C. Various pronunciations

II. Anatomy and Physiology

A. Specialized areas of anatomy
   1. Applied anatomy, or clinical anatomy
   2. Descriptive anatomy, or systematic anatomy
   3. Gross anatomy
   4. Microscopic anatomy
   5. Surface anatomy

6. Developmental anatomy
7. Pathological anatomy
8. Comparative anatomy
B. Specialized areas of physiology
1. Force physiology
2. Electrophysiology
3. Electromyography
4. Auditory physiology
5. Respiratory physiology

III. Building Blocks of Anatomy: Tissues, Organs, and Systems

A. Four basic types of tissue
1. Epithelial tissue
a. Glandular epithelium
b. Beating ciliated epithelia
c. Baseplate (basement membrane)
2. Connective tissue: Supportive tissue
a. Matrix
b. Areolar tissue (loose connective tissue)
c. Adipose tissue
d. Lymphoid tissue
e. Fibrous tissue
f. White fibrous tissue
g. Yellow elastic tissue
h. Blood
i. Plasma
j. Bone
k. Compact bone
l. Spongy bone
3. Muscle tissue
a. Striated muscle
b. Smooth muscle
c. Cardiac muscle
4. Neural tissue

IV. Tissue Combinations

A. Fascia
B. Perimysium
C. Ligaments
1. Visceral ligaments
2. Skeletal ligaments
D. Tendons
1. Aponeurosis
2. Periosteum

E. Cartilage
    1. Hyaline cartilage
    2. Fibrocartilage
F. Joints
G. Operation of muscles
    1. Functional unity
    2. Origin
    3. Insertion
    4. Agonists (prime movers)
    5. Antagonists
    6. Synergists

V. Innervation and Sensation of Muscles

A. Innervation
B. Sensory (afferent) innervation
C. Motor (efferent) innervation
D. Motor nerve
E. Motor unit

VI. Terms of Orientation

A. Anatomical position
B. Sections
    1. Frontal section
    2. Midsagittal section
    3. Sagittal section
    4. Transverse section
C. Relative positioning
    1. Anterior
    2. Ventral
    3. Posterior
    4. Dorsal
    5. Rostral
    6. Caudal
    7. Peripheral
    8. Superficial
    9. Deep
    10. External
    11. Internal
    12. Distal
    13. Medial (mesial)
    14. Superior
    15. Inferior
    16. Prone
    17. Supine

18. Lateral
19. Proximal
D. Axis
  1. Axial skeleton
  2. Appendicular skeleton
  3. Neuraxis (axis of the brain)
E. Joint movement
  1. Flexion
  2. Extension
  3. Hyperextension
  4. Dorsiflexion
  5. Plantar flexion
  6. Plantar grasp reflex
  7. Inversion
  8. Eversion
  9. Pronation
  10. Supination

VII. Terms for Regions of the Body

A. Thorax
B. Abdomen
C. Dorsal trunk
D. Pelvis
E. Cranium
F. Upper extremity
G. Lower extremity

VIII. Systems of Verbal Communication

A. Nervous system
B. Respiratory system
C. Phonatory system
D. Articulatory system
E. Auditory system

TERMINOLOGY OF ANATOMY AND PHYSIOLOGY

The human body and its parts have been studied for centuries, and a rich vocabulary has developed as a result. Many terms will seem foreign at first, but you will want to make this vocabulary your own. A good medical dictionary will help you develop your knowledge. In this chapter, we present the basic elements to prepare you for your study of the anatomy and physiology of speech, including a broad picture of the field of anatomy and the basic tissues of the human body. We also set the stage for your understanding of the new and foreign terminology of anatomy.

UNDERSTANDING LATIN AND GREEK TERMS

The names of muscles, bones, and other organs were mostly set down at a time in history when medical people spoke Latin and Greek as universal languages. The intention was to name parts unambiguously rather than to make things mysterious. Many of the Latin and Greek morphemes are worth learning separately. When you come across a new term, you will often be able to determine its meaning from these components. For instance, when a text mentions an "ipsilateral" course for a nerve tract, you can see *ipsi* ("same") and *lateral* ("side") and conclude that the nerve tract is on the same side as something else.

While you are studying the nomenclature of the field, do not let the formation of plurals confuse you. A few general rules will assist you in sorting through terminology. If a singular word ends in "-a," the plural is most likely "-ae" (*pleura, pleurae*). If the word ends in "-us" the plural word ends with "-i" (*locus, loci*). (The pronunciation some-times changes as well. For instance, *locus* is pronounced with a hard "c," while *loci* changes to a soft "c.") When the singular form ends in "-um" (as in *datum* or *stratum*), the plural ends with "-a" (*data* or *strata*). Often you will hear the Anglicized version of plurals (*hiatuses*), but they are technically incorrect. A common example is *data* as a singu-lar noun, as in "the data *is* inconclusive," rather than the correct usage of "the data *are* inconclusive."

Many terms use a possessive form, denoting ownership (the geni-tive case, in linguistic jargon): *corpus*, "body," *corporum*, "of the body." The English pronunciation of these forms is unfortunately less predictable; the pronunciation presented in the dictionary often does not agree with the pronunciations common among medical personnel. Even among health professionals, though, pronunciation varies widely. Be prepared to adapt to the environment in which you work!

TERMINOLOGY OF ANATOMY

The study of anatomy is extremely hierarchical—what you learn today will be the basis for what you learn tomorrow. The terms are the bedrock for understanding anatomical structures and by mastering terms as they are presented, you will gain the maximum benefit from new material.

Terms of Orientation

Specific terminology lets us communicate relevant information concerning location and orientation of body parts and organs. In the **anatomical position**, the body is erect and the palms and arms face forward, as shown in Figure 1-1. Anytime we discuss terms of direction, we are referring to this position.

Some terms are relevant to the physical orientation of the body (such as *vertical* and *horizontal*). Other terms (such as *frontal, coronal,* and *longitudinal*) refer to **planes** or **axes** of the body and are therefore not relevant to the position of the body.

With the anatomical position in mind, let us turn to planes of reference. You may think of the following planes as referring to sections of a standing body, but they are actually defined relative to imaginary axes of the body.

If you were to divide the body into front and back sections you would have a **frontal section**, or frontal view. A frontal section is also called a coronal section because the coronal suture of the skull divides the head roughly into front and back halves. If you cut the body into left and right halves you would have **midsagittal sections**. A **sagittal** section is any cut that divides the body into left and right portions, and the cut is in the **sagittal plane**. A **transverse section** produces upper and lower halves of a body. Figure 1-1 illustrates these sections.

Note that these are midline sections, which provide equal halves. Sections can also be made off of midline. Armed with these basic planes of reference, you could rotate a structure in space and still discuss the relative orientation of its parts.

The next group of items describes the position of parts of the body in relation to other parts. **Anterior** means "in front of" and is used to describe the front surface of the human body. We also use it to describe the relative position of one organ or structure to another, such as "the central incisors are anterior to the tongue." (Those of you who play cards may say "ante up," meaning, "Put your money up front!" You may also know the term *antebellum*, meaning "before the war.") **Ventral** also refers to the front surface of the human body. Ventral and anterior are synonymous for the standing human, but

Anatomical position: The body is erect and the palms and arms face forward.

Plane: A flat or relatively smooth surface.

Axes: The real or imaginary line running through the center of a body or structure.

Frontal section: Section that divides the body into front and back portions.

Midsagittal section: Section that cuts the body into left and right halves.

Sagittal section: Section that divides the body into left and right parts.

Sagittal plane: Plane created by a sagittal section.

Transverse section: Section that divides the body into upper and lower halves.

Anterior: In front of.

Ventral: The front surface of a body.

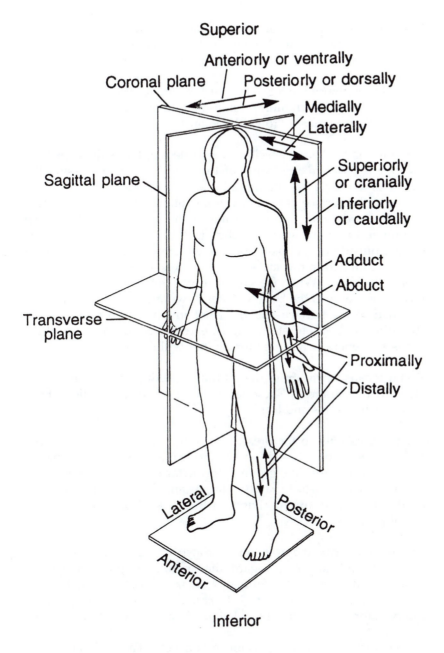

FIGURE 1-1. Terms of orientation and planes of reference.

have different meanings for animals that walk on four legs (quadrupeds). The ventral aspect of a standing dog includes its abdominal wall, which happens to be directed toward the ground.

Posterior: Toward the back; behind.

Dorsal: The back surface of a body.

Rostral: Toward the head.

Caudal: Toward the tail.

Peripheral: Away from the center of the body.

Superficial: Confined to the surface.

Deep: Closer to the central axis of the body.

External: Outside of a cavity or body.

Internal: Within a cavity or body.

Distal: Away from midline.

Medial, mesial: Toward midline.

Superior: Above, farther from the ground.

Inferior: Below, closer to the ground.

Prone: Lying on the belly.

Supine: Lying on the back.

Lateral: To the side.

Proximal: Near a body or structure.

Axial skeleton: The portion of the skeleton that is the head and trunk, with the spinal column being the axis.

Appendicular skeleton: The portion of the skeleton that includes only the lower and upper limbs.

Neuraxis: The axis of the nervous system, including spinal cord, brainstem, and cerebrum.

Posterior is the opposite of anterior, meaning "toward the back" for dogs and humans. **Dorsal** refers to "back," as in "dorsal fin" on a fish. For humans dorsal is synonymous with posterior.

Rostral is often used to mean "toward the head." If it is used to refer to structures in the cranium, *rostral* refers to a structure anterior to another. **Caudal** means "toward the tail."

These terms are "body-specific": Regardless of the body's position, anterior is "toward the front" of that body. When discussing the course of a muscle, we often need to clarify its orientation with reference to the surface of the body. A **peripheral** structure is one that is that placed *away* from the center of the body. For instance, the "peripheral nervous system" refers to the portion of the nervous system outside of the skull bone or vertebral column. **Superficial** means "confined to the surface." **Deep** means "closer to the central axis of the body." When we say one organ is "deep to another," we mean it is closer to the body's center. A wound that is superficial is confined to the surface and does not involve deep structures. A structure can also be referred to as **external** or **internal**, but these terms are generally reserved for cavities within the body.

Distal means "away from the midline." **Medial,** or **mesial,** means "toward the midline." These terms are used for appendicle structures, such as arms and legs.

A few terms refer to the present position of an actual body rather than a description based on the anatomical position. **Superior** (above, farther from the ground) and **inferior** (below, closer to the ground) are used when gravity is important. The terms **prone** (lying on the belly) and **supine** (lying on the back) describe the present actual position.

Often we describe the orientation of a structure relative to another structure, and so we disregard the anatomical position. **Lateral** means "to the side," as in football's "lateral pass." **Proximal** means "near," as in "approximate." *Lateral* and *proximal* are usually reserved for discussion of the relationship between limbs and trunk.

The concept of axis is important to add here. The body and brain (and many other structures) are said to have axes or midlines. The **axial skeleton** is the head and trunk, with the spinal column being the axis. The **appendicular skeleton** includes only the lower and upper limbs. The **neuraxis**, or axis of the brain, is slightly less straightforward, due to morphological changes of the brain during development. The embryonic nervous system is essentially tubular, but as the cerebral cortex develops, a flexure occurs and the telencephalon (the region that will become the cerebrum) folds forward. As a result, the neuraxis takes a T-formation. The spinal cord and brainstem have dorsal and ventral surfaces corresponding to those of the surface of the body. Because the cerebrum folds forward, the dorsal surface is also the superior surface, and the ventral surface is the inferior surface. Most anatomists avoid this confusion by referring to the superior and inferior surfaces.

There are specialized terms associated with movement. **Flexion** refers to bending at a joint, usually toward the ventral surface. That is, flexion usually results in two ventral ("belly") surfaces coming closer together. Sit-ups are an act of flexion, because you are bending at the waist. **Extension** is the opposite of flexion, being the act of pulling two ends farther apart. Again, having completed a sit-up, you return to the extended condition. **Hyperextension**, as in arching your back at the end of your sit-up, is sometimes called **dorsiflexion**. It occurs when extension continues to the point where the dorsal surfaces approach each other.

Use of flexion and extension with reference to feet and hands is a little more complex. **Plantar** refers to the sole of the foot, the flexor surface. If you rise on your toes, you are extending your foot, but the gesture is referred to as **plantar flexion**. A **plantar grasp reflex** is one in which stimulation of the sole of the foot causes the toes of the feet to "grasp." The term *dorsiflexion* may be used to denote elevation of the dorsum (upper surface) of the foot. You may turn the sole of your foot inward, in **inversion**. A foot turned out is in **eversion**. **Palmar** refers to the palm of the hand, that is, the ventral (flexor) surface. A **palmar grasp reflex** is elicited by lightly stimulating the palm of the hand. The response is to flex the fingers to grasp. The side opposite the palm is the dorsal side.

If the hand is rotated so that the palmar surface is directed inferiorly, it is **pronated**. Remember that in the prone position one is lying on the stomach or ventral surface. **Supination** refers to rotating the hand so that the palmar surface is directed superiorly.

Terms for Regions of the Body

The human body can be defined in terms of regions. The **thorax** is the chest region. The **abdomen** is the region represented externally as the front (anterior) abdominal wall. Together these two components

Flexion: Bending at a joint, usually toward the ventral surface.

Extension: The act of pulling two ends farther apart; the opposite of flexion.

Hyperextension: Extension that continues to the point where the dorsal surfaces approach each other.

Dorsiflexion: Hyperextension.

Plantar: Referring to the sole of the foot, the flexor surface.

Plantar flexion: Extension of the toes.

Plantar grasp reflex: Reaction to stimulation of the sole of the foot that causes the toe of the feet to "grasp."

Inversion: Turning the sole of the foot inward.

Eversion: Turning the foot outward.

Palmar: Referring to the palm of hand.

Palmar grasp reflex: Reaction to stimulation of the palm that causes the fingers to grasp.

Pronation: Rotation of the hand so the palmar surface is directed inferiorly.

Supination: Rotation of the hand so the palmar surface is directed superiorly.

Thorax: The chest region.

Abdomen: The region represented externally as the front (anterior) abdominal wall.

Dorsal trunk: *The region commonly referred to as "the back."*

Pelvis: *The area of the hip bones.*

Cranium: *The part of the skull that houses the brain.*

Upper extremity: *The region consisting of the arm, forearm, wrist, and hand.*

Arm: *The region from the shoulder to the elbow.*

Lower extremity: *The region including the thigh, calf, ankle, and foot.*

make up the trunk, or torso. The **dorsal trunk** is the region we commonly refer to as "the back" (*dorsal* refers to back). The area of the hip bones is known as the **pelvis**. The head, or caput, rests atop the trunk. The **cranium** is the part of the skull that houses the brain. The upper and lower extremities are appended to the trunk. The **upper extremity** consists of the **arm** (from the shoulder to the elbow), forearm, wrist, and hand. The **lower extremity** is made up of the thigh, calf, ankle, and foot. These and other useful terms and their definitions are in the glossary at the end of the book.

Summary

- The axial skeleton consists of the trunk and head, whereas the appendicular skeleton is the upper and lower extremities.
- The trunk consists of the abdominal and thoracic regions.
- Anatomical terminology is the specialized set of terms used to define position and orientation of structures.
- A frontal section divides the body into front and back halves, whereas a midsagittal section divides the body into right and left halves.
- A transverse section divides the body into upper and lower portions.
- *Anterior* and *posterior* refer to the front and back surfaces of a body, as do *ventral* and *dorsal* for the erect human.
- *Superficial* refers to the surface of a body, and *deep* refers to directions away from the surface.
- *Superior* means "above," whereas *inferior* is closer to the ground.
- *Prone* means on the belly, and *supine* means on the back.
- *Lateral* refers to the side, *proximal* means close to the central axis, *distal* means farther from the center, and *medial* refers toward the midline of a free extremity.
- *Flexion* and *extension* refer to bending at a joint, where *flexion* refers to bringing ventral surfaces closer together and *extension* is moving them farther apart.
- *Plantar* refers to the sole of the foot, and *palmar* refers to the palm of the hand, both ventral surfaces.
- The axial skeleton is the head and trunk, with the spinal column being the axis.
- The appendicular skeleton includes only the lower and upper limbs.
- The neuraxis, or axis of the brain, is slightly less straightforward, because of morphological changes of the brain during development.

ANATOMY AND PHYSIOLOGY

The term **anatomy** refers to the study of the structure of an organism. **Physiology** refers to the function of an organism and its parts. Many disciplines focus on specialized areas of anatomy. **Applied anatomy**, also known as **clinical anatomy**, is the study of anatomy for diagnosis and treatment of disease as it relates to surgical procedures. **Descriptive anatomy**, also known as **systemic anatomy**, is involved in the description of individual parts of the body without reference to disease conditions. Descriptive anatomy views the body as a composite of systems that function together. **Gross anatomy** studies structures visible without the aid of microscopy. **Microscopic anatomy** examines structures not visible to the unaided eye. **Surface anatomy** is the study of the form and structure of the surface of the body, especially with reference to the organs beneath the surface. **Developmental anatomy** deals with development of the anatomy of the organism from conception to adulthood. **Pathological anatomy** concerns study of diseased tissue. **Comparative anatomy** examines anatomical structures across species.

Physiology has similarly specialized areas. **Force physiology** studies forces exerted by muscles. **Electrophysiology** measures the electrical activity of single cells or groups of cells, including muscle and nervous system tissue. **Electromyography** is the study of electrical activity related to muscle function. **Auditory physiology** includes procedures involved in measurement of auditory function. **Respiratory physiology** is concerned with all processes involved in breathing.

We rely heavily on descriptive anatomy to guide our understanding of the physical mechanisms of speech and to aid our discussion of its physiology. We call on pathological anatomy as we deal with the results of conditions, such as emphysema, that change how systems work. We call on microscopic anatomy to reveal the effect of disease on structures invisible to the unaided eye.

Summary

- Anatomy is the study of an organism's structure, whereas physiology is the study of function.
- Several subspecializations of anatomy interact to provide the detailed knowledge required to understand the anatomy and physiology of speech.
- Descriptive anatomy relates the individual parts of the body to functional systems.

Anatomy: The study of structure of an organism.

Physiology: The study of function of an organism.

Applied, or clinical anatomy: The subdiscipline of anatomy concerned with diagnosis, treatment, and surgical intervention.

Descriptive, or systemic, anatomy: The description of individual parts of the body without reference to disease.

Gross anatomy: The study of structures visible without the aid of microscopy.

Microscopic anatomy: The study of structures not visible to the unaided eye.

Surface anatomy: The study of the form and structure of the surface of the body, especially with reference to the organs beneath the surface.

Developmental anatomy: The study of development of the organism's anatomy from conception to adulthood.

Pathological anatomy: The study concerned with diseased tissue.

Comparative anatomy: The study of anatomical structures across species.

Force physiology: The study of forces exerted by muscles.

Electrophysiology: Measurement and study of the electrical activity of cells.

Electromyography: The study of forces exerted by muscles.

Auditory physiology: The procedures involved in measurement of auditory function.

Respiratory physiology: The study of all processes involved in breathing.

■ Pathological anatomy relates to changes in structure as they relate to disease.
■ Gross and microscopic anatomy refer to levels of visibility of structures under study.
■ Developmental anatomy studies the growth and relevant changes of the organism.

In the sections that follow, we present the building blocks of the human physical system. These blocks include the basic tissues and organs, the structures made up of the tissues, and the systems made up of the organs.

BUILDING BLOCKS OF ANATOMY: TISSUES, ORGANS, AND SYSTEMS

Introduction

Epithelial tissue: Tissue that provides a protective lining for the surface of the body and internal surfaces of cavities.

Connective tissue: Tissue that supports and connects other tissue.

Muscular tissue: Tissue that is capable of contraction.

Neural tissue: Tissue that is specialized to transmit information.

Depending on the type of cell, every human cell is specialized to perform different functions. Cells combine to form tissues.

Four basic tissues comprise the human body: **epithelial, connective, muscular,** and **nervous. Epithelial tissue** provides a protective lining for the surface of the body and internal surfaces of cavities. **Connective tissue** is supportive, and **muscular tissue** is capable of contraction. **Neural tissue** is specialized to transmit information. The subcategories of these tissues are shown in Table 1-1.

Table 1-1. Tissues, Descriptions, and Locations

I. Epithelial

  A. Simple Epithelium: Single layer of cells

    Squamous (pavement) epithelium: Flat; linings of blood vessels, heart, alveoil, lymph vessels

    Cuboidal (cubical) epithelium: Cube-shaped; secretory function in some glands, such as thyroid

    Columnar epithelium: Cylindrical; inner lining of stomach, intestines, gallbladder, bile ducts

    Ciliated epithelium: Cylindrical with cilia; lining of nasal cavity, larynx, trachea, bronchi

  B. Compound Epithelium: Different layers of cells

    Stratified epithelium: Flattened; on bed of columnar cells; epidermis of skin, lining of mouth, pharynx, esophagus, conjunctiva

    Transitional epithelium: Pear-shaped; lining of bladder

(continues)

Table 1-1. *(continued)*

II.Connective

  A. Areolar: Elastic; supports organs, between muscles

  B. Adipose: Cells with fat globules; between muscles and organs

  C. White Fibrous: Strong, closely packed; ligaments binding bones; periosteum covering bone; covering of organs; fascia over muscle

  D. Yellow Elastic: Elastic; in areas requiring recoil, such as trachea, cartilage, bronchi, lungs

  E. Lymphoid: Lymphocytes; make up lymphoid tissue of tonsils, adenolds, lymph nodes

  F. Cartilage: Firm and solid

   1. Hyaline: Bluish white; smooth; on articulating surfaces of bones, costal cartilage of ribs, larynx, trachea, bronchial passageway

   2. Fibrocartilage: Dense, white, flexible; intervertebral discs, between surfaces of knee joints

   3. Yellow (elastic): Firm; pinna, epiglottis

  G. Blood: Corpuscles (cells: red, white), platelets, blood plasma

  H. Bone: Hardest connective tissue

   1. Compact: Has haversian canal, lamellar structure

   2. Cancellous (spongy): Spongy appearance, larger haversian canal, red bone marrow producing red and white blood cells and plasma

III. Muscular

  A. Striated: Skeletal, voluntary muscle

  B. Smooth: Muscle of internal organs, involuntary

  C. Cardiac: Combination of striated and smooth, involuntary

IV. Nervous

  A. Neurons: Transfer information; communicating tissue

  B. Glial cells: Nutrient transfer; blood-brain barrier

Source: Adapted from *Foundations of Anatomy and Physiology* (pp. 1–32), by J.S. Ross and J. W. Wilson, 1966, Baltimore: Williams & Wilkins.

Tissues

Epithelial Tissue

Epithelial tissue is composed of the superficial layer of mucous membranes and the cells that comprise the skin. Epithelial tissue has little material between the epithelial cells so that it forms a tight,

Glandular epithelium:
Epithelium that secretes fluids.

Baseplate (basement membrane): Thin, membranous subsurface of epithelial tissue that serves structural, functional, and developmental purposes depending on its location.

Beating ciliated epithelia: Cells with hairlike protrusions that actively beat to remove contaminants from the epithelial surface.

Matrix: Intercellular material of connective tissue.

Areolar tissue (loose connective tissue): Supportive connective tissue.

Adipose tissue: Areolar tissue that is richly impregnated with fat cells.

Lymphoid tissue: Specialized connective tissue in tonsils and adenoids.

Fibrous tissue: Tissue that binds structures together.

White fibrous tissue: Connective tissue that is strong, dense, and highly organized.

Yellow elastic tissue: Connective tissue in cartilage.

Blood: Connective tissue that contains plasma and blood cells.

Plasma: Fluid component of blood.

compact sheet. It is protective, keeping whatever is covered from seeping out and keeping some foreign material from getting in. There may be many layers of epithelium for added protection. Some forms of epithelium secrete fluids, and these are called **glandular epithelium**.

A **baseplate**, or **basement membrane**, made predominantly of collagen underlies epithelial tissue, providing a number of functions, depending on the location of the epithelium. Basement membrane may serve as a filter (for instance, in the kidneys) or stabilize the epithelial tissue (as in the juncture of connective tissue with epithelium). The basement membrane is important in the process of directing growth patterns for epithelial cells.

Other types of epithelium have cilia, which are hairlike protrusions that actively beat to remove contaminants from the epithelial surface (**beating ciliated epithelia**). Epithelial tissue lines nearly all of the cavities of the body as well as the tubes that connect them.

Connective Tissue

Connective tissue is perhaps the most complex type of tissue. The body has a great deal of connective tissue, which provides support for other structures. Connective tissue is made up mostly of intercellular material, known as the **matrix**, within which the cells of connective tissue are bound. Connective tissue may be solid, liquid, or gel-like. The major types of connective tissue are as follows. **Areolar tissue** (also known as **loose connective tissue**) is supportive. Areolar fibers join to form an area like an elastic woven mat. They form a thin sheet between muscles and organs and fill the space between organs. **Adipose tissue** is areolar tissue that is richly impregnated with fat cells. **Lymphoid tissue** is specialized connective tissue found in tonsils and adenoids. **Fibrous tissue** binds structures together, and it may contain combinations of fiber types. **White fibrous tissue** is strong, dense, and highly organized. It is found in ligaments that bind bones together, as well as in the fascia that encase muscle. **Yellow elastic tissue** is found in cartilage.

Blood is a connective tissue. Blood cells (including red and white corpuscles) are suspended in blood **plasma**, which is the liquid matrix of this connective tissue. Plasma has numerous functions, among them the precipitation of clotting when cells are damaged. The blood cells develop in the marrow of another type of connective tissue, bone.

Osteoporosis

Osteoporosis is a condition wherein bone becomes increasingly porous due to loss of calcium. The reduction in calcium may be the result of aging, vitamin D deficiency, disuse, as found in individuals confined to bed during illness, or other causes. Osteoporosis makes a person susceptible to bone fractures. Breaks of osteoporotic bones may go undetected. For example, an elderly person may "fall and break a hip," when actually the hip might have been broken before the fall, due to the fragility and porousness of the bone. An individual with osteoporosis can break ribs while coughing. Osteoporosis can be localized, as seen in the skull bones of a person with Paget's disease (osteitis deformans).

Bone is the hardest of the connective tissues. The hardness comes from the inorganic salts that make up a large portion of it. Bone is generally described as **compact** or **spongy**. Compact bone has a sheetlike (lamellar) structure, and spongy bone appears porous. Spongy bone contains the marrow that produces both blood cells and blood plasma.

Bone: Dense, inelastic connective tissue.

Compact bone: Sheetlike bone.

Spongy bone: Porous bone.

Muscle Tissue

Muscle fibers can be stimulated to contract. Muscle is generally classified as striated, smooth, or cardiac (Figure 1-2). **Striated muscle** is named for the striped appearance of the tissue when viewed through a microscope. Striated muscle is also known as skeletal because it is the muscle used to move skeletal structures. It is also known as voluntary or somatic muscle because it can be moved in response to conscious, voluntary stimulation. **Smooth muscle** includes the muscular tissue of the digestive tract and blood vessels, and it is sheetlike, with spindle-shaped cells. **Cardiac muscle** is composed of cells that interconnect like a net. Smooth and cardiac muscle are generally outside of voluntary control and are controlled through the autonomic (involuntary) nervous system.

Striated muscle: Skeletal muscle, voluntary muscle.

Smooth muscle: Includes the muscular tissue of the digestive tract and blood vessels not under voluntary control.

Cardiac muscle: Muscle of the heart, composed of cells that interconnect like a net.

Neural Tissue

Neurons, which take on a variety of forms, are specialized for communication. They transmit information from one neuron to another, from neuron to muscle, and from sensory receptors to other neural structures.

Neurons: Cells specialized for communication.

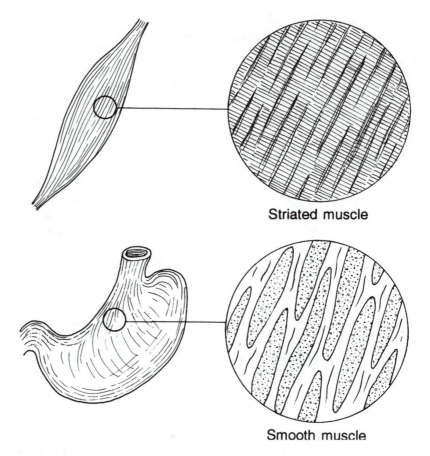

FIGURE 1-2. Striated (*upper*) and smooth muscle (*lower*).

Summary

- Four types of tissue comprise the human body: epithelial, connective, muscular, and neural (nervous).
- Epithelial tissue includes the surface covering of the body and linings of body cavities and passageways.
- Connective tissue varies as a function of the intercellular material (matrix) surrounding it.
- Areolar connective tissue is loose and thin, and adipose tissue is areolar tissue with significant fat deposits.
- White fibrous connective and yellow elastic tissue is found in ligaments, tendons, and cartilage.
- Blood is a fluid connective tissue, whereas bone is a dense, inelastic connective tissue.

- Muscle tissue consists of voluntary (striated), involuntary (smooth), and cardiac muscle.
- Neural tissue is specialized for communication.

Tissue Combinations

The four basic types of body tissue (epithelial, connective, muscular, and nervous) combine to provide structure to the body. Here are some structures that are formed from basic connective tissues.

A **fascia** (pl. fasciae) is a sheetlike membrane of connective tissue that surrounds organs. Fasciae may take many forms, but the fibers are typically woven together for **compressive strength**. Compressive strength is the ability of a material to resist being crushed. **Perimysium** is a special type of fascia that surrounds muscle.

Ligaments are bands of connective tissue that are responsible for binding structures together. **Visceral ligaments** bind organs together and hold structures in place. **Skeletal ligaments** bind bone to bone and must withstand great pressure. Ligaments generally do not stretch.

Tendons are bands of connective tissue that are part of the muscle; they are the means by which muscle is attached to bone or cartilage (see Figure 1-3). The fibers of tendons run longitudinally (as opposed to interwoven or matted, as in fascia). This gives them great

Fascia: Sheetlike membrane of connective tissue that surrounds organs.

Compressive strength: The ability of a material to resist crushing.

Perimysium: Special fascia surrounding muscle.

Ligaments: Bands of connective tissue responsible for binding structures together.

Visceral ligaments: Connective tissue that binds organs together or holds structures in place.

Skeletal ligaments: Connective tissue that binds bone to bone.

Tendons: Connective tissue bands that are part of the muscle and attach muscle to bone or cartilage.

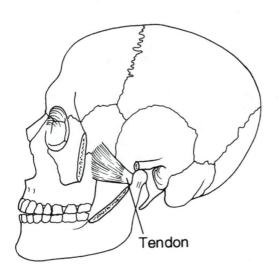

FIGURE 1-3. Tendon attaching muscle to bone.

Tensile strength: The ability of a material to resist being pulled apart.

Morphology: Form.

Aponeurosis: Sheetlike tendon.

tensile strength but reduced compressive strength. Tensile strength gives a material resistance to being pulled apart. Tendons tend to have the **morphology** (or form) of the muscles they serve. Compact, tubular muscles tend to have long, thin tendons. Flat muscles, such as the diaphragm, have flat tendons. An **aponeurosis** is a sheetlike tendon.

Periosteum: Fibrous membrane covering of a bone.

Bones are dense connective tissue providing the structure for most of the body. Bones are broadly characterized by length (long or short) and shape (flat) or are irregular. The **periosteum** is the fibrous membrane covering of a bone that extends along its entire surface except where there is cartilage. The outer periosteum layer is tough and fibrous but the inner layer of periosteum contains cells that facilitate bone repair.

Cartilage: Connective tissue that is elastic.

Elasticity: Having the ability and tendency to return to original position

Articulate: Join together.

Cartilage is a particularly important connective tissue combination. Cartilage has three qualities that make it ideally suited for some structural purposes: great tensile strength, great compressive strength, and **elasticity**, which means that when it is moved or displaced it will tend to return to its original position. Bones often have a cartilaginous portion in areas where they need to have flexibility, such as in the nose, or in areas where two bones **articulate** (join together). Cartilage is smoother than bone, so many joints between bones have cartilage on the two surfaces so they can glide across each other with reduced friction.

Hyaline cartilage: Smooth, glassy, blue cartilage for surfaces of bones that come together in joints

Fibrocartilage: Smooth cartilage with a glassy, blue cast.

Yellow (elastic) cartilage: Cartilage that has greater elasticity than other forms of cartilage.

There are three basic subtypes of cartilage. **Hyaline cartilage** is smooth and has a glassy, blue cast. It gives a smooth surface for mating of bones that come together in joints. It is also a primary form of cartilage for the larynx, trachea, and bronchial passageway. It makes up the cartilaginous portion of the rib cage. **Fibrocartilage** contains collagen fibers that provide the cushion between bones. For instance, it makes up the discs between the vertebrae, as well as the mating surface for the temporomandibular joint between the lower jaw and the skull. Fibrocartilage is a shock absorber and provides a relatively smooth surface for gliding. **Yellow (elastic) cartilage** has less collagen but more elastic fibers. It is found in the pinna (the visible portion of the ear), the nose, and the epiglottis.

Joints

Diarthrodial, or synovial, joints: Highly mobile joints lubricated with synovial fluid.

A joint is the means by which two bones articulate. Although there is a wide variety of joints, we discuss only one type in this overview. **Diarthrodial**, or **synovial, joints** are highly mobile and have a cavity in which synovial fluid, a lubricating substance, is found. Hyaline cartilage covers the surface of each bone of the joint, providing a smooth, strong mating surface.

Summary

- Tissues combine to form larger structures.
- Fascia is a sheetlike membrane surrounding organs.
- Ligaments bind organs together and hold bone to bone or cartilage.
- Tendons attach muscle to bone or to cartilage, and a flat tendon is referred to as an aponeurosis.
- Bones and cartilage provide the structure for the body, articulating by means of joints.
- Cartilage has both tensile and compressive strength and is elastic (fibers of cartilage resist being torn apart or crushed, and cartilage tends to return to its original shape after being deformed).
- Hyaline cartilage is smooth, while fibrocartilage provides a cushion between structures.
- Yellow cartilage is very elastic.
- Diarthrodial (synovial) joints are highly mobile and lubricated by synovial fluid.

Muscles

You can look at muscles in terms of either their anatomy or their physiology. The role of muscle is to move the structures to which it is attached closer together. Anatomically, muscles are groups of muscle fibers with a single functional purpose (**functional unity**). The form of the muscle (morphology) varies widely, depending on its function. Fibers of wide, flat muscles tend to radiate from a broad point of origination to a more focused insertion. More cylindrical muscles have single points of attachment on either end.

Functional unity: Groups of tissues working for a single functional purpose.

Muscle fiber can only actively shorten. A muscle can contract to approximately one half its original length, so long muscles can contract greater distances than short muscles. The diameter of a muscle is directly related to its strength. The more fibers a muscle has, the greater the force the muscle can exert to do work. Muscles can contract only in a straight line, with the exception of sphincter muscles, which act like a drawstring on a purse.

Origin: The point of attachment of a muscle that is immobile when a muscle contracts.

Insertion: The point of attachment of a muscle that is mobile when a muscle contracts.

Agonists (prime movers): Muscles that move a structure.

Antagonists: Muscles that oppose a prime mover or agonist.

Synergists: Muscles used to stabilize structures.

Innervation: Distribution of nervous tissue to serve communication between brain and muscles.

Muscles are attached to some structures at both ends. The point of attachment that is immobile when a muscle contracts is the **origin**. The point of attachment that moves as a result of muscle contraction is the **insertion**. When referring to limbs, the insertion point is more distant from the body. Muscles that move a structure are referred to as **agonists** or **prime movers**. Muscles that oppose a given movement are **antagonists**. Muscles used to stabilize structures are **synergists**.

A muscle attached closer to a joint will move the bone farther and faster than one attached farther from the joint, and it will provide greater range of movement. A muscle attached farther from the joint will be able to exert more force through its range because of the greater leverage and will have an advantage for lifting (see Figure 1-4).

Innervation and Sensation of Muscles

Innervation is communication between neurons or between neurons and muscle. Muscle innervation provides the means for a muscle to contract. Sensory information is also transmitted by neurons,

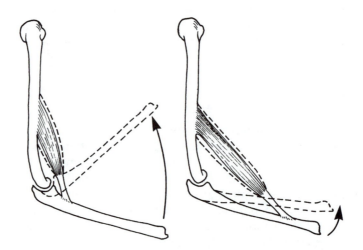

FIGURE 1-4. Mechanical advantage derived from point of insertion. *Left,* the muscle inserts closer to the point of rotation and the movable point will undergo a greater excursion on contraction of the muscle. *Right,* the muscle is attached a greater distance from the point of rotation so that the bone will move a smaller distance, but the muscle is capable of exerting greater force in the direction of movement.

so regions or structures of the body receive afferent (sensory) innervation. Muscles are innervated by a single nerve that is responsible for activating the muscle. Another nerve is responsible for monitoring the muscle's length and state of tension.

Innervation is either **sensory** (generally termed **afferent**) or **motor** (**efferent**, or **excitatory**). A sensory nerve from a muscle sends information about the state of the muscle (for instance, how much it has been stretched) to the central nervous system. A **motor nerve** sends impulses from the nervous system to muscles to make them contract. A **motor unit** consists of one motor nerve fiber and the muscle fibers to which it attaches.

Sensory (afferent) innervation: Innervation that provides the central nervous system with information about the state of the body or tissues.

Motor (efferent/excitatory) innervation: Innervation that causes muscles to contract or glands to secrete.

Motor nerve: Nerve that activates muscle or glands.

Motor unit: Tissue consisting of one motor nerve fiber and the muscle fibers to which it attaches.

Neuromuscular Diseases

A host of neuromuscular conditions prey on the muscular system and the nerve components that supply it with energy. Amyotrophic lateral sclerosis (ALS, or Lou Gehrig's disease) is a condition in which the myelin sheath of the nerve axon is progressively destroyed, resulting in loss of muscle function. Similar myelin destruction occurs in multiple sclerosis (MS), although the course and severity of MS are markedly different from that of ALS. Myasthenia gravis is a condition in which the nerve-to-muscle junction is destroyed as a result of an immune system response. The result is weakness and loss of muscle range because nerve and muscle cannot communicate.

Summary

- Muscle is contractile tissue, with muscle bundles capable of shortening to about half their length.
- The point of attachment with the least movement is the muscle's origin, and the insertion is the point of attachment of relative mobility.
- Muscles that move a structure are agonists and those that oppose movement are antagonists.
- Muscles that stabilize structures are synergists.
- A muscle is innervated by a single nerve.
- Motor nerves communicate excitatory impulses to muscle fibers.
- Sensory nerves communicate sensation from regions of the body to the central nervous system.
- A motor unit is the motor nerve fiber and the muscle fibers it innervates.

SYSTEMS OF VERBAL COMMUNICATION

Verbal communication is a very complex process that capitalizes on the anatomical systems of the body. The systems of verbal communication are defined according to function, and the systems combine organs and structures in a unique fashion. A classical categorization of the systems of verbal communication includes the nervous, respiratory, phonatory, articulatory, resonatory, and auditory systems. In this text, we combine the articulatory and resonatory systems.

The definition of systems of verbal communication is really just a convenience, because no system operates in isolation. Speech and hearing require the integrated action of all of the systems. The nervous system for communication includes the motor and sensory control of all the various structures involved in speech. This is the most essential communication system because without it we would have neither hearing nor speech. The respiratory system for communication is a precise match with the anatomical respiratory system, including the respiratory passageway and lungs. The phonatory system is the system involved in production of voiced sound through vibration of vocal folds (or vocal cords). This system uses components of the respiratory system (the larynx and other structures). The articulatory system is the combination of structures that are used to shape the sounds of speech. It includes parts of the digestive and respiratory systems (the tongue, lips, teeth, soft palate, etc.). The resonatory system includes the nasal cavity and soft palate and portions of the anatomically defined respiratory and digestive systems. It is responsible for one component of articulation, the use of the nasal cavity to produce sounds of speech. Although some speech scientists view the resonatory system as separate from the articulatory system, we take an alternative view in this text and combine the two systems as the articulatory-resonatory system of verbal communication. The auditory system includes the outer, middle, and inner ears, as well as the auditory pathways to the brain. This system provides a mechanism for processing auditory verbal information that we receive.

Summary

- In the discipline of speech pathology, there are five functionally defined systems of speech production: respiratory, phonatory, articulatory-resonatory, auditory, and nervous systems.
- The nervous system includes sensory and motor control of the various structures involved in speech.
- The respiratory system is concerned with respiration.

- The phonatory system is made up of the components of the respiratory and digestive systems associated with production of voiced sounds (the larynx).
- The articulatory-resonatory system includes the structures of the face, mouth, and nose.
- The auditory system is responsible for receiving and processing auditory stimuli.

CHAPTER SUMMARY

Anatomy and physiology are the study of the structure and function of an organism. Subspecializations of anatomy interact to provide the detailed knowledge required to understand the anatomy and physiology of speech. Descriptive anatomy relates the individual parts of the body to functional systems and pathological anatomy relates to changes in structure from disease.

The four basic types of tissue of the human body are epithelial, connective, muscular, and nervous. Epithelial tissue comprises the surface covering of the body and the linings of cavities and passageways. Connective tissue includes the variety of tissues linking structures together, including ligaments, tendons, cartilage, bone, and blood. Muscular tissue is contractile, comprised of striated, smooth, and cardiac. Nervous tissue is specialized for communication.

Tissues combine to form structures and organs. Fascia surrounds organs, ligaments bind bones and cartilage, tendons attach muscle to bone or to cartilage, and bones and cartilage provide the structure for the body. Diarthrodial, or synovial, joints are those in which lubricating synovial fluid is contained in a capsule.

Muscle bundles can shorten to about half their length. The origin of a muscle is the point of attachment with the least movement, and the muscle's insertion is the relatively mobile point of attachment. Agonists are muscles that move a structure, antagonists oppose movement, and synergists stabilize a structure. Muscles are innervated by a single nerve, and innervation can be sensory or motor. A motor unit is the motor nerve fiber and the muscle fibers it innervates.

The axial skeleton supports the trunk and head, and the appendicular skeleton refers to the extremities. Anatomical terminology relates position and orientation of the body and its parts. A frontal plane cuts the body into front and back halves, a sagittal plane divides the body into left and right halves, and a transverse plane divides the body into upper and lower halves. *Anterior* and *posterior* refer to front and back of a body, as do ventral and dorsal for the human. *Peripheral* refers to a direction toward the surface or superficial region, while *deep* refers to direction away from the surface. *Distal* means away from a central structure, and *proximal* means to the side of a structure. *Superior* and *inferior* refer to upper and lower regions. *Lateral* means to the side, and *medial* refers to the midline. *Flexion* refers to bending ventral surfaces toward each other at a joint, and *extension* is moving those surfaces farther apart. *Plantar* and *palmar* refer to ventral surfaces of the feet and hands, respectively.

The discipline of speech pathology includes five functionally defined systems of speech production: respiratory, phonatory, articulatory-resonatory, auditory, and nervous. The respiratory system is concerned with respiration. The phonatory system is made up of the components of the respiratory and digestive systems associated with production of voiced sounds (the larynx). The articulatory system includes the structures of the face, mouth, and nose. The auditory system is responsible for receiving and processing auditory stimuli. The nervous system includes the sensory and motor control of the various structures involved in speech.

Study Questions

1. _____ is the study of the structure of an organism.

2. _____ is the study of the function of a living organism and its parts.

3. _____ anatomy is anatomical study for diagnosis and treatment of disease.

4. _____ anatomy is involved in the description of individual parts of the body without reference to disease, viewing the body as a composite of systems that function together.

5. Skin and mucous membrane are made up of _____ tissue.

6. _____ is a particularly important connective tissue because it is both strong and elastic.

7. _____ is contractile tissue.

8. _____ bind organs together or hold bones to bone or cartilage.

9. _____ is a sheetlike membrane surrounding organs.

10. _____ attach muscle to bone or to cartilage.

11. The relatively immobile point of attachment of a muscle is the _____ .

12. The relatively mobile point of attachment of a muscle is the _____ .

13. Identify the anatomical systems from their definitions:

    A. _____ This system includes smooth, striated, and cardiac muscle of the body.

    B. _____ This system includes the bones and cartilages that form the structure of the body.

    C. _____ This system includes the passageways and tissues involved in gas exchange with the environment, including the oral, nasal, and pharyngeal cavities, the trachea and bronchial passageway, and the lungs.

    D. _____ This system includes the esophagus, liver, intestines, and associated glands.

    E. _____ This system includes the nerve tissue and structures of the central and peripheral nervous systems.

14. Identify the systems of speech from their definitions:

    A. _____ This system includes the passageways and tissues involved in gas exchange with the environment, including the oral, nasal, and pharyngeal cavities, the trachea and bronchial passageway, and the lungs.

    B. _____ This system is involved in production of voiced sound and uses components of the respiratory system (the laryngeal structures).

    C. _____ This system is the combination of structures used to alter the sounds of speech, including parts of the anatomically defined digestive and respiratory systems (the tongue, lips, teeth, soft palate, etc.).

    D. _____ This system includes the nasal cavity and soft palate and portions of the anatomically defined respiratory and digestive systems.

15. On the figure, identify the descriptive terms indicated.

A. _____ plane

B. _____ plane

C. _____ plane

D. _____ aspect

E. _____ aspect

F. _____ (movement away from midline)

G. _____ (movement toward midline)

H. _____ (located away from midline)

I. _____ (located near midline)

J. _____ (related to the side)

K. _____ (above)

L. _____ (below)

16. As our field has developed, the professionals working with speech and language became known as "speech-language pathologists." Reflecting on the terminology you have just reviewed, to what does the term *pathologist* refer?

REFERENCES

Barnett, H. L. (1972). *Pediatrics*. New York: Appleton-Century-Crofts.

Basmajian, J. V. (1975). *Grant's method of anatomy*. Baltimore: Williams & Wilkins.

Bateman, H. E. (1977). *A clinical approach to speech anatomy and physiology*. Springfield, IL: Charles C. Thomas.

Bateman, H. E., & Mason, R. M. (1984). *Applied anatomy and physiology of the speech and hearing mechanism*. Springfield, IL: Charles C. Thomas.

Duffy, J. R. (1995). *Motor speech disorders*. St. Louis, MO: Mosby.

Fink, B. R., & Demarest, R. J. (1978). *Laryngeal biomechanics*. Cambridge, MA: Harvard University Press.

Gosling, J. A., Harris, P. F., Humpherson, J. R., Whitmore, I., Willan, P. L. T. (1985). *Atlas of human anatomy*. Philadelphia: J. B. Lippincott.

Gray, H., Bannister, L. H., Berry, M. M., & Williams, P. L. (Eds.) (1995). *Gray's anatomy*. London: Churchill Livingstone.

Grobler, N. J. (1977). *Textbook of clinical anatomy* (Vol. 1). Amsterdam: Elsevier Scientific.

Kaplan, H. (1960). *Anatomy and physiology of speech*. New York: McGraw-Hill.

Kuehn, D. P., Lemme, M. L., & Baumgartner, J. M. (1991). *Neural bases of speech, hearing, and language*. Boston: Little, Brown.

Moore, K. L., Persaud, T. V. N., & Chabner, D.-E.B (2003). *The developing human*. Philadelphia: W. B. Saunders.

Rahn, H., Otis, A., Chadwick, L. E., & Fenn, W. (1946). The pressure-volume diagram of the thorax. *American Journal of Physiology, 146*, 161–178.

Ross, J. S., & Wilson, K. J. W. (1966). *Foundations of anatomy and physiology*. Baltimore: Williams & Wilkins.

Zemlin, W. R. (1998). *Speech and hearing science: Anatomy and physiology* (4th ed.). Needham Heights, MA: Allyn & Bacon.

CHAPTER

2

Anatomy and Physiology of Respiration

OUTLINE

I. Introduction

A. Respiration is exchange of gas between an organism and its environment

B. Pressure is force distributed over area

C. Boyle's law

D. Pressure increase and decrease

II. Support Structure for Respiration

    A. Vertebral column
        1. Five vertebral segments form a strong but flexible column
        2. Vertebrae labels are based on their levels: C1 to C7 (cervical), T1 to T12 (thoracic), L1 to L5 (lumbar), S1 to S5 (sacral)
        3. Coccyx
        4. Spinous and transverse processes
        5. Vertebral column houses the spinal cord
        6. Spinal nerves
        7. Ribs articulate with the spinal column

III. Pelvic and Pectoral Girdle

    A. Pelvic girdle
        1. Ilium
        2. Sacrum
        3. Pubic bone
        4. Ischium
    B. Pectoral girdle
        1. Scapula
        2. Clavicle
        3. Sternum

IV. Ribs and Rib Cage

    A. Total of 12 ribs: 7 true ribs, 3 false ribs, and 2 floating ribs
    B. Cartilaginous attachment of ribs to the sternum
    C. Elevation of rib cage
    D. Sternum

V. Soft Tissue of the Thorax and Respiratory Passageway

    A. Right and left lung
    B. Trachea and bronchial tree
    C. Oxygen and carbon dioxide exchange
    D. Cleansing action of beating epithelia

VI. Movement of Air through the System

    A. Pleural linings of lungs
    B. Association between the pleurae and the diaphragm
    C. Action of diaphragm in respiration

VII. Diaphragm

A. Primary muscle of inspiration
B. Interaction of diaphragm and central tendon

VIII. Accessory Muscles of Inspiration

A. Anterior thoracic muscles of inspiration
    1. External intercostal
    2. Interchondral portion, internal intercostal
B. Posterior thoracic muscles of inspiration
    1. Levatores costarum (brevis and longis)
    2. Serratus posterior superior
C. Accessory muscles of the neck
    1. Sternocleidomastoid
    2. Scalenes (anterior, middle, posterior)

IX. Muscles of Upper Arm and Shoulder

A. Pectoralis major
B. Pectoralis minor
C. Serratus anterior
D. Levator scapulae
E. Rhomboideus major
F. Rhomboideus minor
G. Trapezius

X. Muscles of Forced Expiration

A. Muscles of thorax: anterior/lateral thoracic muscles
    1. Internal intercostal (interosseous portion)
    2. Transversus thoracis
B. Posterior thoracic muscles
    1. Subcostals
    2. Serratus posterior inferior
C. Abdominal muscles of expiration
    1. Anterolateral abdominal muscles
        a. Transversus abdominis
        b. Internal oblique abdominis
        c. External oblique abdominis
        d. Rectus abdominis
    2. Posterior abdominal muscles: quadratus lumborum
D. Muscles of upper limb: latissimus dorsi

XI. Physiology of Respiration

A. Measurement of respiration
1. Flow, volumes, and capacities
2. Pressure
3. Volume measured in liters, milliliters, and cubic centimeters

B. Respiration for life
1. Respiratory cycle
a. Adults, 12–18 cycles per minute
b. Adults quiet respiration, about 500 cc per cycle
2. Developmental processes of respiration
a. Conducting airway complete at birth
b. As they grow, the lungs are stretched to fill the thorax

C. Volumes
1. Tidal volume (TV)
2. Inspiratory reserve volume (IRV)
3. Expiratory reserve volume (ERV)
4. Residual volume (RV)
5. Dead space air

D. Capacities
1. Vital capacity (VC)
2. Functional residual capacity (FRC)
3. Total lung capacity (TLC)
4. Inspiratory capacity (IC)

E. Pressures of the respiratory system
1. Alveolar pressure
2. Intrapleural pressure
3. Subglottal pressure
4. Intraoral pressure
5. Atmospheric pressure

F. Pressures during respiration
1. Oral pressure
2. Subglottal pressure
3. Alveolar pressure
4. Intrapleural pressure

G. Pressures generated by the tissue
1. Contracting musculature deforms cartilage and connective tissue
2. Recoil forces

H. Effects of Posture on Speech
  1. Reclining position
  2. Force of gravity on the abdomen

I. Pressures of Speech
  1. During speech, we modify our respiratory activities to balance bodily needs and communication needs
  2. Respiration cycle and speed
  3. Checking action
  4. Expiratory reserve volume for speech

INTRODUCTION

The human body depends on regular oxygen exchange to stay alive. As communicating organisms, humans have "hijacked" the respiratory system to provide the energy source for oral communication. As you will see in our discussion of respiratory physiology, we exercise a great deal of external control over the respiratory mechanism while working within the bounds of the biological requirements for life. First, we will discuss respiration, which is essential to sustain life.

Respiration is defined as the exchange of gas between an organism and its environment. We bring oxygen to the cells of the body to sustain life by breathing in (**inspiration**) and eliminate waste products by breathing out (**expiration**). A close look at the mechanics of gas exchange will provide an understanding of how a deficit in this area can impair speech.

Gas exchange happens in the alveoli, the minute air sacs located deep in the lungs, only after gas has been drawn into the system. The basic mechanism of inspiration can be likened to that of a hypodermic needle. If the plunger on the hypodermic needle in Figure 2-1 is pulled down, whatever is near the opening will enter the tube and be drawn into the awaiting chamber. If you envision the respiratory system as a hypodermic needle, with your mouth or nose as the tip of the needle, you will realize that pulling on the plunger (your diaphragm) causes air to enter the chamber (your lungs). Although the rest of this chapter is devoted to the structures and functions of the respiratory process, let us first examine in more detail the physical principles involved.

Respiration: *Exchange of gas between an organism and its environment.*

Inspiration: *The process of bringing air into the lungs for respiration.*

Expiration: *The process of eliminating air from the lungs for respiration.*

air pressure

FIGURE 2-1. Comparison of the action of the diaphragm with that of a plunger on a hypodermic needle. As the diaphragm pulls down, air enters the lungs, just as it enters the chamber of the hypodermic needle.

Before we can talk about the forces that drive respiration, you need an intuitive feel for what air pressure really is. Air pressure is the force exerted on walls of a chamber by molecules of air. Because of their molecular charge, air molecules tend to keep their distance from other air molecules. If the chamber is open to the atmosphere, the pressure exerted on the inner walls of the chamber is the same as that exerted on the outer walls.

The action starts when you close the chamber and change the air volume. Making the chamber smaller does not change the forces that are keeping molecules apart. Rather, it lets those forces be manifest on the walls of the chamber. Although the forces have not changed, the area on which they can exert themselves has, and that results in increased pressure on the walls. That is, Pressure is Force exerted on Area, or $P = F/A$. You have just increased pressure by decreasing area.

Muscle Weakness and Respiratory Function

Many disease processes reduce respiratory function, which can have a remarkable effect on other systems as well. Diseases that produce spasticity can result in paradoxical contraction of the muscles of expiration during inspiration, greatly reducing the vital capacity. Likewise, some individuals have flaccid or hypotonic (low muscle tone) conditions that reduce the degree and strength of muscular contraction. When you think about it, it makes perfect sense that diseases that cause muscular weakness can reduce respiratory capacity.

We must be cautious about quickly blaming the muscles of respiration for apparent deficits in vital capacity, inspiratory reserve, and so forth. When observing an individual with a compromised motor system, remember that you are observing the whole system. An individual with weak labial (lip) muscles might have difficulty getting an adequate seal around the mouthpiece of the spirometer or manometer, so that readings from these instruments will imply respiratory deficits when, in reality, the problem is with the articulatory system! Likewise, insufficiency of the soft palate, whether due to muscular weakness or inadequate tissue, can result in nasal leakage during respiratory tasks. Again, this can result in an apparent respiratory deficit.

Boyle's law states that given a gas of constant temperature, if you increase the volume of the chamber in which the gas is contained, pressure will decrease. When volume increases, pressure decreases, and natural air will flow to equalize that pressure. Thus, air flows into the chamber, in our case, the lungs.

Boyle's law: Given a gas of constant temperature, increasing the volume of the chamber in which the gas is contained will cause a corresponding decrease in pressure.

Figure 2-2 shows the same effect graphically. Each chamber has 11 molecules in it. On the left, the volume of the chamber has been reduced, the 11 molecules are much closer together, and the pressure has increased (known as positive pressure). Likewise, when you pull the plunger back so the molecules are farther apart than the forces dictate, the pressure decreases, and the pressure is now referred to as negative pressure. The beauty of this arrangement is that it provides all the principle we need to discuss respiratory physiology at the macroscopic and microscopic levels. The forces that

Positive Pressure   Negative Pressure

FIGURE 2-2. The piston on the left has been depressed, compressing the air in the chamber and increasing the air pressure. On the right, the piston has been retracted, increasing the space between the molecules and creating a relatively negative pressure.

draw air into the lungs also are responsible for drawing carbon dioxide out.

Summary

- Pressure is defined as force distributed over area.
- Boyle's law tells us that as the volume of a container increases, the air pressure in the container decreases.
- This relatively negative pressure will cause air to enter the container until the pressure is equalized.
- If volume is decreased, pressure increases and air flows out until the pressure inside and outside are equal.
- This principle forms the basis for movement of air into and out of the lungs.

THE SUPPORT STRUCTURE FOR RESPIRATION

The respiratory system consists of a gas-exchanging mechanism supported and protected by a bony cage. Gas exchange is carried out by the lungs while the rib cage protects them.

The lungs are housed in rib cage in the thorax, an area bounded in the superior aspect by the first rib and clavicle and in the inferior by the twelfth rib (see Figure 2-3). The lateral and anterior aspects are composed of the ribs and sternum. The entire thorax is suspended from the vertebral column (spinal column), a structure that doubles as the conduit for the spinal cord.

Vertebral Column

The functional unit of the vertebral column is the vertebra (plural, vertebrae), or spinal column segment. The vertebral column consists of five divisions: cervical, thoracic, lumbar, sacral, and coccygeal

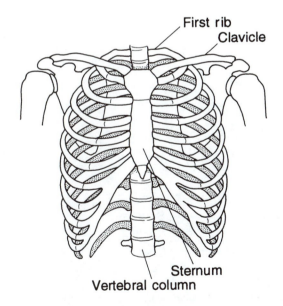

First rib
Clavicle
Sternum
Vertebral column

FIGURE 2-3. Anterior view of the thorax.

(see Figure 2-4). The vertebral column is composed of 33 segments of bone. There are 7 cervical vertebrae, 12 thoracic vertebrae (paralleling the 12 ribs of the thorax), 5 massive lumbar vertebrae, 5 sacral

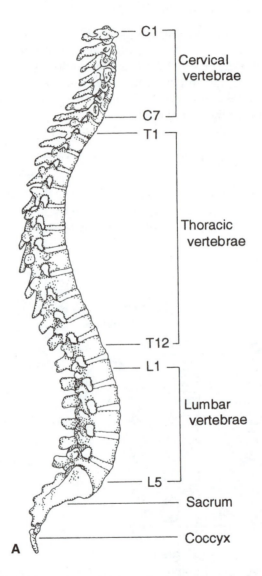

FIGURE 2–4. **A.** Components of the vertebral column, consisting of 7 cervical (C), 12 thoracic (T), and 5 lumbar (L) vertebrae, as well as the 5 fused vertebrae of the sacrum (S), and the coccyx. *(continues)*

C1

C7
T1

T12

B   Posterior   Anterior   Lateral

FIGURE 2-4. (*continued*) **B.** Articulated cervical and thoracic vertebrae.

vertebrae, and 3 (or 4) fused coccygeal vertebrae. The vertebrae are numbered sequentially from superior to inferior by section, so that the uppermost cervical vertebra is C1, the second is C2, and so forth to C7. Likewise, the first thoracic vertebra is T1 and the last is T12. Lumbar vertebrae include L1 through L5, sacral vertebrae include

S1 through S5, and the coccygeal vertebrae are considered a fused unit, known as the coccyx.

The general structure of the vertebrae includes a prominent *spinous process* and *transverse processes* on both sides (see Figures 2-5 and 2-6).

FIGURE 2-5. Superior and lateral views of cervical vertebra.

The *corpus* of the vertebra makes up the anterior, with a prominent hole or *vertebral foramen* just posterior to that. The tracts of the nervous system (spinal cord) that supply the body's periphery pass through the vertebral foramen. The spinal nerves exit and enter the spinal cord through the *intervertebral foramina* on either side of the vertebra. Vertebral segments ride one atop another to form the vertebral

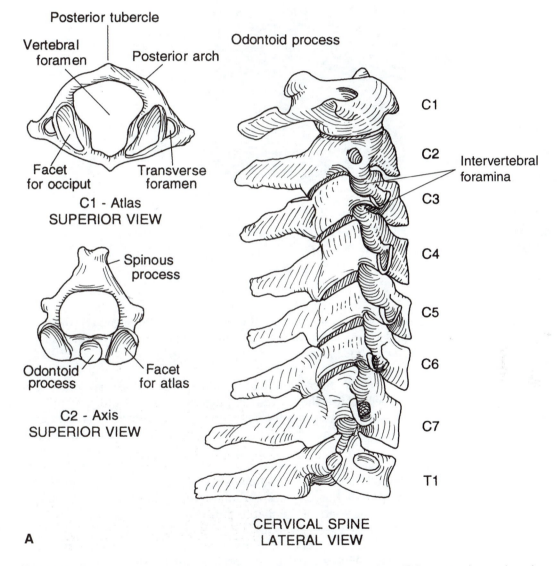

FIGURE 2-6. A. Cervical vertebrae. On left are atlas (C1, *upper*) and axis (C2, *lower*). On the right are the articulated cervical vertebrae. *(continues)*

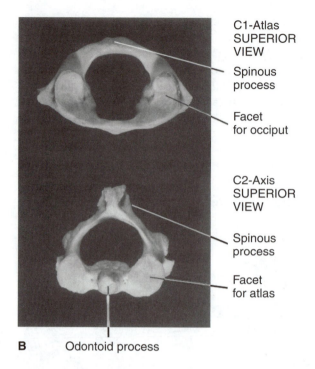

C1-Atlas
SUPERIOR
VIEW

Spinous
process

Facet
for occiput

C2-Axis
SUPERIOR
VIEW

Spinous
process

Facet
for atlas

B   Odontoid process

FIGURE 2-6. *(continued)* **B.** Superior view
of atlas and axis.

column, and this articulation is completed by means of the *superior*
and *inferior articular facets*. The uppermost cervical vertebra, C1, is the
atlas and C2 is the *axis*.

The twelve thoracic vertebrae are the base of the respiratory framework because they form the posterior point of attachment for the
ribs of the bony thorax. The superior and inferior costal facets are
the points of attachment for the ribs, as seen in Figures 2-7 and 2-8.

The five lumbar vertebrae are quite large compared with those of the
thoracic and cervical regions. They provide direct or indirect attachment for a host of back and abdominal muscles, as well as for the
posterior fibers of the diaphragm.

The five sacral vertebrae are actually a fused mass known as the
sacrum. The sacrum and its ossified intervertebral discs retain ves-
tiges of the vertebrae from which they are formed, with remnants of

spinous and transverse processes. The *coccyx* is composed of the fused *coccygeal vertebrae*, and it articulates with the inferior sacrum by means of a small disc (see Figure 2-9).

Summary

- The vertebral column is composed of vertebral segments combined to form a strong but flexible column.
- Vertebrae are labeled, based on their level: C1 to C7 (cervical), T1 to T12 (thoracic), L1 to L5 (lumbar), S1 to S5 (sacral).
- The fused coccygeal vertebrae are referred to as the coccyx.
- The spinal column provides the points of attachment for numerous muscles by means of the spinous and transverse processes.
- The spinal column houses the spinal cord, with spinal nerves emerging from and entering the spinal cord through spaces between the vertebrae.
- The ribs of the rib cage articulate with the spinal column in a fashion that permits the rib cage limited movement for respiration.

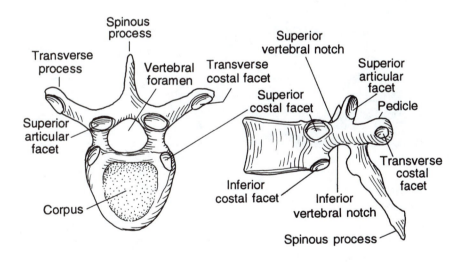

A   SUPERIOR VIEW   LATERAL VIEW

FIGURE 2-7. A. Superior and lateral views of thoracic vertebra. *(continues)*

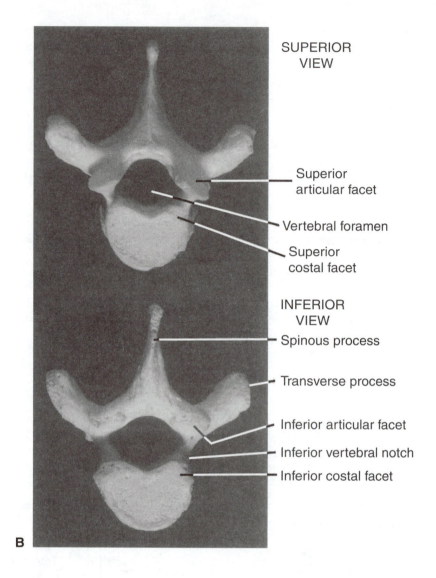

SUPERIOR
VIEW

Superior
articular facet

Vertebral foramen

Superior
costal facet

INFERIOR
VIEW

Spinous process

Transverse process

Inferior articular facet

Inferior vertebral notch

Inferior costal facet

B

FIGURE 2-7. *(continued)* **B.** Superior *(upper)* and inferior *(lower)* views of thoracic vertebra.

Pelvic Girdle

The pelvic girdle provides a strong structure for attaching the legs to the vertebral column (see Figure 2-10). The pelvic girdle is made up of the ileum, sacrum, pubic bone, and ischium. The ilium is a large,

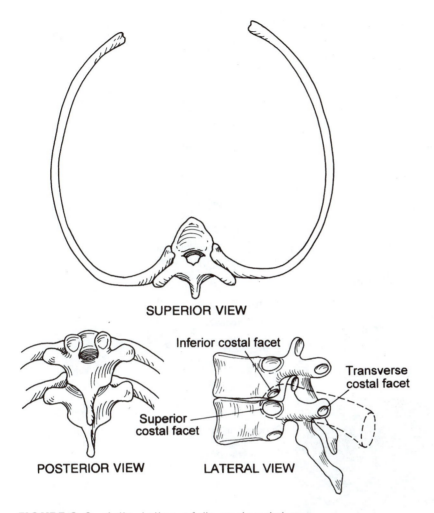

SUPERIOR VIEW

Inferior costal facet

Transverse
costal facet

Superior
costal facet

POSTERIOR VIEW   LATERAL VIEW

FIGURE 2-8. Articulation of rib and vertebrae.

winglike bone (similar in this way to the scapula, or shoulder blade, of the upper body) that provides the bulk of support for the abdominal musculature and the prominent hip bone. The iliac bones articulate with the sacrum laterally, forming the sacroiliac joints.

Pectoral Girdle

The pectoral, or shoulder, girdle includes the scapula and clavicle. The clavicle, also known as the collarbone, is attached to the superior sternum, running laterally to join the scapula. The clavicle provides

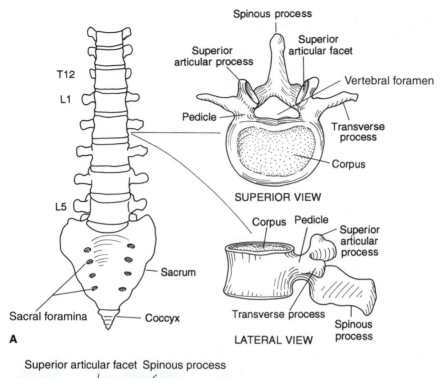

SUPERIOR VIEW

LATERAL VIEW

A

Lumbar Vertebra
SUPERIOR VIEW

B

FIGURE 2-9. A. Lumbar vertebrae articulated with sacrum and coc-cyx (*left*). Upper right shows superior view of lumbar vertebra, and lower right shows lateral view. **B.** Superior view of lumbar vertebra.

the anterior support for the shoulder by its articulation with the scapula (see Figure 2-11). The scapula has its only skeletal attachment via the clavicle, which in turn has its only skeletal attachment at the sternum. From the scapula are slung several muscles that hold it in a dynamic tension that facilitates flexible upper body movement while not compromising strength.

Summary

- The bony support structure of the respiratory system is composed of the rib cage and vertebral column.
- At the base of the vertebral column is the pelvic girdle, composed of the ilium, sacrum, pubic bone, and ischium.
- The pectoral girdle comprises the scapula and clavicle, which attach to the sternum, and is the superior counterpart to the pelvic girdle.

Ribs and Rib Cage

Ribs are capable of a degree of movement, so that the rib cage can rock up in front and flare out via lateral rotation, hinged on the

A

FIGURE 2-10. A. Pelvic girdle, consisting of the ilium, pubis, and ischium. (*continues*)

Iliac crest

Ilium

Acetabulum

Sacrum

Pubic symphysis

Coccyx

Pubic bone

Ischium

Inguinal ligament

B

FIGURE 2-10. *(continued)* **B.** Anterior view of pelvis. Lower view shows location of the inguinal ligament.

vertebral articulation with the rib cage. The rib cage is made up of 12 ribs, with all but the lowest two attached by means of cartilage to the sternum in the front aspect of the rib cage.

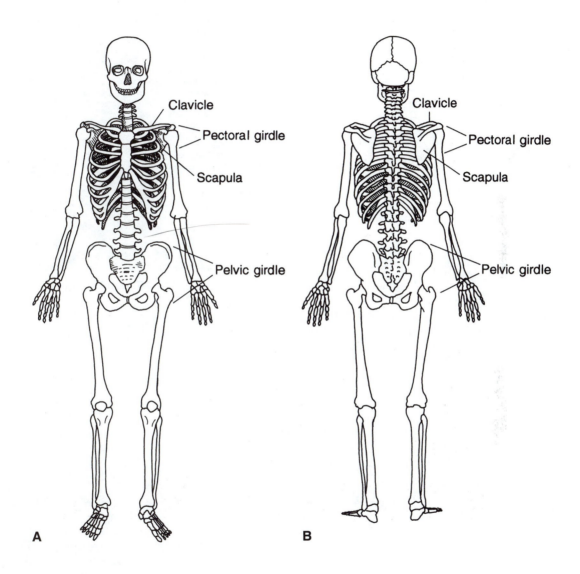

FIGURE 2-11. A. Anterior view of skeleton, showing components of pelvic and pectoral girdle. **B.** Posterior view. *(continues)*

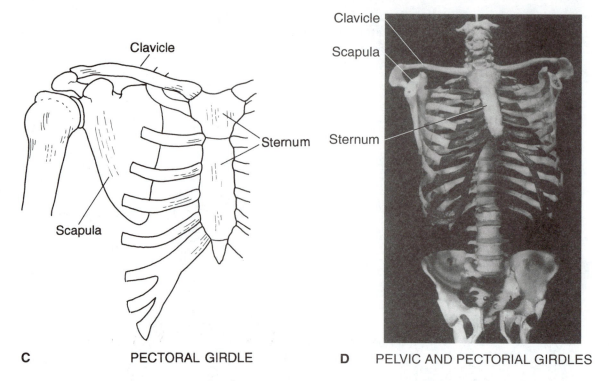

C   PECTORAL GIRDLE   D   PELVIC AND PECTORIAL GIRDLES

FIGURE 2-11. *(continued)* **C.** Isolated pectoral girdle. **D.** Articulated thorax with pelvic and pectoral girdles.

The rib cage tends to slant down in front, as shown in Figure 2-12. With the mobility of the rib cage granted by the articulation of the vertebrae and ribs, the rib cage is quite capable of elevating during inspiration to increase the size of the thorax.

Ribs are of three general classes: true ribs, false ribs, and floating ribs. The *true ribs* consist of ribs 1 through 7, all of which form more or less direct attachment with the sternum. Their actual attachment is by means of a cartilaginous union through the cartilaginous (*chondral*) portion of the rib (see Figure 2-13). The *false ribs* (ribs 8, 9, and 10) also are attached to the sternum through cartilage, although this chondral portion must run superiorly to attach to the sternum. The *floating,* or *vertebral, ribs* (ribs 11 and 12) articulate only with the vertebral column.

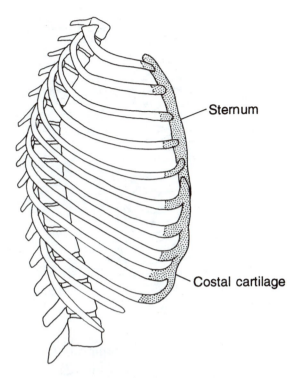

FIGURE 2-12. Lateral view of rib cage showing relationships among ribs and sternum. Note that the rib cage slants down in the front.

The chondral attachment is particularly useful because the elastic properties of cartilage permit the ribs to be twisted on the long axis (**torqued**) without breaking. Thus, the rib cage is quite strong (being made predominantly of bone) but capable of movement (being well-endowed with resilient cartilage).

The rib cage provides the basis for respiration, and the general structure of the "barrel" deserves some attention here. The ribs make their posterior attachment along the vertebral column. The ribs course posterolateral and then arch around to the anterior aspect of the body. This provides the bony structure for most of the posterior, lateral, and anterior aspects of the thorax. The ribs slope downward when the rib cage is inactive and at equilibrium.

FIGURE 2-13. Schematic of relationships among true, false, and floating ribs.

The posterior attachment of the rib is made through a *gliding* (arthrodial) *articulation* with the thoracic vertebrae. This permits the rib to rock up in both lateral and anterior directions during inspiration.

Sternum

The sternum has three components: the *manubrium sterni*, the *corpus* (body), and the *xiphoid*, or *ensiform, process* (see Figure 2-14). The clavicle and first rib are attached to the manubrium sterni, and the second rib articulates at the juncture of the manubrium and corpus, known as the *manubrosternal angle*. The next five ribs (3 through 7) articulate directly with the corpus, and the remaining

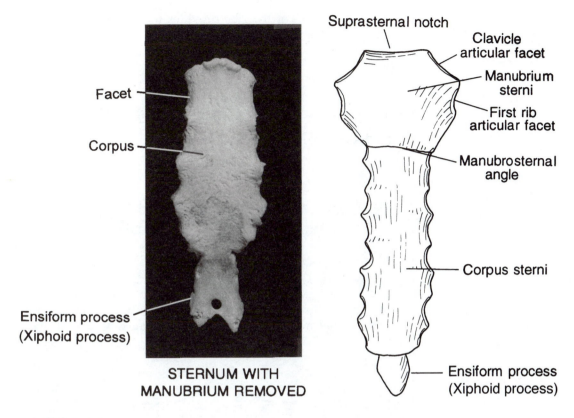

Facet

Corpus

Ensiform process
(Xiphoid process)

**STERNUM WITH
MANUBRIUM REMOVED**

Suprasternal notch

Clavicle
articular facet

Manubrium
sterni

First rib
articular facet

Manubrosternal
angle

Corpus sterni

Ensiform process
(Xiphoid process)

FIGURE 2-14. Schematic and photo of sternum. Note that the manubrium has been removed from the sternum on the left.

(false) ribs (8, 9, and 10) are attached by means of more indirect costal cartilage. The floating ribs (11 and 12) are free in the anterior.

Summary

- The rib cage is composed of 12 ribs (7 true ribs, 3 false ribs, and 2 floating ribs).
- The cartilaginous attachment of the ribs to the sternum permits the ribs to rotate slightly during respiration, allowing the rib cage to elevate.

- The construction of the ribs provides the characteristic curved barrel shape of the rib cage.
- At rest the ribs slope downward, but they elevate during inspiration.

SOFT TISSUE OF THE THORAX AND RESPIRATORY PASSAGEWAY

Turbulence and Respiration

The respiratory passageway offers relatively low resistance to airflow, a fact that works in favor of efficient respiration with little effort. As resistance to airflow increases, the effort required to draw air into the lungs increases as well, causing rapid fatigue. You may remember the exhaustion you felt the last time you had a respiratory infection that caused excessive secretions in your respiratory passageway. Part of the fatigue you felt was caused by the turbulence produced by the mucus in the passageway. The extra drag caused by these elements has to be overcome to keep the body oxygenated, and the muscles of respiration have to work overtime to do the task.

Deep inside the rib cage lies the core of respiration. Gas exchange for life occurs within the lungs, which are spongy, elastic tissue that is richly perfused with vascular supply and air sacs. Healthy, young lungs are pink; older lungs that have undergone the stresses of modern, polluted life are gray. The lungs communicate with the external environment by means of the respiratory passageway, which includes the oral and nasal cavities, larynx, trachea, and bronchial tubes.

Bifurcates: Divides into two parts.

The trachea is a flexible tube composed of a series of 16 to 20 hyaline cartilage rings that are open in the posterior aspect. This tube runs from the inferior border of the larynx for about 11 cm, where it **bifurcates** (divides) to become the left and right mainstem bronchi (or bronchial tubes), which serve the left and right lungs, respectively (see Figure 2-15).

The cartilaginous rings of the trachea are particularly well suited for the task of air transport. Because the process involves drawing air into the lungs and expelling it, pressures (negative and positive) must be generated to get that gas moving, but the same pressures will tend to collapse or expand tissue that is not reinforced for strength. On the other hand, a strictly rigid tube would restrict body movements. Thus, the trachea must be both rigid and flexible. In response to this need, the trachea is built of hyaline cartilage rings

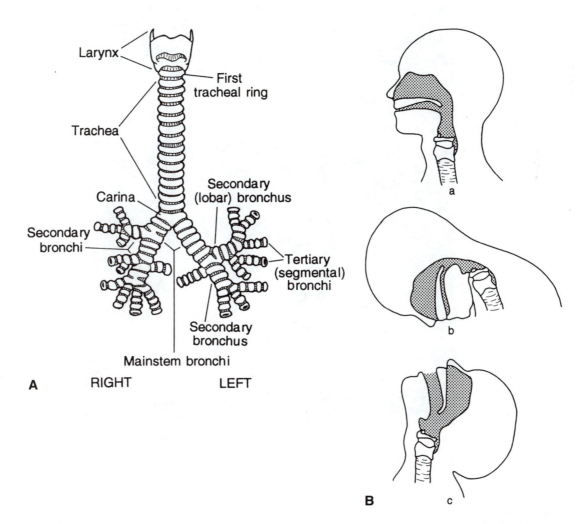

FIGURE 2-15. A. Bronchial passageway, including trachea, mainstem bronchi, secondary (lobar) bronchi, and tertiary (segmental) bronchi. **B.** Effect of head posture on airway patency (modified from data and views of Moser and Spragg, 1982). *(continues)*

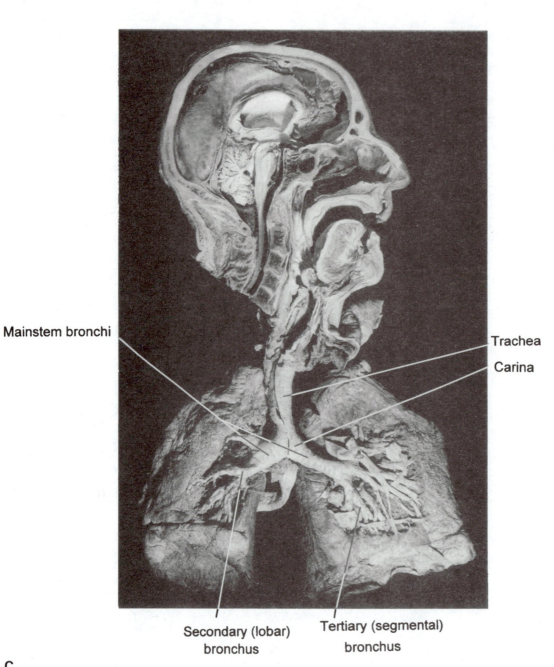

Mainstem bronchi

Trachea

Carina

Secondary (lobar)
bronchus

Tertiary (segmental)
bronchus

C

FIGURE 2-15. *(continued)* **C.** Respiratory passageway from oral cavity to segmental bronchi. Note that lungs have been dissected to reveal the bronchi within.

connected by fibroelastic membrane. The cartilage provides support while the membrane permits freedom of movement.

Posterior to the trachea is the esophagus. The *esophagus* is a long, collapsed tube that runs behind and adjacent to the trachea and is the conduit to the digestive system.

The lungs are a composite of tissues, including blood, arterial and venous network, connective tissue, respiratory pathway, and tissue specialized for gas exchange. The bronchial tree is characterized by increasingly smaller tubes as it progresses into the depths of the lungs. The *mainstem bronchi* serve the left and right lungs, and the *lobar* (intermediate) *bronchi* supply the lobes of the lungs. Further branchings occur, down to the final *terminal respiratory bronchioles.*

The right lung is composed of three lobes, separated by fissures. The left lung has only two lobes (see Figure 2-16). The right mainstem bronchus divides to supply the superior, middle, and inferior lobes of the right lung. The left mainstem bronchus bifurcates to serve the superior and inferior lobes of the left lung, and there is a vestigial middle lobe (called the lingula). The space vacated by the missing lobe is taken up by the heart and mediastinum, or "middle space," structures (see Figure 2-17).

Pneumothorax

Pneumothorax (*pneumo* = air) is aggregation of air in the pleural space between the lungs and the chest wall with subsequent loss of the negative intrapleural pressure. It can arise through one of several means, but the product is always a "collapsed" lung. In "open" pneumothorax, air is introduced into the space through a breech of the thoracic wall, typically by means of a puncture wound (e.g., knife wound, automobile accident, etc.). Air introduced into the intrapleural space causes a loss of the constant negative intrapleural pressure. If you recall that this pressure maintains the close bond between the visceral pleural lining of the lungs and that of the inner thorax, it may not surprise you to learn that when that bond is broken by the open wound, the lungs collapse. This collapse occurs because the lungs are in a state of constant distension, due to the difference between the size of the thorax and the smaller lungs.

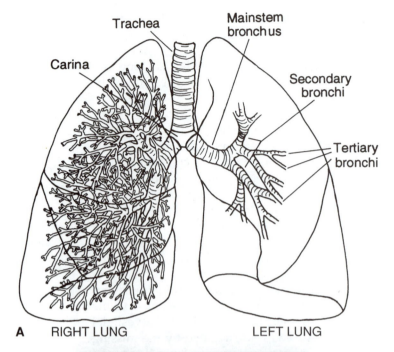

A   RIGHT LUNG   LEFT LUNG

B

FIGURE 2-16. A. Bronchial tree within lungs (modified from data and view of DesJardins, 1984). **B.** Lung dissected to reveal bronchial passageway.

The next level of branching serves the segments of each lobe. At this level of division, the bronchi divide repeatedly into smaller and smaller cartilaginous tubes, with the final tube being the terminal (end) bronchiole (see Figure 2-18).

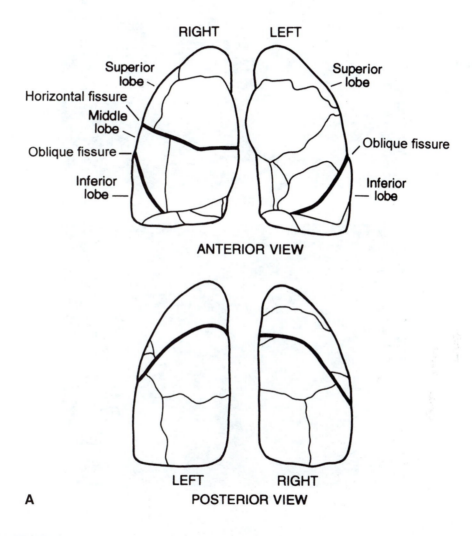

FIGURE 2-17. A. Schematic representation of lungs, showing lobes and segments. *(continues)*

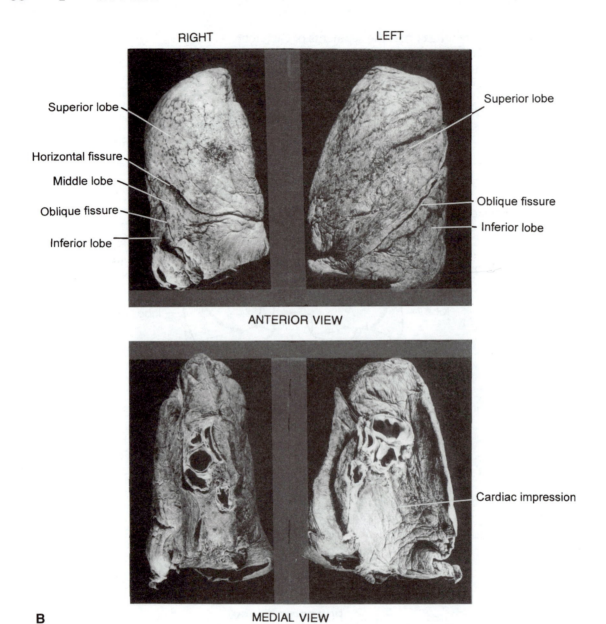

RIGHT   LEFT

Superior lobe

Horizontal fissure

Middle lobe

Oblique fissure

Inferior lobe

Superior lobe

Oblique fissure

Inferior lobe

ANTERIOR VIEW

Cardiac impression

B   MEDIAL VIEW

FIGURE 2-17. *(continued)* **B.** Anterior and medial view of lungs.

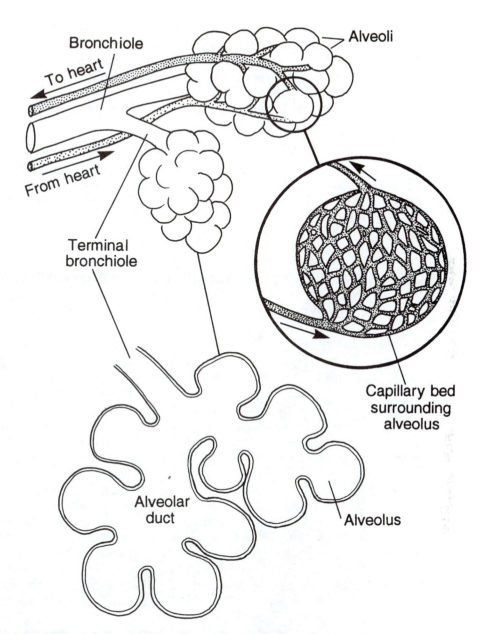

Bronchiole

Alveoli

To heart

From heart

Terminal
bronchiole

Capillary bed
surrounding
alveolus

Alveolar
duct

Alveolus

FIGURE 2-18. Schematic representation of cluster of alveoli with capillary bed. Lower portion shows a cross section through alveoli and terminal bronchiole.

This repeated branching has an important effect on respiratory function. There are 28 generations of subdivisions in the respiratory tree, providing a truly amazing amount of surface area for respiration. Although the cross-sectional area of the trachea is about 5 cm^2 (about the diameter of a quarter), the cross-sectional area of the 300,000,000 alveoli would equal 70 M^2, or the area of a rug large enough to cover a 10 ft. × 4 ft. room!

The terminal bronchiole is small (about 1 mm in diameter), and at its end becomes the alveolar duct, which in turn communicates with the alveolus. The alveoli are extremely small (approximately $\frac{1}{4}$ mm in diameter) but extremely plentiful. There are approximately 300 million alveoli in mature lungs.

Muscular Weakness and Respiration

Individuals with diseases that weaken the muscles of inspiration are at significant respiratory risk for a number of reasons. Although gravity is the friend of respiration in a person with normal function, inspiration requires muscular effort, and that effort is aimed very specifically at overcoming gravity.

Individuals in the later stages of demyelinating diseases such as amyotrophic lateral sclerosis (ALS) suffer from extreme muscular weakness as a result of the disease but are still faced with the oxygenation demands typically met with respiratory work. If a person with such a disease is placed in the supine position (on the back), gravity will conspire against his or her respiratory effort, and this "resting" position will actually put the person at risk for respiratory distress. Here's why: When supine, gravity is pushing on the abdominal viscera, forcing the viscera toward the person's back. When the individual attempts to inhale, the abdomen should protrude, but with compromised muscular strength, that will require more effort than the person can accomplish. When supine, the abdominal viscera are one more thing to overcome, and that is one thing too many.

To overcome this, people in the later stages of ALS often remain in a semireclined position to permit rest but capitalize on gravity to assist with respiration. By the way, this might also give you a clue as to why individuals with weakened musculature are more prone to pneumonia than healthy individuals. It takes a great deal of work to clear the lungs and to keep them clear.

The **alveoli** at this terminal point do the real work of respiration by virtue of their architecture and relationship with the vascular supply (see Figure 2-18). The alveolus is an extremely thin membrane (about one third the thickness of a red blood cell) that is permeable to both oxygen and carbon dioxide in the proper circumstances.

Alveoli: Air sacs in the lungs.

The rich investment with alveoli make the lungs spongy because the surfactant (a substance that lowers surface tension) at that level promotes inflation of the alveoli. Each alveolus is richly supplied with blood for gas exchange from more than 2,000 capillaries. A little multiplication will reveal that there are more than 600,000,000,000 (600 billion) capillaries involved in gas exchange, reminding us of the amount of vascular tissue in the lungs. The lungs also have an intricate lacework of cartilage; the bronchial tree is invested with this supportive tissue and most branches of this tree contain cartilage. At the terminal point in the bronchial tree the marvel of gas exchange takes place. Attached to the final cartilaginous bronchiole is the alveolus, or air sac, the point at which oxygen and carbon dioxide are transferred to and from the bloodstream.

The respiratory pathway has multiple filtering functions to safeguard the lungs against pollutants. The nostril hairs are the first line of defense, catching most particulate matter greater than 10 microns (a micron is one millionth of a meter) before they enter the trachea. The moist mucous membrane of the upper respiratory system provides another receptacle for foreign matter. Goblet cells in the mucosal lining and submucosal glands secrete lubricant into the respiratory tract that traps pollutants as they enter the trachea and larynx. The respiratory passageway from the nose to the beginning of the bronchi is lined with tall columnar epithelium covered by cilia (hairlike processes) that beat more than 1,000 times per minute. In the lower pathway, the beating action drives pollutants upward, and beating drives nasal-passage contaminants posteriorly.

The beating epithelia progressively move the material up the bronchi to the level of the vocal folds in the larynx, at which time the breathing person feels the stimulation of secretion at the vocal folds and "clears her throat." That "ahem" is just enough force to blow the mucus off the folds (mucus is the dense fluid product of mucous membrane tissue), where it can be swallowed without further ado. Unfortunately, these beating epithelia can be damaged by pollutants such as cigarette smoke, resulting in the failure of this system. Particles in the 2 to 10 micron range will settle on the walls of the bronchi, where they are eliminated by these beating epithelia. If a particle is smaller than 2 microns, it will generally reach the alveolus but will be eliminated by microphages, the cells that destroy foreign matter.

The lymphatic system provides a final cleaning stage for the respiratory tissue. The upper respiratory passageway effectively removes normal levels of particulate pollution down to diameters of approximately 5 microns, but smaller particles are not filtered. These particles down to the level of the terminal bronchiole are eliminated by the lymphatic system. Pollutants are suspended in mucus and through coughing migrate to the bronchioles, where they can be eliminated by the lymphatics and macrophages.

The respiratory passageway also protects the lungs by warming and humidifying the air as it enters. The mucous membrane is highly vascularized, permitting rapid transfer of heat from blood to air.

Summary

- The respiratory system is composed of right and left lungs, which have three and two lobes, respectively.
- Communication between the external and internal environments is by means of the trachea and bronchial tree.
- Repeated subdivisions of this bronchial tree ends with the alveoli, the site of gas exchange.
- These highly vascularized alveoli provide the mechanism by which oxygen enters the bloodstream and carbon dioxide is removed.
- Pollutants entering the respiratory tract are removed through the cleansing action of beating epithelia that line the bronchial passageway.

MOVEMENT OF AIR THROUGH THE SYSTEM

Recall that the cavity holding the lungs is supported by muscle and bone, which cover every centimeter of the thoracic wall. Likewise, the bottom of the thoracic cavity is completely sealed by the diaphragm, making the thorax almost impervious to the outside world, were it not for the respiratory passageway. The only way air can normally enter or leave the lungs is through the tubes connected to them (the bronchial tree, continuous with the upper respiratory passageway).

Now comes the tricky part. The lungs are simply placed inside this cavity, not held to the walls by ligaments or cartilage. It is as if you placed a too-small sponge in a too-large bottle, because the thoracic volume is greater than that of the lungs at rest.

The lungs and inner thoracic wall are completely covered with a *pleural lining* (see Figure 2-19), and this lining is a smooth contact for rough tissue, as well as a mechanism for translating the force of thorax enlargement into inspiration. The lungs are encased in linings referred to as the *visceral pleurae*, and the thoracic linings are the *parietal pleurae*. The visceral and parietal pleurae are actually continuous with each other. These wrappings completely encase both the lungs and inner thorax. This continuous sheet provides the airtight seal required to permit the lungs to follow the movement of the thorax.

To understand how these pleurae help us breathe will take a little thought. You have probably experienced the difficulty involved in separating two pieces of plastic food wrap, especially if there is fluid between the two sheets. There is a degree of surface tension arising from the presence of fluid and highly conforming surfaces that helps keep the sheets together. Likewise, cuboidal cells in the pleural lining produce a mucous solution that is released into the space between the parietal and visceral pleurae. This surfactant reduces the surface tension in the lungs and provides a slippery interface between the

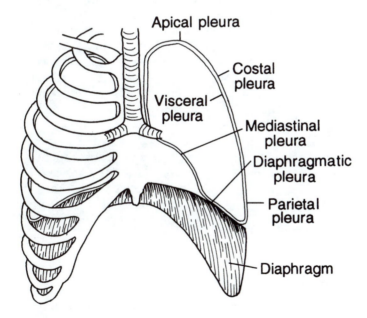

FIGURE 2-19. Pleural linings of the lungs and thorax. Parietal pleurae include costal, diaphragmatic, mediastinal, and apical pleurae. Visceral pleurae line the lungs.

lungs and the thoracic wall, permitting easy, low-friction gliding of the lungs within the thorax. The lung and rib cage surfaces conform to each other as a result of the fluid bond between them, and a negative pressure is maintained by lack of contact with the outside atmosphere. When you contract the diaphragm, the pleural lining of the diaphragm (diaphragmatic pleura) maintains its contact with the visceral pleurae of the two lungs above it, and the lungs expand.

Spinal Cord Injury

The spinal cord is well protected by the osseous vertebral column because the vertebrae fit together like a partial lock-and-key to inhibit motion. The vertebral column is richly bound by ligaments and surrounded by muscles of the back.

Despite this redundant protection, the spinal cord is frequently traumatized. The most frequent cause of spinal cord injury is vehicle accidents, especially those in which the occupant is not properly restrained. When a person is ejected from a vehicle, the vertebral column can undergo rotatory stresses that can tear the spinal cord, and impact can compress the vertebral column (typically the compression occurs in the corpus, implying hyperflexion of the neck), which can result in distension of the spinal cord. Significant transverse forces can cause a shearing of the spinal cord as well.

The result of spinal cord injury is often loss of motor and sensory function to the area below the injury, with subsequent paraplegia (legs paralyzed) or quadriplegia (both arms and both legs paralyzed). For an exhaustive review of spinal cord injury see Mackay, Chapman, and Morgan (1997).

Mediastinal: *Referring to the mediastinum of the thorax.*

The heart is encased in the **mediastinal** pleurae, along with nerves, blood vessels, thymus gland, the esophagus, and lymph vessels (see Figure 2-20). The mediastinum is the most important and best protected region of the body.

Pericardium: *The membranous sac enclosing the heart.*

The left and right *phrenic nerves* serving the diaphragm pass along the lateral surfaces of the **pericardium** (the membranous sac enclosing the heart) to innervate the diaphragm.

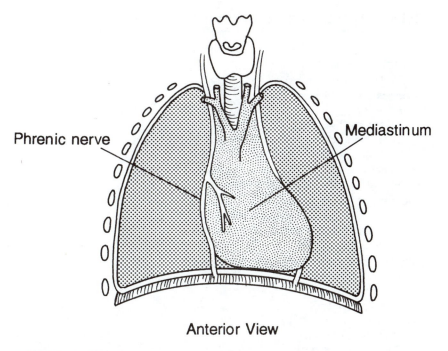

Phrenic nerve

Mediastinum

Anterior View

FIGURE 2–20. Relationships among mediastinum, diaphragm, and lungs. Note the phrenic nerve innervation of the diaphragm.

Summary

- The lungs are covered with pleural linings that, in conjunction with the lungs, provide the mechanism for air movement through muscular action.
- When the diaphragm contracts, the lungs are pulled down due to the association between the pleurae and the diaphragm.
- Diaphragmatic contraction expands the lungs, drawing air into them through the bronchial passageway.

MUSCLES OF INSPIRATION

As with many voluntary bodily functions, inspiration is a graded activity. Depending on your body's needs, you are capable of quiet inspiration, which requires only one muscle, and forced inspiration, which calls on many more muscles. We enlist the help of increasingly larger numbers of muscles as our respiratory needs increase. Refer to Table 2-1 for a summary of the muscles of respiration.

Table 2–1. Muscles of Respiration

Inspiration

Primary of Thorax
    Diaphragm

Accessory of Thorax
    Anterior
    External intercostal
    Interchondral portion, internal intercostal
    Posterior
    Levatores costarum (brevis and longis)
    Serratus posterior superior

Muscles of Neck
    Sternocleidomastoid (superficial neck)
    Scalenus (anterior, middle, posterior)
    Trapezius

Muscles of Thorax, Back, and Upper Limb
    Pectoralis major
    Pectoralis minor
    Serratus anterior
    Subclavius
    Levator scapulae
    Rhomboideus major
    Rhomboideus minor

Expiration

Muscles of Thorax, Back, and Upper Limb
    Anterior
    Internal intercostal (interosseous portion)
    Transversus thoracis
    Posterior
    Subcostal
    Serratus posterior inferior
    Innermost intercostal
    Latissimus dorsi

Abdominal Muscles
    Anterolateral
    Transversus abdominis
    Internal oblique abdominis
    External oblique abdominis
    Rectus abdominis
    Posterior
    Quadratus lumborum

Palpation of Sternal Landmarks

Palpation of structures (feeling them with your hands) on your own body will improve your awareness of these structures and their organization into systems. First, palpate the sternal notch. To identify its location, find your "Adam's apple," the prominence of the larynx about which you will learn a great deal in future chapters. Now draw your finger down until you reach a prominent horizontal ledge. That ledge is the sternal notch. Now draw your finger to either side and you will feel a significant bump. This is the clavicle.

Now move your fingers laterally to feel the clavicle itself as it projects to its union with the scapula. Identify the lower margin of the clavicle at the sternoclavicular joint; if you press deeply into the muscle at that point, you may be able to palpate the first rib. Move your fingers back to the sternal notch, and then draw them down the sternum about an inch. You should easily feel a prominent ridge, the manubrosternal angle or joint. Placing one finger on your sternal notch and another on the manubrosternal angle will show you the upper and lower limits of the manubrium sterni.

If you draw your finger down another couple of inches below the manubrosternal angle, you will feel the lower margin of the corpus sterni, and beneath this the xiphoid or ensiform process.

The union of the sternum and clavicle is the sternoclavicular joint, and it occurs at the manubrium sterni, lateral to the sternal notch.

Palpation: Feeling a structure using one's hands.

Primary Inspiratory Muscle of Thorax: The Diaphragm

The primary muscle of inspiration is the *diaphragm*. As seen in Figure 2-21, the diaphragm completely separates the abdominal and thoracic cavities (with the exception of vascular and esophageal hiatuses). This striated muscle takes the form of a large inverted bowl. The edges of this irregular bowl attach along the inferior boundary of the rib cage and xiphoid process and to the vertebral column in the posterior aspect. The intermediate region is made up of a large, leafy aponeurosis called the *central tendon*. When the muscle contracts, muscle fibers shorten and the diaphragm pulls the central tendon down and back (see Figure 2-22).

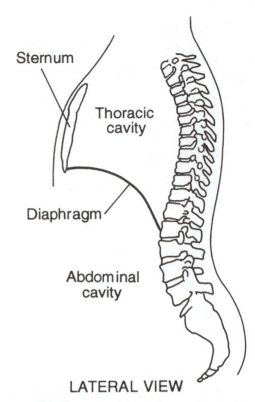

Sternum

Thoracic cavity

Diaphragm

Abdominal cavity

LATERAL VIEW

FIGURE 2-21. Lateral view schematic of diaphragm and thorax. Notice that the diaphragm courses markedly down from the sternum to the vertebral attachment, completely separating the thorax from the abdomen.

Palpation of Rib Cage

Although you cannot palpate your diaphragm, you can identify its margins easily enough. First, find your xiphoid process. This point marks part of the origin of the rectus abdominis, but the diaphragm attaches on the inner surface. Place your fingers on the xiphoid process and the muscle below, and breathe deeply in and out once. You can feel the rectus abdominis being stretched during inspiration. Now place the fingers of both hands at the bottom of the rib cage on both sides of the sternum, so that your fingers are pressing into your abdominal muscles. Breathe out as deeply as you can and hold that posture while you bend slightly forward. Your fingers are marking the margin of the diaphragm, although you are palpating abdominal muscles.

Bring your fingers up to feel your ribs. Place your fingers between the ribs, with your little finger of each hand on the abdominal muscles below the rib cage. Breathe in a couple of times and feel the abdominal muscles first draw in and then tighten up as you reach maximum inspiration. Feel your rib cage elevate as you do this.

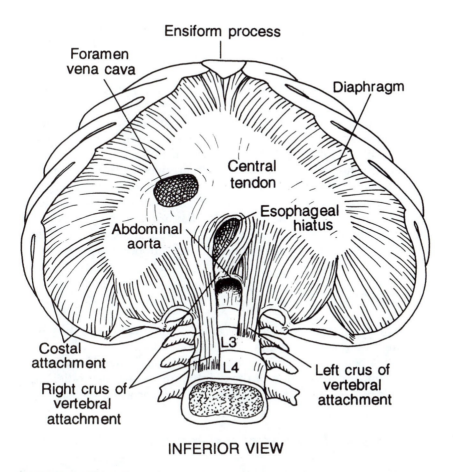

FIGURE 2–22. Inferior view schematic of diaphragm, as seen from the abdominal cavity.

The muscle fibers of the diaphragm radiate out from the central tendon, forming the sternal, costal, and vertebral attachments. The anterior-most *sternal attachment* is made at the xiphoid process, with fibers coursing up and back to insert into the anterior central tendon. Lateral to the xiphoid, the fibers of the diaphragm attach to the inner borders of ribs 7 through 12 and to the costal cartilages to form the *costal attachment*. In the posterior aspect, the *vertebral diaphragmatic* attachment is made with the lumbar vertebrae.

The actual muscle fibers of the diaphragm radiate out from the imperfect center formed by the central tendon. Careful examination of the forces of muscular contraction will be most helpful in later discussion of muscular contraction and action. Remember that muscle can perform only one task, and that is to shorten. If a muscle is attached to two points, shortening tends to bring those two points closer together or simply tense the muscle if neither point is capable of moving. Although the principles of muscle action and result still hold, movement of the diaphragm will not make a great deal of sense until you realize where the points of attachment really are.

Contraction of the diaphragm has the result of pulling the central tendon down. It is directly analogous to placing someone in the middle of a blanket while a host of friends pull on the corners of the blanket. When the friends pull together, the person in the middle flies up. Because the diaphragm has the shape of an inverted bowl, pulling on the edges (muscular contraction) draws the center down (see Figure 2-23). Innervation of the diaphragm is by means of the phrenic nerve. The diaphragm can be placed under voluntary control, but it is under primary control of the autonomic system.

Summary

- The primary muscle of inspiration is the diaphragm, the dividing point between the thorax and the abdomen.
- The fibers of the diaphragm pull on the central tendon, resulting in downward motion of the diaphragm during inspiration, and this movement expands the lungs in the vertical dimension.

Accessory Muscles of Inspiration

Although the diaphragm is the major contributor to inspiration, it needs help to meet your body's needs for forced inspiration. If you take a look at Figure 2-24A, you will see the rib cage from the side. Direct your attention first to the way the ribs run. They are directed distinctly downward as they make their path to the front of the skeleton. Next, imagine raising the ribs in front. When you do that, the front of the rib cage expands as a result. Swinging those ribs up means that they will swing out a bit, thereby increasing the volume of the rib cage.

To put this function in everyday terms, look at Figure 2-24B showing venetian blinds from the side. When they are closed, they are similar to the rib cage at rest, and when they are opened, they are similar to ribs being elevated. That elevation brings the ribs more nearly horizontal, just like the blinds, and that change increases the overall front-to-back dimension. We will differentiate these muscles that are responsible for elevation based on their locations.

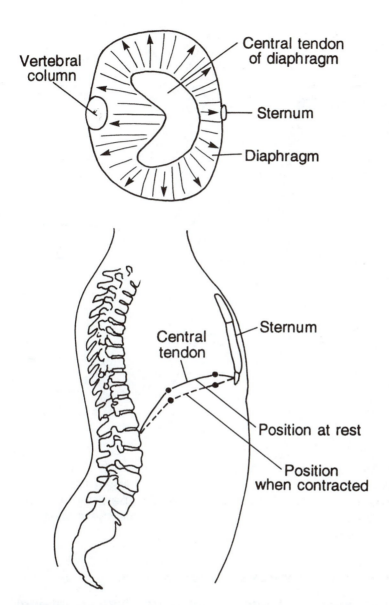

FIGURE 2-23. *Top:* Schematic of transverse view of the diaphragm with central tendon. The arrows depict the direction of force on contraction of the diaphragm. *Bottom:* This lateral view of the diaphragm shows that contraction of the diaphragm pulls the central tendon down.

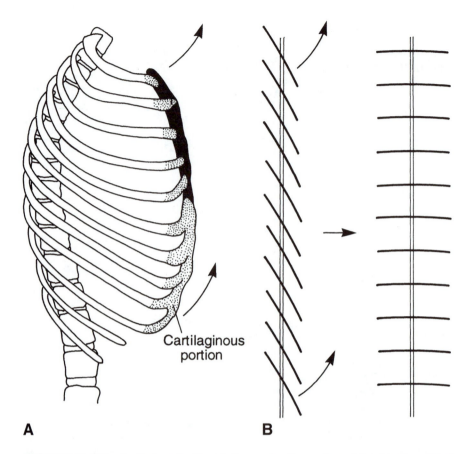

Cartilaginous
portion

A   **B**

FIGURE 2–24. A. Schematic of rib cage from the side. Notice that the ribs slant down as they run forward. During inspiration the rib cage elevates, as shown by the arrows. **B.** On the right side, the venetian blinds shown from the side demonstrate the change in volume achieved by elevation of the rib cage.

Anterior Thoracic Muscles of Inspiration

External Intercostal and Interchondral Portion, Internal Intercostal Muscles. The *external intercostal* muscles are among the most significant respiratory muscles for speech. They not only provide a significant proportion of the total respiratory capacity, but they also perform functions that are uniquely speech-related.

As you can see in Figure 2-25, the 11 external intercostal muscles reside between the 12 ribs of the thorax, providing the ribs with both unity and mobility. The external intercostal muscles originate on the lower surface of each rib (except rib 12) and course downward and

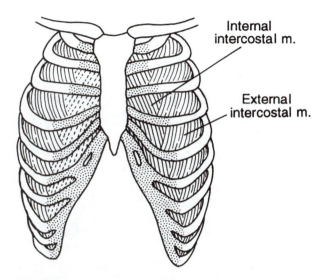

Internal intercostal m.

External intercostal m.

FIGURE 2-25. Rib cage with external and internal intercostal muscles. On the left rib cage the fascia covering the internal intercostals has been removed, whereas it remains present and translucent on the right. External intercostals are absent near the sternum, and thus one can see the deeper internal intercostals in that region.

inward to insert into the upper surface of the rib immediately below. These muscles provide a unified surface of diagonally slanting striated muscle on all costal surfaces of the rib cage with the exception of the region near the sternum. Contraction of external intercostal fibers in that region would provide little benefit (and perhaps some negative effect) to the job of increasing cavity size.

The internal intercostal muscles are predominantly muscles of expiration, with the exception of the chondral portion. The **parasternal** ("near the sternum") portion of the internal intercostal muscles encompassing the chondral aspect of the ribs is active during forced inspiration.

Parasternal: Near the sternum.

The external intercostal muscles elevate the rib cage. As the rib cage is elevated, the flexible coupling of the costosternal attachment permits the chondral portion of the ribs to rotate. The net result is that the sternum remains relatively parallel to the vertebral column even as the rib cage expands, increasing the anterior dimension and thus the volume of the lungs. The effort involved in raising the ribs twists (torques) the elastic cartilaginous portion of the ribs; when that force is relaxed, the cartilage returns to its original form. Innervation of the external intercostal muscles is achieved by the intercostal nerves arising from T1 through T11.

Keeping the Airway Open in Respiratory Emergency

Sometimes in a respiratory emergency it is necessary to ensure that the respiratory pathway remains patent ("open"). In a conscious patient, the normal head and neck orientation places the mouth at a 90° angle to the airway above the larynx (pharynx). If an unconscious individual's head drops forward (see Figure 2-15B(b)), the airway can become occluded and limit respiration.

In some cases, there is concern that the vocal folds or airway above that level will not remain open, so an emergency tracheostomy is performed (*tracheo* = trachea; *stoma* = mouth). This medical procedure involves opening an artificial passageway into the trachea.

If the risk of head movement is minimal (i.e., there appears to be no cervical spine trauma), a trauma patient will receive an endotracheal tube (be intubated) to provide respiratory support for the patient.

Although the external intercostals account for most of the second dimensional change (the anterior-posterior dimension), there are other muscles that help. Any muscle that attaches to the rib cage or sternum could feasibly elevate either the rib cage or sternum. Some other possible assistants in respiration are the *levatores costarum* (*brevis* and *longis*) and *serratus posterior superior*, as shown in Figure 2-26. You can imagine that they would elevate the rib cage on contraction, as would the serratus posterior superior.

Posterior Thoracic Muscles of Inspiration

Levatores Costarum. Shortening the levatores costarum (brevis and longis) tends to elevate the rib cage. Although these muscles would appear to be muscles of the back, they are considered thoracic muscles. The brevis ("brief") portions of the levator costarum originate on the transverse processes of vertebrae C7 through T11, for a total of 12 levator costarum brevis muscles. Fibers course obliquely down and out to insert into the tubercle of the rib below.

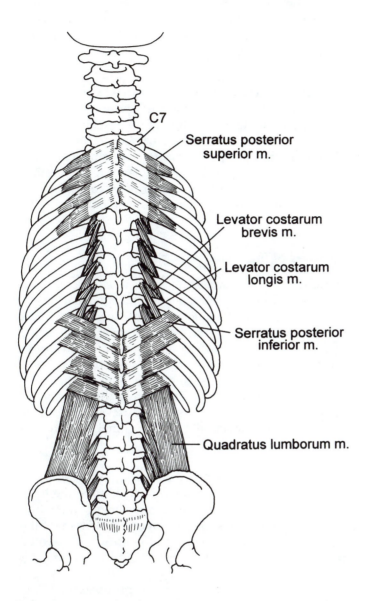

FIGURE 2-26. Posterior thoracic muscles of inspiration. Note that the levatores costarum are present on all ribs but in the superior aspect they are deep to the serratus posterior muscles.

The longis portions originate on the transverse processes of T7 through T11, with fibers coursing down and obliquely out. The fibers bypass the rib below the point of origin, inserting instead into the next rib. You can see that the longis portion will have a greater effect on elevation of the rib cage. The levatores costarum are innervated by the intercostal nerves.

Serratus Posterior Superior. In Figure 2-26, you can see that, given their course, contraction of the serratus posterior superior muscles could easily contribute to elevation of the rib cage. The serratus posterior superior muscles have their origins on the spinous processes of C7 and T1 through T3. Fibers from these muscles course down and laterally to insert just beyond the angles of ribs 2 through 5. Innervation of the serratus posterior superior is completed by means of the ventral intercostal portion of the spinal nerves T1 through T4 or T5.

Accessory Muscles of the Neck

Sternocleidomastoid. The *sternocleidomastoid muscle* courses from origin on the mastoid process of the temporal bone to its insertion at the sternum (sterno) and clavicle (cleido) (see Figure 2-27). When a sternocleidomastoid is contracted separately, it will rotate the head toward the side of contraction. When both left and right sternocleidomastoid muscles are contracted simultaneously, the thoracic cavity will be the beneficiary because these muscles have the capacity to elevate the sternum and subsequently the anterior rib cage. The sternocleidomastoid and trapezius muscles derive their innervation from the eleventh cranial nerve, spinal branch (XI) accessory.

Scalenus Anterior, Middle, and Posterior. The *scaleni*, or scalenes, are muscles of the neck that provide stability to the head and facilitate rotation and, by virtue of their attachment on the first and second ribs, can increase the superior-inferior dimension of the thorax (see Figure 2-27). Neck stability and control are essential ingredients for normal development of speech.

The *anterior scaleni* originate on the transverse processes of vertebrae C3 through C6, with fibers coursing down to insert into the superior surface of the first rib. The *middle scaleni* take their origin on transverse processes of vertebrae C2 through C7, also inserting into the first rib. The *posterior scaleni* insert into the second rib, having coursed from the transverse processes of C5 through C7. The scaleni anterior are innervated by spinal nerves C4 through C6.

Gastroesophageal Reflux

The esophageal orifice is situated in the inferior laryngopharynx and is enveloped by the musculature of the inferior pharyngeal constrictors. The cricopharyngeus muscle, which is actually part of the inferior constrictor, controls the size of the orifice by contracting to constrict the opening.

Esophageal reflux is a condition in which digestive acids are expelled into the region above the superior orifice of the esophagus, causing irritation to the delicate laryngeal tissue. Gastroesophageal reflux disease (GERD) refers to the chronic reintroduction of gastrointestinal contents into the esophagus and respiratory passageway. In adults GERD can lead to swallowing difficulties, inflammation of laryngeal tissues, and even aspiration pneumonia if the esophageal contents enter the lungs. In newborns and very young children, a weak esophageal sphincter can result in reflux and the inability to retain nourishment. This is life-threatening because of the potential for malnutrition and aspiration. The condition is not uncommon among children with cerebral palsy, and often results in frequent vomiting, loss of nutrition, and aspiration pneumonia.

There are numerous nonsurgical interventions for GERD, including diet change, medications, and position changes. If less invasive procedures fail to alleviate the condition, the size of the esophageal opening may be reduced surgically through a procedure known as Nissen fundoplication ("sling"), thereby inhibiting regurgitation of stomach contents. Nissen fundoplication involves surgical narrowing of the esophageal opening by releasing a flap of tissue from the stomach, followed by elevation and suturing of the flap to the esophageal orifice. The child may receive nutrition through a tube run through the nasal cavity into the esophagus (nasogastric tube; *naso* = nose; *gastric* = stomach) or through orogastric (oral feeding tube) feeding, again via tube. These are both types of *gavage*, or getting food to the stomach through a tube.

Surgical placement of a gastronomy tube may be required if reflux cannot be controlled adequately to guarantee nutrition. This procedure, referred to as gastronomy, results in surgical placement of a feeding tube into the stomach wall. Similarly, jejunostomy is placement of a feeding tube into the small intestine. For a more detailed discussion, see Langley and Lombardino (1991).

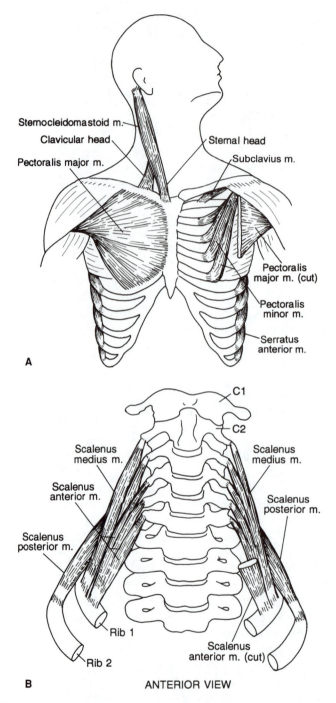

FIGURE 2-27. A. Schematic of pectoralls major, pectoralls minor, sternocleidomastoid, subclavius, and serratus anterior muscles. **B.** Schematic of scalenus anterior, medius, and posterior muscles.

Muscles of Upper Arm and Shoulder

The accessory muscles of the arm may assist the external intercostal in elevation of the thorax by virtue of their attachment to the sternum and ribs. Although not confirmed through physiological study, the action of each of the following muscles has the potential to increase the anterior-posterior dimension of the thorax.

Pectoralis Major and Minor. The *pectoralis major* muscle is a large, fan-shaped muscle that originates from two heads (see Figure 2-27). The *sternal head* attaches along the length of the sternum at the costal cartilages, and the *clavicular head* arises from the anterior surface of the clavicle. The muscle converges at the crest of the greater tubercle of the humerus. In respiration, the pectoralis major elevates the sternum and thus increases the transverse dimension of the rib cage.

The *pectoralis minor* originates on the anterior surface of ribs 2 through 5, with fibers coursing up to converge on the coracoid process of the scapula. As with the pectoralis major, respiratory function would involve elevation of the rib cage, although this function has not been verified for either muscle. Both pectoralis major and minor are innervated by the pectoral nerves, arising from the brachial plexus.

Serratus Anterior. Fibers of the *serratus anterior* muscle arise from ribs 1 through 9 along the side of the thorax, coursing up to converge on the inner vertebral border of the scapula. Contraction may elevate the ribs to which it is attached and subsequently the rib cage (see Figure 2-27). The serratus anterior receives innervation by spinal nerves C5 through C7.

Back Muscles of Inspiration

Levator Scapulae. The *levator scapulae* muscle provides neck support secondarily as a result of its function as an elevator of the scapula. This muscle originates from the transverse processes of C1 through C4 and courses down to insert into the medial border of the scapula (see Figure 2-28). The levator scapulae derives its innervation from the brachial plexus.

Rhomboideus Major and Minor. The *rhomboids* (*major* and *minor*) lie deep to the trapezius, originating on the spinous processes of T2 through T5 (*rhomboideus major*) and from C7 and T1

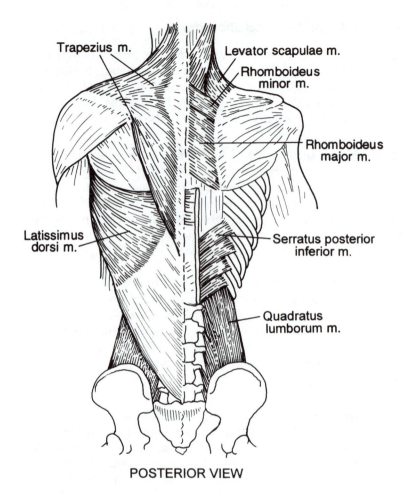

POSTERIOR VIEW

FIGURE 2-28. Accessory muscles of respiration: Trapezius, levator scapulae, rhomboideus minor, rhomboideus major, serratus posterior inferior, latissimus dorsi, and quadratus lumborum.

(rhomboideus minor). The rhombhoid muscles course down and laterally to insert into the medial border of the scapula. Primary speech function of the rhomboids is the support they provide for the upper body, especially the shoulder girdle. The rhomboids receive their innervation from the dorsal scapular nerves arising from spinal C5.

Trapezius. The *trapezius* (Figure 2-28) is a massive muscle making up the superficial upper back and neck, originating along the spinous processes of C2 to T12. Fibers of this muscle fan laterally to insert into the acromion of scapula and superior surface of clavicle. Contraction of this muscle clearly plays a significant role in elongation of the neck and in head control. The trapezius muscle is innervated by the XI Accessory.

Summary

- The diaphragm is an exceptionally important muscle of inspiration, but many accessory muscles of inspiration and expiration also serve respiration.
- Generally, muscles of the thorax and neck that elevate the rib cage serve an accessory function for inspiration.

Muscles of Forced Expiration

Active expiration requires muscles to act on the lungs indirectly to "squeeze" the air out of them. This is achieved in two ways. The front-to-back dimension of the rib cage is reduced when the rib cage is pulled down by the internal intercostal muscles, the innermost intercostal muscles, and the transversus thoracis muscles. The second means of reducing the volume of the thorax is by reducing the superior-inferior dimension. We can forcefully expire by contracting the muscles of the abdominal region which, in turn, squeeze the abdomen and force the viscera upward, reducing the size of the thorax. The abdominal muscles of expiration (see Figure 2-29) are very much like a cummerbund, wrapping the abdomen front, side, and back of into a neat package.

The layers of abdominal muscles provide excellent support for the rib cage during lifting and other body movements. These movements virtually force immobilization of the thorax by inflating the lungs and closing off the vocal folds, and the abdominal muscles help to compress the viscera while simultaneously stabilizing the thorax.

Muscles of Thorax: Anterior/Lateral Thoracic Muscles

Internal Intercostal, Interosseous Portion. The *interosseous portion* of the *internal intercostal* muscles is a significant contributor to forced expiration. The internal intercostal muscles are pervasive in the thorax, originating on the superior margin of each rib and running up and medially to insert into the inferior surface of the rib

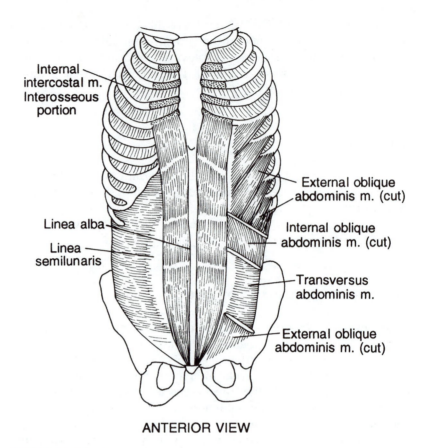

Internal intercostal m. Interosseous portion

Linea alba

Linea semilunaris

External oblique abdominis m. (cut)

Internal oblique abdominis m. (cut)

Transversus abdominis m.

External oblique abdominis m. (cut)

ANTERIOR VIEW

FIGURE 2–29. Accessory muscles of expiration and landmarks of the adominal aponeurosis.

above. They are absent in the posterior aspect of the rib cage near the vertebral column. Because the external intercostal muscles run at nearly right angles to the internals, these two sets of muscle provide significant support for the rib cage and protection of the ribs, as well as maintenance of rib spacing.

The internal intercostal muscles also provide a mechanism for depressing the rib cage. As you can see from the schematic of Figure 2-30, when the interosseous portion of the internal intercostal contracts and shortens, the direction of movement is down, and the expanded rib cage becomes smaller. The internal intercostals muscles are innervated by the intercostal nerves.

Transversus Thoracis. As the name implies, the *transversus thoracis* ("transverse muscles of thorax") muscles are found on the inner

Sternum

Effect of contraction
of internal intercostal muscles

FIGURE 2-30. Effects of contraction of the interosseous portion of the internal intercostals is to pull the rib cage down, thereby decreasing the volume of the lungs.

surface of the rib cage. The muscles originate on the margin of the sternum, with fibers coursing to the inner chondral surface of ribs 2 through 6. Contraction of the muscles decreases the volume of the thoracic cavity. The thoracic intercostal nerves innervate the transverses thoracis.

Posterior Thoracic Muscles

Subcostals. The *subcostal muscles* are widely variable but generally take a course parallel to the internal intercostal and thus can serve expiration. The subcostals are on the inner posterior wall of the thorax. Unlike the intercostal muscles, the subcostals can span more than one rib. The subcostals are innervated by the intercostal nerves of the thorax.

Serratus Posterior Inferior. The *serratus posterior inferior* muscles originate on the spinous processes of T11, T12, and L1 through L3 and course up and laterally to insert into the lower margin of the lower five ribs. Contraction of these muscles pulls the rib cage down for expiration. The serratus posterior inferior is innervated by the intercostal and subcostal nerves.

Abdominal Muscles of Expiration

If you consider the human skeleton and imagine placing muscles in the region between the rib cage and the pelvis, you will realize that there are few places from which muscles can originate. To deal with this, nature has provided a tendinous structure, the abdominal aponeurosis. Figure 2-31 shows a schematic representation of the abdominal aponeurosis from the front, as well as in the transverse section. The *linea alba* ("white line") runs from the xiphoid process to the pubic symphysis, forming the midline structure for muscular attachment. In the transverse view, you can see that as the linea alba progresses laterally, it differentiates into two sheets of aponeurosis, between which is placed the rectus abdominis. This aponeurotic wrapping comes back together to form another band of tendon, the *linea semilunaris*. This tendon once again divides, but this time into three sheets of aponeurosis, which provide a way to attach three more muscles to this structure.

In the posterior aspect, the fascia join to form the *lumbodorsal fascia*. This structure connects the three abdominal muscles (transversus abdominis, internal and external oblique abdominis) with the vertebral column. The *external oblique aponeurosis* communicates directly with the fascia covering the rectus abdominis, forming a continuous layer of connective tissue from the linea alba to the external oblique muscle.

Anterolateral Abdominal Muscles.   The abdominal muscles of expiration function by compression of the abdominal viscera. This compression function not only is useful in respiration, but also aids in defecation, vomiting, and childbirth (with vocal folds tightly adducted).

Transversus Abdominis.   The transversus abdominis (see Figure 2-31) runs laterally, originating in the posterior aspect at the vertebral column via the thoracolumbar fascia of the abdominal aponeurosis. Its anterior attachment is to the transversus abdominis aponeurosis, as well as to the inner surface of ribs 6 through 12. Its inferior-most attachment is at the pubis. Contraction of the transversus significantly reduces the volume of the abdomen. Innervation of the transversus abdominis is via the thoracic and lumbar nerves.

Internal Oblique Abdominis.   The *internal oblique abdominis* is located between the external oblique abdominis and the transversus abdominis. As seen in Figure 2-31, this muscle fans out from its origin on the inguinal ligament and iliac crest to the cartilaginous

A   TRANSVERSE VIEW

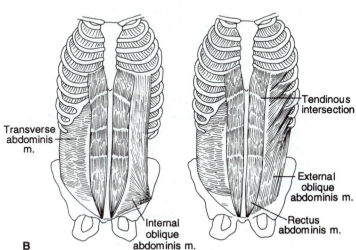

B

FIGURE 2–31. **A.** Schematic of abdominal aponeurosis as related to the abdominal muscles of expiration. **B.** Transversus abdominis, rectus abdominis, external and internal oblique abdominis muscles.

portion of the lower ribs and the portion of the abdominal aponeurosis lateral to the rectus abdominis, and thus, by association, inserts into the linea alba. Contraction of the internal oblique abdominis assists in rotation of the trunk when unilaterally contracted or flexion of the trunk when bilaterally contracted. Innervation of the rectus abdominis is via the thoracic and lumbar nerves.

External Oblique Abdominis. The *external oblique abdominis* muscles are the most superficial of the abdominal muscles, as well as the largest of this group. These muscles originate along the osseous portion of the lower seven ribs and fan downward to insert into the iliac crest, inguinal ligament, and abdominal aponeurosis (lateral to rectus abdominis). Bilateral contraction of these muscles flexes the vertebral column, and unilateral contraction results in trunk rotation. These muscles receive innervation from the thoracoabdominal nerve arising from T7 through T11 and subcostal nerve from T12.

Rectus Abdominis. The *rectus abdominis* muscles are the prominent midline muscles of the abdominal region, with inferior origin at the pubis (see Figure 2-31). The superior attachment is at the xiphoid process of sternum and the cartilage of the last true rib (rib 7) and the false ribs. These "rectangular" (i.e., rectus) muscles are manifest in a series of four or five segments connected (and separated) by tendinous slips known as tendinous intersections. Contraction draws the chest closer to the knees and compresses the abdominal contents. Innervation of the rectus abdominis is by means of the intercostal and subcostal nerves.

Posterior Abdominal Muscles

Quadratus Lumborum. As seen in Figure 2-31, the *quadratus lumborum* are located in the dorsal aspect of the abdominal wall. These muscles originate along the iliac crest and fan up and into the transverse processes of the lumbar vertebrae and inferior border of the twelfth rib. Unilateral contraction of the quadratus lumborum assists lateral movement of the trunk, whereas bilateral contraction fixes the abdominal wall in support of abdominal compression. These muscles are innervated by the lowest thoracic nerve, T12, and the first four lumbar nerves.

Muscles of Upper Limb

Latissimus Dorsi. The *latissimus dorsi* muscle (see Figure 2-28) originates from the lumbar, sacral, and lower thoracic vertebrae, with fibers rising fanlike to insert into the humerus. Its primary role is in movement of the upper extremity, but it clearly plays a role in chest stability, and perhaps expiration. With the arm immobilized, contraction of the latissimus dorsi stabilizes the posterior abdominal wall, performing a function similar to that of the quadratus lumborum. Innervation for this muscle arises from the posterior branch of the brachial plexus.

Summary

- To inflate the lungs, you need to expand the cavity that holds them so air can rush in.
- To do this, you can either increase the long dimension fairly easily by contracting the diaphragm or you can elevate the rib cage with just a little bit more effort.
- Forced expiration reverses this process by pulling the thorax down and in and by forcing the diaphragm higher into the thorax.

PHYSIOLOGY OF RESPIRATION

Respiration requires muscular effort, and the degree to which an individual can control that musculature determines, in large part, the efficiency of respiration. Respiratory function (physiology) changes as we exercise, age, or suffer setbacks in health. Considering its importance in speech, it is no wonder that as the respiratory system goes, so goes communication. We are capable of both quiet and forced expiration.

The process of expiration eliminates the waste products of respiration. Attend to your own respiratory cycle to learn an important aspect of quiet expiration. Close your eyes while you breathe in and out ten times, quietly and in a relaxed manner. Pay particular attention to the area around your diaphragm, including your rib cage and your abdomen. What you experienced is the active contraction of the diaphragm, followed by a simple relaxing of the musculature. You actively contract to breathe in, and then simply let nature take its course for expiration. It is a little like blowing up a balloon, because the balloon will deflate as soon as you let go of it. The forces on the balloon that cause it to lose its air are among those that cause your lungs to deflate. The forces we need to talk about are torque, elasticity, and gravity.

Aspiration

Aspiration refers to entry of liquid or solid materials into the lungs, but it can also refer to the removal of materials from the lungs (more commonly referred to as suctioning). Fluid or solids can enter the lungs as a result of some failure in muscular strength, coordination, sensation, or awareness.

Aspiration of foreign matter into the lungs is a very real danger in cases of neurological deficit, and the individual suffering from stroke or traumatic brain injury is particularly vulnerable. Sometimes a patient loses sensation in the laryngeal region, so that a protective cough or "clearing" response does not occur when food or liquid contacts the larynx. If a patient has muscular weakness, he or she might also demonstrate diminished or ineffective (nonproductive) cough and reduced elevation of the larynx during swallow.

Because the client with neurological deficit may not be aware or competent to seek help, it is wise to know the symptoms of aspiration. If the client's voice sounds wet or gurgly or if the client has a history of respiratory illnesses, the client is at risk for aspiration pneumonia. Likewise, the client may have a weak, breathy vocalization or cry, indicating laryngeal muscle weakness and the possibility of inadequate protective function.

Torquing: Twisting of a shaft while one end does not move.

Torquing refers to the twisting of a shaft while one end does not move. Take the end of a plastic ruler in one hand, and with the other hand grasp the other end of the ruler and twist it around its long axis (see Figure 2-32). When you let go of one end, the ruler returns to its original state, the product of a restoring force contributed by the elastic qualities of the material from which the ruler is made.

Think of the "shafts" we could twist in the rib cage. If you thought "rib," you thought right. Unfortunately, bone is poorly designed in the area of restoring forces (forces that return a body to its original position) because it is quite inelastic. There is an elastic element, however, in the chondral portion of the rib cage, and we do take advantage of that.

The second element that drives passive expiration is elasticity. There is elasticity in both the muscles and the lungs. Return to our earlier

FIGURE 2–32. When the rib cage is elevated the cartilage of the ribs is torqued, or twisted. Because cartilage is highly elastic it tends to return to its original condition after being torqued.

discussion of the elevation of the rib cage by the external intercostals and the accessory muscles of inspiration. When those muscles pull the rib cage up and out, the anterior cartilage comes under some torquing strain. As soon as the muscles stop pulling on the rib cage, it returns to its original shape thanks to the restoring forces of elastic cartilage, and that causes the rib cage to drop back down to its resting state.

Recall that the lungs are highly elastic, porous tissue. They are sponge-like and when they are compressed (as in forced expiration), they tend to expand. Likewise, if you were to grab a sponge by its edges and stretch it, when you release it, the sponge would return to its original shape and size.

During early human development, the lungs completely fill the thorax so that they are not stretched to fit the relaxed rib cage. As the child develops, the rib cage grows at a faster rate than the lungs, and the pleural linings and increased negative intrapleural pressure provide a means for the lungs to be stretched out to fill that space.

The result of this stretching is greatly increased capacity and reserve in adults, but not in infants. Because the infant's thorax and lungs are equal in size, an infant must breathe two to three times as often as an adult for adequate respiration. The adult's lungs are stretched out and never completely compressed, so there is always a reserve of air in them that is not undergoing gas exchange.

Upon increasing the thorax size, the lungs expand just as if you had grabbed them and stretched them out. When the muscles expanding the rib cage relax, the lungs tend to return to their original shape and size. In addition, when you inhale and your abdomen protrudes, you are stretching the abdominal muscles. Relaxing the inspiratory process lets those muscles return to their original length; that is, the abdominal muscles tend to push your abdominal viscera back in and to force the diaphragm up.

One final force that supports passive expiration is gravity. When a person stands or sits erect, gravity is acting on the ribs to pull them back after they have been expanded through the effort of the accessory muscles of inspiration. Gravity also works in favor of maximizing your overall capacity because it pulls the abdominal viscera down, leaving more room for the lungs. We will talk about this more because body position becomes a significant issue in the efficiency of respiration.

Summary

- We are capable of quiet respiration as well as forced inspiration and expiration.
- Quiet inspiration uses the diaphragm and often the external intercostals, but forced inspiration uses many of the accessory muscles.
- Expiration can be passive, driven by the forces of torque, elasticity, and gravity.
- We also can use muscles that reduce the size of the thorax by compressing the abdomen or pulling the rib cage down, and this forces air out of the lungs beyond that which is expired in passive expiration.

Protection against Trauma

The lungs are obviously important for life function, and seem to be designed with damage control in mind. The two lungs are encased in separate pleural linings, so that if one lung is penetrated by an object (e.g., a lung is punctured by a broken rib), the other lung continues to function. Likewise, the segmented nature of lungs is a protective device. If a lung is punctured, the extremely rich vascular bed bleeds significantly and dangerously. The segmented nature of the lungs provides some protection against total lung failure. Bleeding in one segment is isolated to that segment, at least until the bronchial tree is filled with blood.

Measurement of Respiration

The quantity of air processed through respiration is dictated primarily by bodily needs, and speech physiology operates within these limits. We will discuss respiration in terms of rate of air flow, volume and lung capacities, and pressure.

Respiratory flow, volumes, and capacities are measured with a **spirometer** (see Figure 2-33). The classic wet spirometer involves a tube connected to a container that is open at the bottom. This container is placed inside another container that is full of water. To measure lung volume, an individual breathes into the tube, causing a volume of water to be displaced. The amount of water displaced gives an accurate estimate of the amount of air that was required to displace it.

Spirometer: Device that measures volume of air expelled or inspired.

The classic U-tube **manometer** is one means of measuring pressure, as shown in Figure 2-34. A subject is asked to place the tube in his or her mouth and to blow. The force of the subject's expiration is exerted on a column of water that is pushed down the tube, around the U-bend and up the other end of the tube. The more force the person uses, the higher the column rises. We can measure the effects of that force in inches or in centimeters of water (i.e., barometric pressure is often reported in millimeters of mercury, which refers to how many millimeters of mercury were elevated by the pressure). Because water is considerably less dense than mercury, the same amount of pressure will elevate a column of water much higher than a similar column of mercury. For this reason we measure the rather small pressures of respiration with the water standard, although mechanical and electronic techniques are eliminating the waterfilled tube.

Manometer: Device that measures pressure.

WET SPIROMETER

FIGURE 2-33. Wet spirometer used to measure lung volumes. When the individual exhales into the tube, gas entering the air chamber displaces the water, causing the chamber to rise. These changes are charted on the recording drum.

FIGURE 2-34. U-tube manometer for measurement of respiratory pressure.

Emphysema

Emphysema is generally considered to be a product of a modern society that has not solved its pollution problems. Often the disease results from tobacco smoking, but it can arise from living in an industrial environment. Its progression is slow and may be arrested to some degree by altering the respiratory environment.

The mechanism for emphysema appears to be as follows. Recall that the bronchial passageway is richly infused with ciliated epithelia that beat continuously to remove contaminants from the respiratory tract. This continuous waste-removal process is seriously hampered by pollutants that, in the early stages of emphysema, destroy the epithelia.

The absence of epithelia greatly reduces the respiratory system's ability to clean and remove waste products, which allows deposition of pollutants in the alveoli. The alveoli undergo a significant morphological (form) change: The walls of the alveoli break down and alveoli recombine so that clusters of alveoli become one sac. Although this may seem benign, it has a devastating effect in that the surface area for gas exchange is greatly reduced as a result.

A second morphological change arises as a compensation to the first. The individual with emphysema is faced with an ongoing shortage of oxygen and is forced to attempt continually deeper inspirations to accommodate; a characteristic "barrel chest" results from these efforts.

This second change causes a third pathological response. Recall that the lower margin of the rib cage marks the point of attachment of the diaphragm. Because the rib cage is flared out due to emphysema, contraction of the diaphragm (which pulls on the rib cage) causes the rib cage to pull down and in medially, which actually reduces the size of thorax rather than increases it.

The final morphological change arising from this trilogy of tragedy is respiratory failure. The respiratory mechanism is highly compromised, leaving the individual susceptible to respiratory diseases such as pneumonia.

Breathing requires that gas exchange be ongoing. The body has specific needs that must be met continually, so we will need to discuss respiration in terms of the rate of airflow into and out of the lungs (airflow is measured as cubic centimeters per second or minute). We also need to speak of the quantities or volumes involved in this gas exchange (measured in liters [L], milliliters [mL], cubic centimeters [cc], or on occasion, cubic inches).

Respiration for Life

The respiratory process is a direct function of the action of the diaphragm and muscles of respiration. As discussed earlier, contraction of muscles of inspiration causes expansion of the alveoli, resulting in a negative alveolar pressure and air being drawn into the lungs. Understanding the pressure changes in this process is critical.

Respiratory Cycle

A cycle of respiration is defined as one inspiration and one expiration. During *quiet respiration*, adults complete between 12 and 18 cycles of respiration per minute (see Figure 2-35). This quiet breathing pattern, known as quiet tidal respiration (because it can be visualized as a tidal flow of air into and out of the lungs) involves about 500 mL (½ liter) of air with each cycle. A quick calculation reveals that we process something in the order of 6,000 to 8,000 mL (6–8 liters) of air every minute. As work output increases, an adult increases his or her oxygen requirements by a factor of 20.

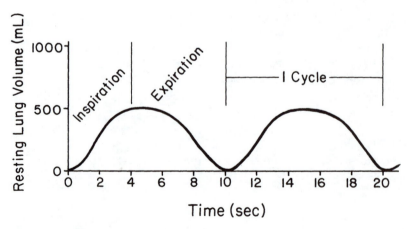

FIGURE 2-35. Volume display of two cycles of quiet respiration.

Pleurisy

Pleurisy is a condition in which the pleural linings of the thoracic cavity are inflamed. When the inflammation results in "dry pleurisy," the patient is experiencing extreme pain upon breathing because the lubricating quality of the intrapleural fluid has been lost. "Adhesions" may result, in which portions of the parietal pleurae adhere to the visceral pleurae. (The patient may experience "breaking up" of these adhesions for quite some time following his or her bout with pleurisy.) Pleurisy can be unilateral or bilateral and may result in movement of excessive fluid (potentially purulent) into the pleural space.

Developmental Processes of Respiration

The lungs undergo a great deal of prenatal development, as seen in Figure 2-36. By the time a healthy infant is born, the cartilaginous conducting airway is complete, although the number of alveoli will increase from about 25 million at birth to more than 300 million by 8 years of age. We retain that number throughout life. The conducting airways grow steadily in diameter and length until thorax growth is complete, although the thorax expands to a greater degree than the lungs. As the thorax expands, the lungs are stretched to fill the cavity, a fact that helps to explain two differences between adults and children. As mentioned earlier, adults breathe between 12 and 18 times per minute while at rest, but a newborn breathes an average of 40 to 70 cycles per minute. By 5 years, the child is down to about 25 **breaths per minute (bpm)**, and that number drops to about 20 bpm at 15 years of age. The adult has a considerable volume of air that is never expelled, but the infant does not have this reserve. In essence, the thorax expands during growth and development and stretches the lungs beyond their natural volume (see Figure 2-37).

Breaths per minute (bpm): The number of complete inhalations and exhalations performed in one minute.

Accessory muscles of inspiration used to augment diminished respiratory support most typically include the anterior, middle, and posterior scalene muscles (to elevate the first and second ribs) and the sternocleidomastoid (to elevate the sternum and increase the anteroposterior dimension of the rib cage). You may have seen people with severe respiratory difficulties stretch their arms in front of

Clavicular Breathing

Clavicular breathing is a form of respiration in which a major source of thorax expansion is elevation of the rib cage via contraction of the accessory muscles of inspiration, most notably the sternocleidomastoid. Clavicular breathing often is an adaptive response by an individual to some previous or present pathological condition (e.g., chronic obstructive pulmonary disease) that prohibits other means to expand the thorax. Because elevation of the sternum results in only a small increase in thorax size, clavicular breathing is a less-than-perfect solution to the problem of respiration.

them and hold onto the back of a chair to breathe: When they do this, they give the pectoralis major muscles something to work against, thus allowing these muscles to increase the anteroposterior dimension. You may have also seen these patients "shrugging," a sure sign that the trapezius muscle is in use to raise the rib cage.

Residual volume: The volume of air that cannot be expelled.

As a result of this expansion, there is a volume of air in the adult lung that cannot be expelled (**residual volume**), and this volume helps to account for the reserve capacity of adults relative to infants. Infant lungs have yet to undergo the proliferation of the alveoli seen during childhood, and infants must breathe more frequently to meet their metabolic needs.

Volumes and Capacities

Volume: In respiration, the displacement of air that represents specifically partitioned components of the respiratory system, measured in cubic centimeters or cubic inches.

Capacity: Functional unit that is a combination of respiratory volumes, used to express physiological limits.

Milliliter (mL): One thousandth of a liter.

Cubic centimeter (cc): A milliliter or one thousandth of a liter.

Respiration is the product of a number of forces and structures, and for us to make sense of them we need to define some volumes and capacities of the lungs. When we refer to **volumes,** we are partitioning off the respiratory system so that we can accurately estimate the amount of air each compartment can hold. **Capacities** are more functional units. Capacities refer to combinations of volumes that express physiological limits. Volumes are discrete, whereas capacities represent functional combinations of volumes.

Both volumes and capacities are measured in **milliliters** (mL, thousandths of a liter) or **cubic centimeters** (cc, which is another name for milliliters). To get an idea of what these volumes and capacities really amount to, look at a 2-liter soda bottle. One liter is 1,000 mL, which is also 1,000 cc. There are five volumes that we should consider. Refer to Figure 2-38 as we discuss these.

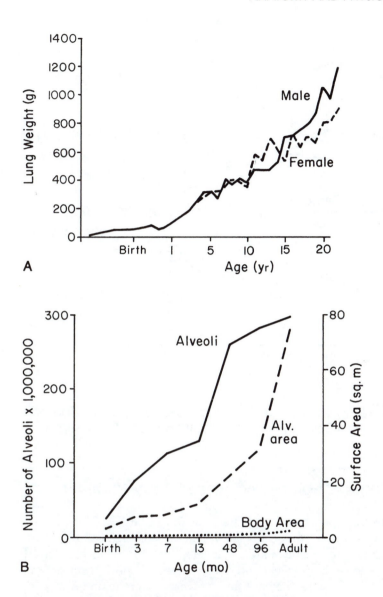

FIGURE 2-36. A. Changes in lung weight as a function of age. Males and females are essentially equivalent in lung weight until puberty, at which time the increased thoracic cavity size of the male is reflected in larger lung weight. **B.** Changes in lung tissue with age. The number of alveoli increases radically through the fourth year of life, and the total alveolar area stabilizes around puberty when the thorax approximates its volume. (Data from *Handbook of Biological Data* by W.S. Spector, 1956, pp. 162, 176–180, 353. Philadelphia: W. B. Saunders.)

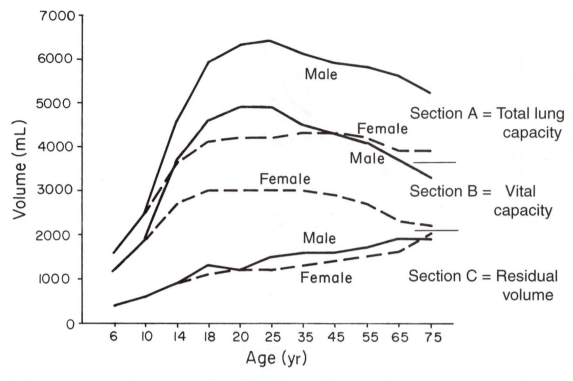

FIGURE 2-37. Vital capacity, total lung volume, and residual volume as a function of age. (Data from *Handbook of Biological Data* by W. S. Spector, 1956, p. 267. Philadelphia: W. B. Saunders.)

Trunk Stability and Upper Body Mobility

Control of speech musculature depends in large part on the development of trunk control. If an infant fails to develop neck extension, he or she will not develop the ability to balance neck extensors and flexors. While the normal neck extension begins developing, the back muscles begin to come under control, again becoming dynamically opposed by anterior trunk muscles. Through this interplay of antagonist and agonist trunk muscles, the infant develops the ability to rotate the trunk, stabilize the hips, and elevate the head in preparation for speech. Once controlled, the infant can rotate his or her head, differentiate mandible movement from head movement, and differentiate tongue movement from mandible movement. All the while, the infant is developing the dynamic aspects of laryngeal control that permit the larynx to descend and the tongue to become controlled.

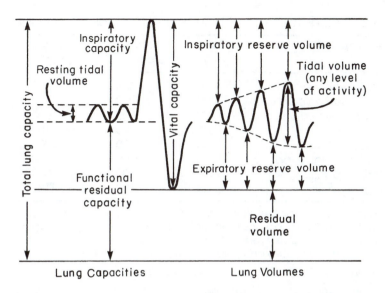

FIGURE 2-38. Lung volumes and capacities displayed on a spirogram. (Modified from data of Pappenheimer et al., 1950)

Tidal Volume. The volume of air that we breathe in during a respiratory cycle is referred to as **tidal volume (TV)**. The average **quiet tidal volume** (tidal volume at rest) for adult males is around 600 cc, and for adult females, approximately 450 cc. This works out to an average of 525 cc for adults, or approximately one quarter of the volume of a 2-liter soda bottle every 5 seconds. You will breathe in the air in three of these bottles every minute. Tidal volume increases markedly as effort increases. You may wish to refer to Table 2-2.

Tidal volume: The volume of air exchanged during one cycle of respiration.

Quiet tidal volume: Tidal volume at rest.

Inspiratory Reserve Volume. The second volume of interest is **inspiratory reserve volume (IRV)**. Inspiratory reserve volume is the volume that can be inhaled after a tidal inspiration. It is the volume of air that is in reserve for use beyond the volume you would breathe in tidally, averaging 2,475 cc for adults.

Inspiratory reserve volume (IRV): The volume of air that can be inhaled after a tidal inspiration (approximately 2,475 cc for adults).

Expiratory Reserve Volume. The parallel volume for expiration is the **expiratory reserve volume (ERV)**. Expiratory reserve volume is the amount of air that can be expired following passive, tidal expiration, amounting to about 1,000 cc (1.0 liter). This volume is referred to as resting lung volume (RLV) also because it is the volume of air in the resting lungs after a passive exhalation.

Expiratory reserve volume (ERV): The volume of air that can be expired following passive, tidal expiration (approximately 1,000 cc for adults).

Table 2–2. Typical Respiratory Volumes and Capacities in Adults

Volume/Capacity	Males* (cc)	Females** (cc)	Average (cc)
Resting tidal volume	600	450	525
Inspiratory reserve volume	3000	1950	2475
Expiratory reserve volume	1200	800	1000
Residual volume	1200	1000	1100
Vital capacity	4800	3200	4000
Functional residual capacity	2400	2700	2550
Inspiratory capacity	3600	2400	3000
Total lung capacity	6000	4200	5100

Note: Volumes and capacities vary as a function of body size, gender, age, and body height. These volumes represent approximate values for healthy adults between 20 and 30 years of age. Vital capacity is estimated by accounting for age (in years) and height (in cm):

*Males: VC in mL = (27.63 − (0.112 × age in yr)) × ht. in cm.

**Females: VC in mL = (21.78 − (0.101 × age in yr)) × ht. in cm.

Source: Data from Baldwin, Cournand, and Richards, (1948) as cited in *An Introduction to Respiratory Physiology* by F. F. Kao, 1972, p. 39. Amsterdam: Excerpta Medica; and *The Mechanical Basis of Respiration* by R. M. Peters, 1969, p. 49. Boston: Little, Brown.

Residual volume (RV): The volume of air in the lungs after a maximum exhalation (approximately 1,100 cc in adults).

Residual Volume. The third volume of interest is **residual volume (RV)**. Residual volume is the amount of air in the lungs after a maximum exhalation. No matter how forcefully you exhale, there is a volume of air (about 1.1 liters) that cannot be eliminated. This volume exists because the lungs are stretched as a result of the relatively expanded thorax. By the way, this does not mean we do not use that air, but rather that it is a volume that is not eliminated during expiration.

Dead air space: The space, representing the conductive passageway of the respiratory system, that contains a volume of air that never undergoes gas exchange (approximately 150 cc in adults).

Dead Air Space. The air in the conducting passageways cannot be involved in gas exchange because there are no alveoli there. The volume that cannot undergo gas exchange in the lungs is **dead air space**, and an adult has a volume of about 150 cc. The volume associated with dead air is included in residual volume because both are volumes associated with air that cannot be expelled.

Vital capacity (VC): The combination of inspiratory reserve volume, expiratory reserve volume, and tidal volume, representing the capacity of air available for speech (approximately 4,000 cc in adults).

The volumes can be combined in a number of ways to characterize physiological needs. Four capacities are useful combinations of air volumes: vital, functional residual, total lung, and inspiratory.

Vital Capacity. Of the capacities, **vital capacity (VC)** is the most often cited in speech and hearing literature because it represents the capacity of air available for speech. Vital capacity is the combination of inspiratory reserve volume, expiratory reserve volume, and tidal volume. That is, vital capacity represents the total volume of air that can be inspired after a maximal expiration. Because VC = IRV + ERV + TV, you can calculate that it is approximately 4,000 cc in the average adult.

Functional residual capacity (FRC): The volume of air in the thorax after a passive exhalation (approximately 2,100 cc in adults).

Total lung capacity (TLC): The total volume of the respiratory system that can undergo gas exchange, equaling the sum of tidal volume, inspiratory reserve volume, expiratory reserve volume, and residual volume (approximately 5,100 cc in adults).

Inspiratory capacity: The maximum inspiratory volume possible after tidal expiration (approximately 3,000 cc in adults).

Functional Residual Capacity. Functional residual capacity (FRC) is the volume of air in the body after a passive exhalation (FRC = ERV + RV). In the average adult, this comes to approximately 2,100 cc.

Total Lung Capacity. Total lung capacity (TLC) is the sum of all the volumes (TLC = TV + IRV + ERV + RV), totaling approximately 5,100 cc. Note that this is different from vital capacity. Vital capacity represents that volume of air that is involved in a maximal respiratory cycle, whereas total lung capacity includes the residual volume. Residual volume serves as a buffer in respiration because it does not immediately interact with the environment.

Inspiratory Capacity. Inspiratory capacity (IC) is the maximum inspiratory volume possible after tidal expiration (IC = TV + IRV). This refers to the capacity of the lungs for inspiration and represents a volume of approximately 3,000 cc in the adult.

Summary

- The volumes of respiration indicate arbitrary partitioning of the respiratory system and include tidal volume (the volume inspired and expired in a cycle of respiration), inspiratory reserve volume (air inspired beyond tidal inspiration), expiratory reserve volume (air expired beyond tidal expiration), residual volume (air that remains in the lungs after maximal expiration), and dead air, which cannot undergo gas exchange.

- Vital capacity is the volume of air that can be inspired after a maximal expiration.

- Functional residual capacity is the air that remains in the body after passive exhalation. Total lung capacity represents the sum of all lung volumes.

- Inspiratory capacity is the volume of air that can be inspired from resting lung volume.

Pressures of the Respiratory System

There are five specific pressures for nonspeech and speech: alveolar, intrapleural, subglottal, intraoral, and atmospheric (see Figure 2-39). The atmosphere in which we live exerts a sizable pressure on the surface of the earth (760 mm Hg; that is, sufficient pressure to elevate a column of mercury 760 mm against gravity). **Atmospheric pressure** (P_{atm}) is actually our reference in discussions of the respiratory system, and so we will treat it as a constant zero against which to compare respiratory pressures. **Intraoral**, or **mouth, pressure** (P_m) is the pressure in the mouth that could be measured, while **subglottal pressure** (P_s) is the pressure below the vocal folds. We can assume that subglottal and intraoral pressures are equal to alveolar pressure during normal respiration with open vocal folds. As we progress more deeply into the lungs, we can estimate **alveolar** or **pulmonic, pressure** (P_{al}), the pressure in the individual alveolus. If we were to measure the pressure in the space between parietal and visceral pleurae, we would refer to it as pleural, or **intrapleural, pressure** (P_{pl}). Intrapleural pressure is negative throughout

Atmospheric pressure (P_{atm}): *Pressure generated as a result of the weight of atmospheric gasses.*

Intraoral (P_m): *Pressure in the oral cavity.*

Subglottal pressure (P_s): *Pressure beneath the level of the vocal folds.*

Alveolar, or pulmonic, pressure (P_{al}): *Pressure in the alveolus.*

Intrapleural pressure (P_{pl}): *Pressure between the visceral and parietal pleurae.*

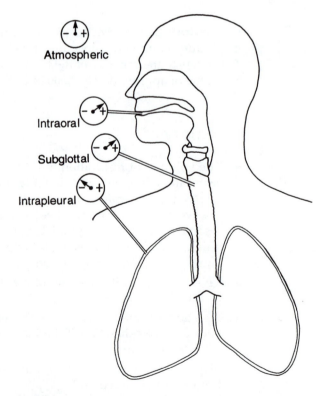

FIGURE 2-39. Pressures of respiration.

respiration. Recall that the lungs, inner thorax, and diaphragm are wrapped in a continuous sheet of pleural lining. When one attempts to separate the visceral from parietal pleurae, a negative pressure ensues.

These pressure measurements are all relative to atmospheric pressure. When we refer to alveolar pressure as being, for instance, +3 cm H_2O, it means that, through muscular effort, we have generated +3 cm H_2O pressure above and beyond atmospheric pressure (if atmospheric pressure is 1,033 cm H_2O, then alveolar pressure would be 1,036 cm H_2O). When the diaphragm is pulled down for tidal inspiration, Boyle's law predicts that alveolar pressure will drop (relative to atmospheric pressure), and it does. In quiet tidal inspiration, alveolar pressure drops to approximately –2 cm H_2O until equalized with atmospheric pressure by inspiratory flow. Likewise, during expiration the pressure at the alveolar level becomes positive with reference to the atmosphere, increasing to +2 cm H_2O during quiet tidal breathing.

"Getting the Wind Knocked Out of You"

Why does a blow to the abdomen result in your losing your breath? Logic would dictate that you would lose your breath from being hit in the chest.

Try to recall what happened the last time you had the wind knocked out of you. First, something hit you in the abdominal region or you fell and landed on your stomach. Remember that forced expiration depends in large part on contraction of the abdominal muscles which, in turn, causes the abdominal viscera to push the diaphragm up and pull the thorax down. Both of these gestures remove air forcefully from the lungs.

This doesn't explain the agony you experience trying to regain respiratory control, however. When large muscles are passively stretched, a reflex is triggered that causes the muscle to contract involuntarily. This contraction increases the effect of being hit in the abdomen because it causes you to forcefully exhale just when you needed to inhale!

Figure 2-40 is a schematic of the alveolar pressures, intrapleural pressures, and change in lung volume during quiet tidal breathing.

This figure shows the alveolar pressure associated with a cycle of respiration and illustrates what we have been talking about. We have placed markers on it so that we can discuss how this whole system of pressures and flows works together.

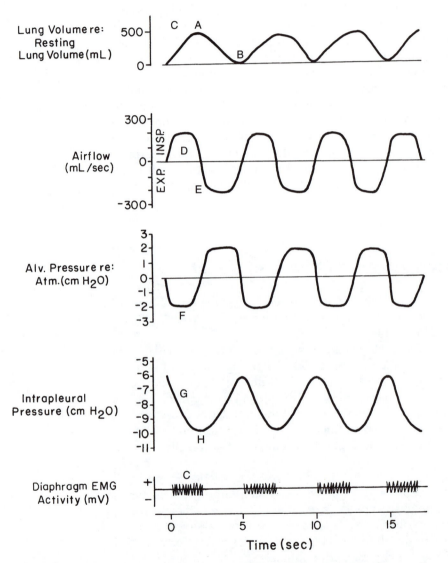

FIGURE 2-40. Relationships of pressures, flows, and volumes to diaphragm activity. Contraction of the diaphragm causes a drop in intrapleural and alveolar pressure, which results in an increase in airflow and lung volume. (Data from *Physiology of Respiration* by J. H. Comroe, 1965. Chicago: Year Book Medical Publishers.)

Look at the curve labeled lung volume; it shows the periodic function that represents tidal respiration. Point A represents the peak of that inspiration, and the lungs have about 500 cc of air in them. Point B represents the end of the expiratory cycle, where our subject has relaxed the forces of inspiration and the lungs have passively evacuated down to resting lung volume. At the bottom of the figure, point C represents the electromyographic activity recorded from the diaphragm as it contracted. Putting these two traces together, you can see that as the diaphragm contracts the volume increases to a maximum at the point where the diaphragmatic contraction is complete.

Let us examine the airflow component. As the diaphragm contracts, there is a fairly steady flow of air into the lungs (measured in mL/sec), indicated by point D. When the inspiratory effort is completed (represented by the termination of the diaphragm activity and the volume peak at A), the flow of air into the lungs ends. That is, when the diaphragm stops contracting, air stops flowing. As air leaves the lungs, the airflow becomes negative at point E (which simply means that the air is flowing in a different direction). Alveolar pressure goes positive (+2 cm H_2O) during expiration. To summarize, when the diaphragm contracts, airflow begins and is fairly steady throughout the inspiratory cycle. When the diaphragm stops contracting, the air begins to flow out of the lungs.

This is a good time to examine the pressures driving this process. If you recall that contraction of the diaphragm causes the alveolar pressure to drop, the point marked F will make sense. When the diaphragm is contracted (C), pressure deep in the lungs drops. At this point, alveolar pressure reaches its maximum negativity during this tidal respiration (–2 cm H_2O relative to atmospheric pressure), because the negative pressure is responsible for airflow into the lungs. Looking at point G will explain why that pressure drops. You will recall that intrapleural pressure is constantly negative relative to atmospheric pressure, and the lungs are in a state of continued expansion in the thoracic cavity. This is reflected in the fact that the highest pressure on the intrapleural plot is negative (–6 cm H_2O).

When the diaphragm contracts, the intrapleural pressure becomes even more negative as the diaphragm attempts to pull the diaphragmatic pleurae away from the visceral pleurae. During the entire period of contraction of the diaphragm, the pressure continues to drop: The diaphragm is pulling farther away from its resting point, and the pressure between the pleurae increases proportionately. As the diaphragm reaches the end of its contraction, intrapleural pressure reaches a maximum negativity (point H), which reverses upon relaxation of the diaphragm. When the diaphragm contracts, the volume (space) between the two pleural linings increases; as Boyle's law predicts, the pressure drops.

Depression of the diaphragm for quiet tidal inspiration results in an intrapleural pressure of approximately -10 cm H_2O, but relaxing the diaphragm during quiet expiration does not return the pressure to atmospheric, but rather returns it to a constant rest pressure of -6 cm H_2O. In the average, healthy individual, intrapleural pressure remains negative at all times, becoming increasingly negative as muscles of inspiration act on the lungs.

The fact that this intrapleural pressure remains negative underscores two important notions. First, the lungs are in a state of continual expansion because the thorax is larger than the lungs that fill it. Second, the lungs are never completely deflated under normal circumstances. During inspiration and expiration, two more pressures are of interest to us. Subglottal pressure is the pressure beneath the level of the vocal folds (*glottis* refers to the space between the vocal folds). Above the vocal folds the respiratory pressure in the oral cavity is referred to as intraoral pressure. When the vocal folds are open, intraoral pressure, subglottal pressure, and alveolar pressure are the same.

The pressure beneath and above the vocal folds is directly related to what is happening in the lungs, as long as the vocal folds are open for air passage. If the lungs are drawing air in, the pressure at both of these locations is negative. If the lungs are in expiration, the pressure is relatively positive. Things get more difficult when the vocal folds are closed.

Supraglottal: The region above the vocal folds.

When we close vocal folds for phonation (voicing), we place a significant blockage in the flow of air through the upper respiratory pathway. Closing the vocal folds causes an immediate increase in the subglottal air pressure as the lungs continue expiration. At the same time, closing the vocal folds causes the intraoral pressure to drop to near atmospheric, resulting in a large difference in pressure between the **supraglottal** (above vocal folds) and subglottal regions. If this increased pressure exceeds 3 cm to 5 cm H_2O, the vocal folds will be blown open and voicing will begin. This turns out to be a critical pressure in itself because it marks the minimal requirement of respiration for speech.

You can now view these critical pressures as a system: We are continually playing the respiratory system against the relatively stable

Use of Abdominal Muscles for Childbirth and Other Biological Functions

Nature has a way of getting the most use out of structures, and the abdominal muscles are a great example. Clearly, we use the abdominal muscles to force air out of the lungs, but they serve several other worthwhile (even vital) functions. The act of vomiting requires evacuation of the gastric contents, and to do so necessitates forceful action from the abdominal muscles.

A less obvious function has to do with thoracic fixation. For the muscles of the upper body to gain maximum benefit, they need to pull against a relatively rigid structure. The thorax can be made rigid by inhaling and then capturing the respiratory charge by closing off the vocal folds. To demonstrate this process, take a very deep breath and hold it. To do this, you must close off the folds.

This thoracic fixing gives leverage for lifting (notice that you "grunt" when you lift because some air is escaping past the vocal folds, having been compressed by your muscular effort), but it also gives leverage in the other direction. Defecation requires compression of the abdomen and increase in abdominal pressure, and that process also demands thoracic fixation for efficiency.

Another not immediately obvious use for abdominal muscle contraction is childbirth. Although you may not have experienced this directly, you are probably familiar with midwives, nurses, or partners whose job it was to remind the mother-to-be to "breathe." It shouldn't surprise you to realize that the mother has not forgotten this basic biological process, but rather she has an overwhelming, deep biological urge to "push." Besides providing supportive encouragement, the person who is cheerleading is doing so to keep the mother from closing the vocal folds (you can't breathe through closed folds) because if she does, she will start pushing the baby to its new home before the time has come (Creasy, 1997).

atmospheric pressure. Contraction of the diaphragm and muscles of inspiration decreases the intrapleural pressure markedly, which, in turn, expands the lungs. When the lungs expand, alveolar pressure drops relative to atmospheric pressure, causing air to enter the lungs. Relaxing the muscles of inspiration permits the natural recoil of the lungs and cartilage to draw the chest back to its original position, and the relaxed diaphragm again returns to its relatively elevated position in the thorax. When this happens, intrapleural pressure increases (but still stays negative), alveolar pressure becomes positive relative to atmospheric pressure, and air leaves the lungs.

Summary

- Volumes and pressures vary as a direct function of the forces acting on the respiratory system.
- With the vocal folds open, oral pressure, subglottal pressure, and alveolar pressure are roughly equivalent.
- Intrapleural pressure remains constantly negative, increasing in negativity during inspiration.
- These pressures are all measured relative to atmospheric pressure.
- During inspiration, expansion of the thorax decreases the already negative intrapleural pressure, and the increased lung volume results in a negative alveolar pressure.
- Air from outside the body flows into the lungs when the pressure in the lungs is negative relative to the atmosphere.
- During expiration, this pressure differential is reversed, with air escaping the lungs to equalize the positive alveolar pressure with the relatively negative atmospheric pressure.

Pressures Generated by Tissue. At this point, we should address the forces of expiration more deeply. Expiration capitalizes on torque, elasticity, and gravity to reclaim some of the energy expended during inspiration. When muscles of inspiration contract, they stretch tissue, torque cartilage of the ribs, and distend the abdomen.

These restoring forces actually generate pressures themselves. Elastic forces govern how much effort is required to inhale. This relationship is described in the curve of Figure 2-41.

The dashed line on this figure is the relaxation point, the point where no pressure is generated because all parts of the system are at equilibrium. The dashed relaxation point of zero pressure represents about 38% of vital capacity. When you relax entirely with open airway, the lungs still have 38% of the total exchangeable volume left, and this could be forcefully exhaled. Said another way, from this point you can actively inhale 62% of your vital capacity.

FIGURE 2-41. Relaxation pressure curve representing pressures generated by the passive forces of the respiratory system.

Summary

- The process of contracting musculature deforms the cartilage and connective tissue, and recoil forces will drive the respiratory system back to equilibrium after inspiration or expiration.
- Relaxing the musculature after inspiration results in a positive alveolar pressure that decreases as volume approaches resting lung volume.
- When the pressure is measured following forced expiration, a negative relaxation pressure is found, increasing to equity at resting lung volume.

Effects of Posture on Speech

Body posture is a significant contributor to efficiency of respiration, and any condition that compromises posture also compromises respiration (see Figure 2-42). As the body is shifted from an erect, sitting to a supine posture, the relationship between the physical structures of respiration and gravity changes. In the sitting posture, gravity is pulling the abdominal viscera down (supporting inspiration), as well

FIGURE 2–42. Pressure–volume relationship for muscular activity by percentage of vital capacity. Pi = pressure from muscles of inspiration; Pe = pressure from muscles of expiration; Pr = pressure from relaxation of muscles of inspiration and expiration. (Based on data from "The Pressure–Volume Diagram of the Thorax" by H. Rahn, A. Otis, L. E. Chadwick, &; W. Fenn, 1946, p. 164. *American Journal of Physiology, 146,* 161–178.)

as pulling the rib cage down (supporting expiration). When the body is in the supine position, gravity is pulling the abdominal viscera toward the spine. The result of this is spread of the viscera toward the thorax and further distension of the diaphragm into the thoracic cavity. When a body is supine, gravity supports neither expiration nor inspiration: Muscles of inspiration must elevate both abdomen and rib cage against gravity.

Although vital capacity is not affected, the ability to completely inflate the lungs is. Because of the shift in viscera and effects of gravity on the rib cage, the lung volume is significantly reduced from approximately 38% of vital capacity in sitting position to 20% in supine.

You may have already realized the danger this poses to a person whose illness requires that he or she stay in bed for long periods of time. Pneumonia is a major complication of conditions that immobilize a person.

Summary

- Posture and body position play important roles in volumes for respiration.
- When the body is reclining, the abdominal contents shift rostrally as a result of the forces of gravity.
- Aside from reducing the resting lung volume, the force of gravity on the abdomen increases the effort required for inspiration.

Pressures of Speech

The respiratory system operates at two levels of pressure virtually simultaneously. The first level is the relatively constant supply of subglottal pressure required to drive the vocal folds. To produce sustained voicing of a given intensity, this pressure is relatively constant. As we will see, the minimum driving pressure to make the vocal folds move would elevate a column of water between 3 cm and 5 cm (3–5 cm H_2O), with conversational speech requiring between 7 cm and 10 cm H_2O. Loud speech requires a concomitant increase in pressure.

The second level of pressure requires microcontrol. Even as we maintain the constant pressure needed for phonation, we are also quite capable of rapidly and briefly changing the pressure for linguistic purposes such as syllable stress. With quick bursts of pressure (and laryngeal adjustments), we can have rapid and brief increases in vocal intensity and vocal pitch. To maintain that constant pressure for speech, we must first charge the system. During normal respiration, inhalation takes up approximately 40% of the cycle and expiration takes up about 60% (see Figure 2-43).

In fact, the respiratory cycle for speech is markedly different. You need a long, drawn-out expiration to produce long utterances, and you need a very short inspiration to maintain the smooth flow of communication. When you breathe in for speech, you spend only 10% of the respiratory cycle on inspiration and about 90% breathing out. This does not change the amount of air we breathe in and out. We still breathe exactly the volume we need for our metabolic processes (too much and we take in too much oxygen, or hyperventilate; too little and we take in too little oxygen and become hypoxic).

Instead of letting the air out through total relaxation when we speak, we let the air out slowly, using muscles to restrain the airflow. If you

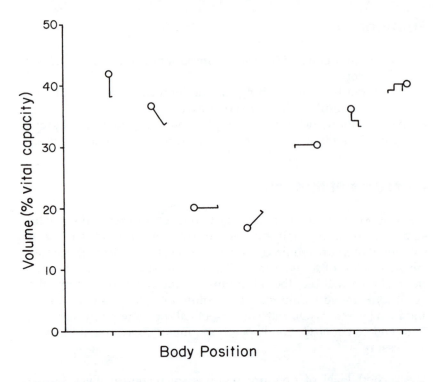

FIGURE 2-43. Vital capacity changes resulting from postural adjustment. (Data from "Kinematics of the Chest Wall During Speech Production: Volume Displacement of the Rib Cage, Abdomen, and Lung," by T. J. Hixon, M. D. Goldman, and J. Mead, 1973. *Journal of Speech & Hearing Research, 16*, 78–115.)

Checking action: Using the muscles of inspiration to impede the outflow of air during expiration.

remember that the lungs are attempting to empty as a result of their being stretched for inspiration, then you might realize that if you were to hold that inspiration position you would impede the outflow of air. This process is called **checking action**. That is, you "check" (impede) the flow of air out of your inflated lungs by means of the muscles that got it there in the first place—the muscles of inspiration.

There is an expiratory parallel to checking action, and that is the process of speaking on expiratory reserve. What happens when we get down to that resting lung volume point of 38% during speech? If we have more to say before we inhale, we have to enlist the muscles of expiration to push beyond that resting lung volume.

Summary

- During speech we modify our respiratory activities to balance bodily needs and communication needs.
- During respiration for speech we spend markedly less time in inspiration than in expiration, thus capitalizing on the positive pressures generated.
- We also meter out that respiratory charge through checking action, using the muscles of inspiration to restrain expiration.
- We use our muscles of expiration to capitalize on the expiratory reserve volume for speech.
- Even as we maintain this relatively constant subglottal pressure through muscles of inspiration and expiration, we also use those muscles to produce small surges in pressure for syllable stress during speech.

Muscular Activity during Respiration

Electromyography is the process of measuring and recording the electrical activity associated with muscular contraction. Figure 2-44 is a schematic representation of some classic data from Draper, Ladefoged, and Whitteridge (1959) showing the electrical activity of musculature during several phases of respiration for speech. The recordings were made directly from muscle fibers rather than through surface electrodes, and muscle activity is represented by spikes of activity during contraction. Note that some muscles are not amenable to recording because it is difficult to make positive identification of deep muscles.

Examination of Figure 2-44 supports the concepts we have been discussing throughout the chapter on respiration. During inspiration there is clear evidence of diaphragmatic and external intercostal activity. It should also be evident that the activity of these muscles continues even during expiration. This is clear evidence of checking action. Look closely at Figure 2-44 and you will see that the diaphragm ceases activity earlier than the external intercostals, but both of these muscles become silent by the time resting lung volume is achieved.

As the speaker continues to speak, he or she is using expiratory reserve and must exert the muscles of forced expiration to capitalize on that reserve. As the speaker reaches deeper and deeper into expiratory reserve, the internal intercostals, external oblique, and rectus abdominis are called into duty in that order. This is an important

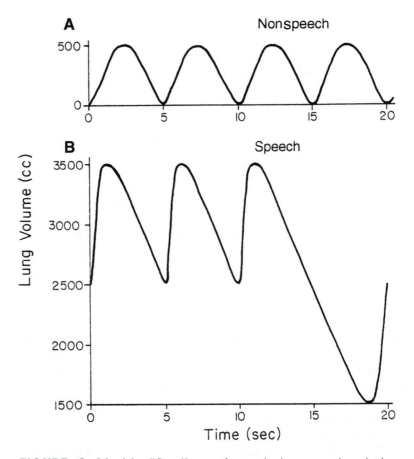

FIGURE 2-44. Modification of respiratory cycle during speech compared with nonspeech respiratory cycle. **A.** This trace represents quiet tidal respiration, with volume related to resting lung volume. **B.** This trace is related to total lung capacity. The speaker rapidly inhales a markedly larger volume than during quiet tidal inspiration and then slowly exhales the air during speech. Note that inspiration occurs with the same timing in both speech and nonspeech, but that the expiratory phase is proportionately longer during speech. In the final portion of the trace, the speaker is called on to speak on expiratory reserve volume.

point. The musculature is recruited as needed to develop increasingly greater abdominal pressure (and, subsequently, alveolar pressure). To plumb the depths of the respiratory system, increasing numbers of expiratory muscles are needed. Remember that not all muscles are represented here.

CHAPTER SUMMARY

Respiration is the process of gas exchange between an organism and its environment. The rib cage, made up of the spinal column and ribs, houses the lungs, which are the primary organs of respiration. By means of the cartilaginous trachea and bronchial tree, air is brought into the lungs for gas exchange within the minute alveolar sacs. Oxygen enters the blood and carbon dioxide is removed, to be expired.

Air is drawn into the lungs through muscular effort. The diaphragm, placed between the thorax and abdomen, contracts during inspiration. The lungs expand when the diaphragm contracts, drawn by pleurae linked through surface tension and negative pressure. When lungs expand, the air pressure in the lungs becomes negative with respect to the outside atmospheric pressure, and Boyle's law dictates that air will flow from the region of higher pressure to fill the lungs. Accessory muscles provide added expansion of the rib cage for further inspiration.

Expiration can occur passively, through the forces of torque, elasticity, and gravity acting on the ribs and rib cage. It also can be forced, by use of muscles of the abdomen and those that depress the rib cage to evacuate the lungs.

Respiration requires the balance of pressures. Decreased alveolar pressure is the product of expansion of the thorax. When the thorax expands, the pressure between the pleurae decreases as the thorax and diaphragm are pulled away from the lungs. The force of the distended lungs increases the negative intrapleural pressure, and the expansion causes a drop in alveolar pressure as well. The relatively lower alveolar pressure represents an imbalance between pressures of the lungs and the atmosphere, and air will enter the lungs to equalize the imbalance. Expiration requires reduction in thorax size, which results in a positive pressure within the alveoli, with air escaping through the oral and nasal cavities. The intrapleural pressure becomes less negative during expiration, but it never reaches atmospheric pressure.

Several volumes and capacities can be identified in the respiratory system. Tidal volume is the volume inspired and expired in a cycle of respiration, and inspiratory reserve volume is the air inspired beyond tidal inspiration. Expiratory reserve volume is air expired beyond tidal expiration, and residual volume is air that remains in the lungs after maximal expiration. Dead air space contains air that cannot undergo gas exchange. Vital capacity is the volume of air that can be inspired after a maximal expiration, and functional residual capacity is the air that remains in the body after passive exhalation. Inspiratory capacity is the volume that can be inspired from resting lung volume. Total lung capacity is the sum of all lung volumes.

For speech we must work within the confines of pressures and volumes required for life. We alter the respiratory cycle to capitalize on expiration time and restrain that expiration through checking action. We also generate pressure through contraction of the muscles of expiration when the lung volume is less than resting lung volume. With these manipulations we maintain a respiratory rate to match our metabolic needs, and even use the accessory muscles of inspiration and expiration to generate small bursts of pressure for syllabic stress.

Study Questions

1. _____ is defined as force distributed over area.

2. _____ pressure causes air to enter the container until the pressure is equalized.

3. How many of each of the following vertebrae are there?

    _____ cervical vertebrae

    _____ thoracic vertebrae

    _____ lumbar vertebrae

    _____ sacral vertebrae (fused)

4. On the following figure identify the indicated landmarks.

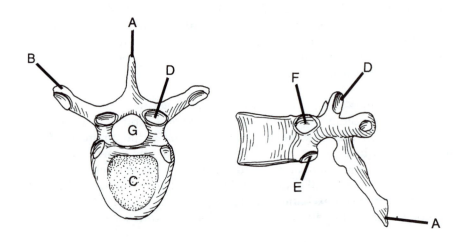

A. _____ process

B. _____ process

C. _____

D. _____ facet

E. _____ facet

F. _____ facet

G. _____ foramen

5. The _____ passes through the vertebral foramen.

6. On the following figure identify the indicated landmarks.

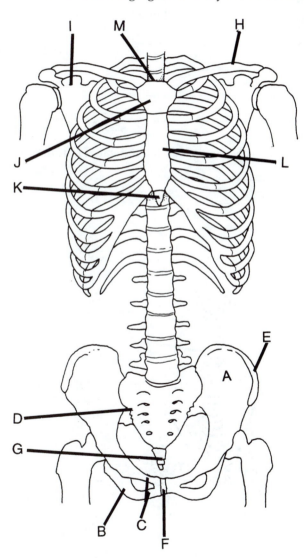

A. _____ (bone)

B. _____ (bone)

C. _____ (bone)

D. _____

E. _____

F. _____

G. _____

H. _____ (bone)

I. _____ (bone)

J. _____

K. _____

L. _____

M. _____

7. On the following figure please identify the indicated landmarks.

A. _____

B. _____

C. _____

D. _____

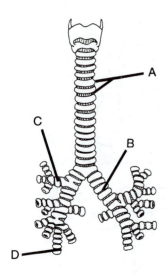

8. On the following figure identify the muscles and indicated structures.

A. _____

B. _____

C. _____

D. _____

E. _____

F. _____ ligament

G. _____

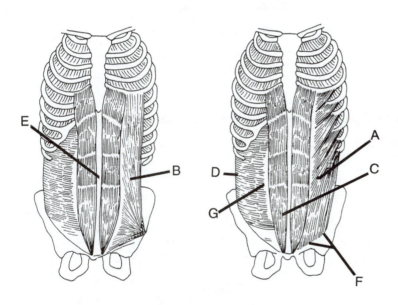

9. On the following figure identify the indicated muscles.

A. _____

B. _____

C. _____

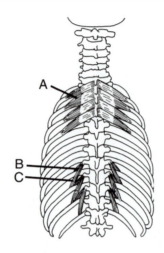

10. Identify the muscles indicated in the following figure.

A. _____

B. _____

C. _____

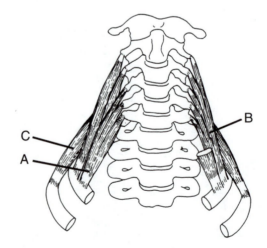

11. Identify the muscles and portions of muscles indicated in the following figure.

   A. _____

   B. _____ head

   C. _____ head

   D. _____

   E. _____

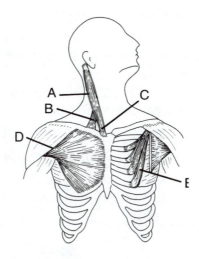

12. Contraction of the diaphragm increases the _____ dimension of the thorax.

13. Contraction of the accessory muscles of inspiration increases the _____ dimension of the thorax.

14. Contraction of the muscles of expiration _____ the volume of the thorax.

15. Passive expiration involves the forces of _____, _____, and _____.

16. Identify the described volumes and capacities.

   A. _____ volume: The volume of air that we breathe in during a respiratory cycle.

   B. _____ volume: The volume that can be inhaled after a tidal inspiration.

   C. _____ volume: The volume that can be exhaled after a tidal expiration.

   D. _____ volume: The volume that remains in the lungs after a maximal exhalation.

   E. _____ capacity: The combination of inspiratory reserve volume, expiratory reserve volume, and tidal volume.

   F. _____ capacity: The volume of air in the body after a passive exhalation.

   G. _____ capacity: The sum of all the volumes.

17. _____ is the volume of air that cannot undergo gas exchange.

18. _____ pressure is the air pressure in the oral cavity.

19. _____ pressure is the air pressure below the vocal folds.

20. _____ pressure is the pressure in the alveolus.

21. _____ pressure is the pressure between the visceral and parietal pleural membranes.

22. When the diaphragm contracts, pressure in the alveolus _____ (increases/decreases).

23. When air pressure in the lungs is lower than that of the atmosphere, air will _____ (enter/leave) the lungs.

24. When the body is reclining, the resting lung volume _____ (increases/decreases).

25. Use of the muscles of inspiration to impede the outward flow of air during speech is termed _____ .

26. Emphysema results in a breakdown of the alveolar wall, resulting in enlargement of alveolar clusters and consequent enlargement of the thorax known as "barrel chest." The result of this is that the diaphragm is pulled down at rest. Discuss the implications of the muscular action of inspiration and expiration on this altered system.

REFERENCES

Agostoni, E., & Mead, J. (1964). Statics of the respiratory system. In W. Fenn, & H. Rahn (Eds.), *Handbook of physiology, respiration* (Vol. 1, Sect. 3). Washington, DC: American Physiological Society.

Arnott, W. M. (1973). *Disorders of the respiratory system.* Oxford, England: Blackwell Scientific.

Baken, R., & Cavallo, S. (1981). Prephonatory chest wall posturing. *Folia phoniatrica, 33,* 193–202.

Baken, R., Cavallo, S., & Weissman, K. (1979). Chest wall movements prior to phonation. *Journal of Speech and Hearing Research, 22,* 862–872.

Baken, R., & Orlikoff, R. F. (1999). *Clinical measurement of speech and voice,* (2nd ed.). San Diego: Singular Publishing Group.

Basmajian, J. V. (1975). *Grant's method of anatomy.* Baltimore: Williams & Wilkins.

Bateman, H. E., & Mason, R. M. (1984). *Applied anatomy and physiology of the speech and hearing mechanism.* Springfield, IL: Charles C. Thomas.

Beck, E. W. (1982). *Mosby's atlas of functional human anatomy.* St. Louis: Mosby.

Bergman, R., Thompson, S., & Afifi, A. (1984). *A Catalog of human variation.* Baltimore: Urban & Schwarzenberg.

Bly, L. (1994). *Motor skills acquisition in the first year.* Tucson, AZ: Therapy Skill Builders.

Burrows, B., Knudson, R. J., & Kettel, L. J. (1975). *Respiratory insufficiency.* Chicago: Year Book Medical Publishers.

Campbell, E. (1958). An electromyographic examination of the role of the intercostal muscles in breathing in man. *Journal of Physiology, 129,* 12–26.

Campbell, E., Agostoni, E., & Davis, J. (1970). *The respiratory muscles, mechanics and neural control.* Philadelphia: W. B. Saunders.

Chusid, J. G. (1985). *Correlative neuroanatomy and functional neurology* (17th ed.). Los Altos, CA: Lange Medical Publications.

Comroe, J. H. (1974). *Physiology of respiration.* Chicago: Year Book Medical Publishers.

Creasy, R. K. (1997). *Management of labor and delivery.* Malden, MA: Blackwell Science.

DesJardins, T., & Burton, G. G. (2001). *Clinical manifestation and assessment of respiratory disease.* Chicago: Mosby.

Draper, M., Ladefoged, P., & Whitteridge, D. (1959). Respiratory muscles in speech. *Journal of Speech and Hearing Research, 2,* 16–27.

Ganong, W. F. (2003). *Review of medical physiology* (21st ed.). New York: McGraw-Hill/Appleton & Lange.

Gordon, M. S. (1972). *Animal physiology: Principles and adaptations.* New York: Macmillan.

Gosling, J. A., Harris, P. F., Humpherson, J. R., Whitmore, I., & Willan, P. L.T. (1985). *Atlas of human anatomy.* Philadelphia: J. B. Lippincott.

Gray, H., Bannister, L. H., Berry, M. M., & Williams, P. L. (Eds.). (1995). *Gray's anatomy.* London: Churchill Livingstone.

Grobler, N. J. (1977). *Textbook of clinical anatomy* (Vol. 1). Amsterdam: Elsevier Scientific.

Hixon, T. J. (1973). Respiratory function in speech. In F. D. Minifie, T. J. Hixon, & F. Williams (Eds.), *Normal aspects of speech, hearing, and language* (pp. 73–126). Englewood Cliffs, NJ: Prentice-Hall.

Hixon, T. J., Goldman, M. D., & Mead, J. (1973). Kinematics of the chest wall during speech production: Volume displacement of the rib cage, abdomen, and lung. *Journal of Speech and Hearing Research, 16,* 78–115.

Hlastala, M. P., & Berger, A. J. (1996). *Physiology of respiration.* New York: Oxford University Press.

Kahane, J. (1982). Anatomy and physiology of the organs of the peripheral speech mechanism. In N. Lass, L. McReynolds, J. Northern, & D. Yoder (Eds.), *Speech, language, and hearing. Vol. 1: Normal processes* (pp. 109–155). Philadelphia: W. B. Saunders.

Kao, F. F. (1972). *An introduction to respiratory physiology.* Amsterdam: Exerpta Medica.

Kaplan, H. (1960). *Anatomy and physiology of speech.* New York: McGraw-Hill.

Kent, R. D. (1997). *The speech sciences.* San Diego: Singular Publishing Group.

Konno, K., & Mead, J. (1968). Measurement of the separate volume changes of rib cage and abdomen during breathing. *Journal of Applied Physiology, 22,* 407–422.

Kuehn, D. P., Lemme, M. L., & Baumgartner, J. M. (1989). *Neural bases of speech, hearing, and language.* Boston: Little, Brown.

Langley, M. B., & Lombardino, L. J. (1991). *Neurodevelopmental strategies for managing communication disorders in children with severe motor dysfunction.* Austin: Pro-Ed.

Lass, N., McReynolds, L., Northern, J., & Yoder, D. (Eds.). (1982). *Speech, language, and hearing. Vol. I: Normal processes.* Philadelphia: W. B. Saunders.

Lee, D. H. K. (1972). *Environmental factors in respiratory disease.* New York: Academic Press.

Logemann, J. (1998). *Evaluation and treatment of swallowing disorders* (2nd ed.). Austin: Pro-Ed.

MacKay, L. E., Chapman, P. E., & Morgan, A. S. (1997). *Maximizing brain injury recovery.* Gaithersburg, MD: Aspen.

McMinn, R. M. H., Hutchings, R. T., & Logan, B. M. (1994). *Color atlas of head and neck anatomy.* London: Mosby-Wolfe.

McReynolds, L., Northern, J., & Yoder, D. (Eds.). *Speech, language, and hearing. Vol. I: Normal processes.* Philadelphia: W. B. Saunders.

Miller, A. D., Bianchi, A. L., & Bishop, B. P. (1997). *Neural control of the respiratory muscles.* Boca Raton, FL: CRC Press.

Mohr, J. P. (1989). *Manual of clinical problems in neurology.* Boston: Little, Brown.

Moser, K. M., & Spragg, R. G. (1982). *Respiratory emergencies.* St. Louis: Mosby.

Murray, J. F. (1976). *The normal lung. The basis for diagnosis and treatment of pulmonary disease.* Philadelphia: W. B. Saunders.

Netter, F. H. (1983a). *The CIBA collection of medical illustrations. Vol. 1. Nervous system: Part I. Anatomy and physiology.* West Caldwell, NJ: CIBA Pharmaceutical Company.

Netter, F. H. (1983b). *The CIBA collection of medical illustrations. Vol. 1. Nervous system: Part II. Neurologic and neuromuscular disorders*. West Caldwell, NJ: CIBA Pharmaceutical Company.

Netter, F. H. (1997). *Atlas of human anatomy*. Los Angeles: Icon Learning Systems.

Pace, W. R. (1970). *Pulmonary physiology*. Philadelphia: F. A. Davis.

Pappenheimer, J. R., Comroe, J. H., Cournand, A., Ferguson, J. K. W., Filley, G. F., Fowler, W. S., Gray, J. S., Helmholtz, H. F., Otis, A. B., Rahn, H., & Riley, R. L. (1950). *Standardization of definitions and symbols in respiratory physiology. Bethesda, MD: Proceedings of the Federation of the American Society for Experimental Biology*, Vol. 9 (pp. 602–605).

Peters, R. M. (1969). *The mechanical basis of respiration*. Boston: Little, Brown.

Rahn, H., Otis, A., Chadwick, L. E., & Fenn, W. (1946). The pressure–volume diagram of the thorax and lung. *American Journal of Physiology, 146,* 161–178.

Rohen, J. W., Yokochi, C., Lutjen-Drecoll, E., & Romrell, L. J. (2002). *Color atlas of anatomy* (5th ed.). Philadelphia: Williams & Wilkins.

Rosse, C., Gaddum-Rosse, P., & Rosse, G. (1997). *Hollinshead's textbook of anatomy*. Philadelphia: Lippincott-Raven.

Scott, J. R., Disaia, P. J., Hammond, C. B., & Spellacy, W. N. (1994). *Danforth's obstetrics and gynecology*, (7th ed.). Philadelphia: J. B. Lippincott.

Snell, R. S. (1978). *Gross anatomy dissector*. Boston: Little, Brown.

Spector, W. S. (1956). *Handbook of biological data*. Philadelphia: W. B. Saunders.

Taylor, A. (1960). The contribution of the intercostal muscles to the effort of respiration in man. *Journal of Physiology, 151,* 390.

Tokizane, T., Kawamata, K., & Tokizane, H. (1952). Electromyographic studies on the human respiratory muscles. *Japan Journal of Physiology, 2,* 232.

Twietmeyer, A., & McCracken, T. D., (1992). *Coloring guide to regional human anatomy* (2nd ed.). Philadelphia: Lea & Febiger.

Zemlin, W. R. (1998). *Speech and hearing science: Anatomy and physiology* (4th ed.). Needham Heights, MA: Allyn & Bacon.

CHAPTER

3

Anatomy and Physiology of Phonation

OUTLINE

I. Introduction to Phonation

    A. Phonation is voicing

    B. Airflow

    C. The Bernoulli principle

    D. Sustained phonation depends on

        1. Subglottal pressure

        2. Tissue elasticity

        3. Constriction of airflow

II. Phonatory Mechanism

A. Framework of the larynx
   1. Cricoid cartilage
   2. Thyroid cartilage
   3. Epiglottis
   4. Arytenoid cartilages
   5. Corniculate cartilages
   6. Cuneiform cartilages

B. Inner larynx
   1. Cavity of the larynx
   2. Ligaments connect cartilages
   3. Valleculae
   4. Cricotracheal ligament
   5. Fibroelastic membrane
   6. Pyriform sinus
   7. Aryepiglottic folds

C. Structure of the vocal folds
   1. Vocal ligament
   2. Aditus
   3. Glottis

D. Structure of the larynx
   1. Cricoid cartilage
   2. Thyroid cartilage
   3. Arytenoid cartilage
   4. Corniculate cartilage
   5. Epiglottis
   6. Cuneiform cartilages
   7. Hyoid bone

E. Movement of the cartilages
   1. Cricothyroid joint
   2. Cricoarytenoid joint

F. Laryngeal musculature
   1. Intrinsic laryngeal muscles
      a. Adductors
         1) Lateral cricoarytenoid
         2) Transverse arytenoid
         3) Oblique arytenoid
      b. Abductor: Posterior cricoarytenoid muscle
      c. Glottal tensors
         1) Cricothyroid muscle
         2) Thyrovocalis muscle
      d. Relaxer: thyromuscularis muscle

2. Extrinsic laryngeal muscles
    a. Hyoid and laryngeal elevators
        1) Digastricus anterior and posterior
        2) Stylohyoid muscle
        3) Mylohyoid muscle
        4) Geniohyoid muscle
        5) Hyoglossus muscle
        6) Genioglossus muscle
        7) Thyropharyngeus and cricopharyngeus muscles
    b. Hyoid and laryngeal depressors
        1) Sternohyoid muscle
        2) Omohyoid muscle
        3) Sternothyroid muscle
        d) Thyrohyoid muscle

III. Physiology of Phonation

  A. Nonspeech laryngeal function
    1. Protective function of the larynx
    2. Coughing
  B. Laryngeal function for speech
    1. Attack
        a. Simultaneous attack
        b. Breathy vocal attack
        c. Glottal attack
    2. Termination of phonation
    3. Sustained phonation
    4. Vocal register
        a. Modal phonation
        b. Falsetto
        c. Glottal fry
        d. Breathy phonation
        e. Whispering
    3. Frequency, pitch, and pitch change
        a. Optimal pitch
        b. Habitual pitch
        c. Average fundamental frequency
        d. Pitch range
        e. Tension of the vocal folds and mass per unit length
        f. Pitch and subglottal pressure

4. Intensity and intensity change
   a. Increased subglottal pressure
   b. Increased adductory force
   c. Increased laryngeal tension
5. Linguistic aspects of pitch and intensity
   a. Suprasegmental elements
   b. Intonation
6. Theories of phonation

Vocal folds (vocal cords): The vibrating component of the larynx used to produce sound.

Spoken communication uses both voiceless and voiced sounds, and this chapter is concerned with that critical distinction. Voiceless phonemes or speech sounds are produced without use of the **vocal folds**, for example, the /s/ or /f/ sounds. Voiced sounds are produced by action of the vocal folds, for example, the /z/ and /v/ sound. Phonation, or voicing, is the product of vibrating vocal folds, and this occurs in the larynx. Just as we referred to respiration as the source of energy for speech, phonation is the source of voice for speech. Respiration is the energy source that permits phonation, and without respiration there would be no voicing.

The vocal folds, or vocal cords, are located in the airstream at the upper end of the trachea. As the airstream passes between the vocal folds, they may be made to vibrate, much as a flag flaps in the wind.

MECHANISMS OF PHONATION

Vocal folds are masses that can be set into vibration. The larynx is the cartilaginous structure that houses the two bands of tissue we call the vocal folds. The paired vocal folds are situated on both sides of the larynx so that they actually intrude into the airstream, as you can see in Figure 3-1. In the view from above, you can see that the vocal folds are bands of tissue that are visible from a point immediately behind your tongue (not shown) looking down toward the lungs. From behind, you can see that the vocal folds also constrict the airway, a critical concept for phonation.

You will remember from our discussion of respiratory physiology that any constriction of the airway greatly increases airway turbulence. The vocal folds are a source of turbulence in the vocal tract. Without them, air would pass relatively unimpeded out of the lungs and into the oral cavity.

A   SUPERIOR VIEW

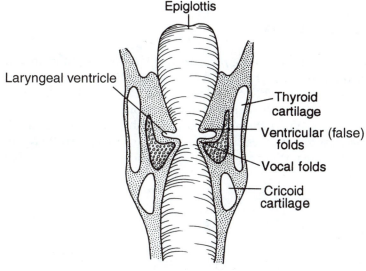

B   POSTERIOR VIEW

FIGURE 3–1. A. Vocal folds from above. **B.** Anterior view of larynx showing constriction of laryngeal space caused by the vocal folds.

Daniel Bernoulli, a seventeenth-century Swiss scientist, recognized the effects of constricting a tube during fluid flow. The **Bernoulli effect** states that given a constant volume flow of air or fluid, at a point of constriction there will be a decrease in air pressure and an increase in velocity of the flow. If you put a constriction in a tube, air will flow faster as it detours around the constriction and the pressure on the wall at the point of constriction will be lower than that of the surrounding area. Let us further examine this statement.

Bernoulli effect (principle): Given a constant volume flow of air or liquid, at a point of constriction there will be a decrease in air pressure perpendicular to the flow and an increase in velocity of flow.

Airflow Increase

If you have placed your thumb over a garden hose, you know that the rate of water flow increases as a result of that constriction. Likewise, if you have been white-water rafting, you will immediately recognize that the white water comes from constriction in the flow of the river, in the form of boulders. As the water flows through the constriction, the rate of flow increases, giving you the thrill as you speed uncontrollably toward your fate.

Air Pressure Drop

To get an intuitive feel for the pressure drop, think about the flow in terms of molecules of air. Look at Figure 3-2. We have drawn it so you can count the number of molecules of air in the tube relative to the tube's length. In the unconstricted regions, you can count 10 molecules of air. Where the tube is narrower, there are fewer air molecules because there is less space for them to occupy, so there are only 5 in that area. Where the constriction ends, you once again see 10 molecules.

FIGURE 3-2. Rate of airflow through the tube increases at the point of constriction, and air pressure decreases at that point.

Biological Functions of the Larynx

Although we capitalize on the larynx for phonation, it has a much more important function. The larynx is an exquisite sphincter in that the vocal folds are capable of a very strong and rapid clamping of the airway in response to threat of intrusion by foreign objects. As evidence of this primary function, there are three pairs of laryngeal muscles directly responsible for either **approximating** (bringing folds into contact) or tensing the vocal folds, although only one pair of muscles is responsible for opening them. The vocal folds are "wired" to close immediately on stimulation by outside agents, such as food or liquids, a response followed quickly by a rapid and forceful exhalation. This combination of gestures stops intrusion by foreign matter and rapidly expels that matter away from the airway's opening.

Approximation: When referring to vocal folds, making contact.

The larynx has other important functions as well. Because the vocal folds provide an excellent seal to the respiratory system, they permit you to hold your breath, thus capturing a significant respiratory charge for such activities as swimming.

Holding your breath also serves other functions. Lifting heavy objects requires you to "fix" your thorax by inhaling and clamping your laryngeal sphincter (vocal folds). This gives the muscles of the upper body a solid framework with which to work. You might remember from Chapter 2 that tightly clamping the vocal folds plays an important role in the labor of childbirth.

When air is forced into a narrow tube, that volume of air has to squeeze into a smaller space. Because each unit mass of air becomes longer and narrower, it covers a longer stretch of the tube's walls. The pressure exerted by this mass, although the same in an overall sense, is now distributed over more of the wall. The result is that each atom of the wall feels less force from the air molecules, and the narrow part of the tube is more likely to collapse. This effect occurs only when the air is forced to move; air without forced movement will sooner or later equalize its pressure everywhere. If you remember that pressure is force exerted on an area ($P = F/A$), a drop in pressure makes perfect sense.

The Bernoulli Effect in Everyday Life

If you are a baseball fan, you will appreciate the amazing curve ball of your favorite pitcher more when you realize that the Bernoulli effect is the driving force behind it. In this case, the pitcher ensures that the ball begins its flight with the smooth surface toward the front and that the seam on the ball rotates to the side of the ball sometime during its brief flight. The seam acts as a constriction; the pressure on the seam side is lower than that on the opposite smooth side, and the ball is "sucked" toward the seam (there are other processes involved, but we'll ignore them here). At least one pitcher has demonstrated the ability to "weave" the ball through a series of fence posts by putting just the right spin on the ball. For an excellent discussion of this effect, see Adair (1995).

The vocal folds are made up of muscle and epithelial tissue. Because these are soft tissues, the folds are capable of moving when sufficient force is exerted on them. In Figure 3-3A the vocal folds are closed. In Figure 3-3B the air pressure generated by the respiratory system is beginning to force the vocal folds open, but there is no transglottal flow because the folds are still making full contact. By part D the vocal folds have been blown open. Because the vocal folds are elastic, they tend to return to the point of equilibrium, which is the point of rest. They cannot return to equilibrium, however, as long as the air pressure is so great that they are kept apart. When they are apart, however, there is a drop in pressure at the point of constriction (the Bernoulli effect), and we already know that if there is a drop in pressure, something is going to move to equalize that pressure.

In parts E, F, and G you can see the result of the negative pressure. The vocal folds are being sucked back toward midline (E) as a result of the negative pressure and tissue elasticity. Parts F and G show the folds again making contact, with airflow completely halted. The vocal folds are, in essence, sucked back to midline by the pressure drop at the constriction. When the vocal folds are pulled back toward midline by their tissue-restoring forces, they completely

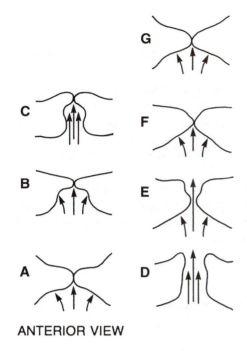

ANTERIOR VIEW

FIGURE 3-3. One cycle of vocal fold vibration seen through a frontal section. **A.** Air pressure beneath the vocal folds arises from respiratory flow. **B.** Air pressure causes the vocal folds to separate in the inferior. **C.** Superior aspect of vocal folds begins to open. **D.** Vocal folds are blown open, flow between the folds increases, and pressure at the folds decreases. **E.** Decreased pressure and elastic quality of vocal folds causes folds to move back toward midline. **F.** Vocal folds make contact inferiorly. **G.** The cycle of vibration is completed.

block the flow of air for an instant as they make contact. When they are in contact, air has stopped flowing briefly, and therefore the negative pressure related to flow is gone also. Instead, there is the force of respiratory charge beneath the folds ready to blow them apart once again. By the way, the minimum subglottal pressure that will blow the vocal folds apart to sustain phonation is approximately 3 cm to 5 cm H_2O, although much larger subglottal pressures are required for louder speech.

What you hear as voicing is the product of the repeated opening and closing of the vocal folds. The motion of the tissue and airflow disturb the molecules of air, causing the phenomenon we call sound.

The act of bringing the vocal folds together for phonation is **adduction**, and the process of drawing the vocal folds apart to terminate phonation is **abduction**. As we will see, both of these movements use specific muscles, but the actual vibration of the vocal folds is the product of airflow interacting with the tissue in absence of repetitive muscular contraction.

Adduction: The process of moving two structures closer together.

Abduction: The process of moving two structures farther apart.

Summary

- Phonation, or voicing, is the product of vibrating vocal folds in the larynx.
- The vocal folds vibrate as air flows past them; the Bernoulli phenomenon and tissue elasticity help maintain phonation.
- The Bernoulli principle states that given a constant volume flow of air or fluid, at a point of constriction there will be a decrease in air pressure perpendicular to the flow and an increase in velocity of the flow.
- The interaction of subglottal pressure, tissue elasticity, and constriction of the airflow caused by the vocal folds produces sustained phonation as long as pressure, flow, and vocal fold approximation are maintained.

A TOUR OF THE PHONATORY MECHANISM

This is a good opportunity to walk you through the vocal mechanism. We will get into details soon enough, but for now let us look at the larger picture.

Framework of the Larynx

The larynx is a structure made of muscle and cartilage located at the superior (upper) end of the trachea. It comprises three unpaired and three paired cartilages bound by ligaments and lined with mucous membrane.

Process: Protrusion of an anatomical structure.

In Figure 3-4 you can see the relation between the trachea and larynx. The *cricoid cartilage* is a complete ring resting atop the trachea and is the most inferior of the laryngeal cartilages. The *thyroid cartilage* is the largest of the laryngeal cartilages, articulating with the cricoid cartilage below by means of paired **processes** that let it rock forward and backward at that joint. With this configuration, the paired *arytenoid cartilages* ride on the high-backed upper surface of the cricoid cartilage, forming the posterior point of attachment for the vocal folds. The *corniculate cartilages* ride on the superior surface of each arytenoid. The inner surface of the thyroid cartilage provides the anterior point of attachment for the vocal folds.

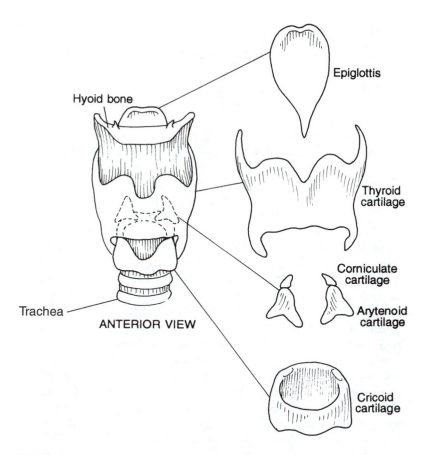

FIGURE 3–4. Larynx *(left)* and cartilages making up the larynx *(right)*.

The thyroid cartilage articulates with the hyoid bone by means of a pair of superior processes. Medial to the hyoid bone and thyroid cartilage is the *epiglottis,* a leaf-shaped cartilage.

Summary

- The larynx is a musculo-cartilaginous structure located at the upper end of the trachea that comprises the cricoid, thyroid, and epiglottis cartilages, as well as the paired arytenoid, corniculate, and cuneiform cartilages.
- The thyroid and cricoid cartilages articulate by means of the cricothyroid joint, which lets the two cartilages come closer together in front.

Laryngectomy

Patients who undergo laryngectomy (surgical removal of the larynx) lose the structures necessary to produce sound. The larynx is removed and the oral cavity is sealed off from the trachea and lower respiratory passageway as a safeguard because the protective function of the larynx is also lost. Laryngectomees (individuals who have undergone laryngectomy) must alter their activities because they now breathe through a tracheostoma, an opening placed in the trachea through a surgical procedure known as a tracheostomy.

Loss of the ability to phonate is but one of the difficulties facing the laryngectomee. This patient has difficulty with expectoration (elimination of phlegm from respiratory passageway) and coughing, and is no longer able to enjoy swimming or other activities that would expose the stoma to water or pollutants. The air entering the patient's lungs is no longer humidified or filtered by the upper respiratory passageway, and a filter must be kept over the stoma to prevent introduction of foreign objects. The flavor of foods is greatly reduced because the patient no longer breathes through the nose, and our perception of food relies heavily on the sense of smell. Depending on pre- and postoperative treatment, laryngectomees may experience extreme dryness of oral tissues arising from damage to salivary glands from radiation therapy.

■ The arytenoid and cricoid cartilages also articulate with a joint that permits a wide range of arytenoid motion.
■ The corniculate cartilages rest on the upper surface of the arytenoids, and the cuneiform cartilages reside in the aryepiglottic folds.

Inner Larynx

The vocal folds are bands of mucous membrane, connective tissue, and muscle that are slung between the arytenoid cartilages and the thyroid cartilage so that they can be moved into and out of the airstream. Muscles attached to the arytenoids perform both adductory and abductory functions.

Laryngeal Membranes

The cavity of the larynx is a constricted tube with a smooth and reasonably aerodynamic surface (see Figure 3-5). The *thyrohyoid membrane* stretches across the space between the *greater cornu* of hyoid and the lateral thyroid cartilage.

Intrinsic ligaments connect the cartilages of the larynx and form the support structure for the cavity of the larynx, as well as that of the vocal folds themselves. The *fibroelastic membrane* of the larynx is composed of the upper quadrangular membranes and *aryepiglottic folds*, the lower *conus elasticus*, and the *vocal ligament*, which is actually the upward free extension of the conus elasticus.

If you will look at the profile of the larynx in Figure 3-6, you will appreciate some of the relationships among the structures. The **aditus** is the entry to the larynx from the pharynx above. View A of Figure 3-7 is looking through the aditus into the vestibule. You can see two "bumps" under the aryepiglottic folds that are caused by the cuneiform cartilages embedded in the folds. The second set of prominences posterior to the first two are from the *corniculate cartilages* on the arytenoids.

Aditus: The entrance of the larynx.

The vestibule is the cavity between the entry to the larynx, or aditus, and the **ventricular**, or vestibular, folds. The ventricular folds are known also as the false vocal folds because they are not used for phonation. The space between the margins of the false vocal folds and the true vocal folds below is the *laryngeal ventricle*, or laryngeal sinus, and the anterior extension of this space is the *laryngeal saccule*. The saccule, or pouch, is endowed with more than 60 mucous glands that secrete lubricating mucus into the laryngeal cavity. These sacs are actually endowed with muscle to squeeze the mucus out for lubrication.

Ventricular: Referring to cavities or passageways to structures.

The **glottis** is the space between the vocal folds, inferior to the ventricle and superior to the conus elasticus. This is the most important laryngeal space for speech because it is defined by the variable sphincter that permits voicing. In adults at rest the length of the glottis is approximately 20 mm from the **anterior commissure** (anterior-most opening) to the **posterior commissure** (between the arytenoid cartilages). The glottis area is variable, depending on the moment-to-moment configuration of the vocal folds. At rest, the posterior glottis is approximately 8 mm wide; this dimension doubles during forced respiration.

Glottis: The space between the vocal folds.

Anterior commissure of glottis: *The anterior-most region of the glottis.*

Posterior commissure of glottis: *The posterior-most region of the glottis.*

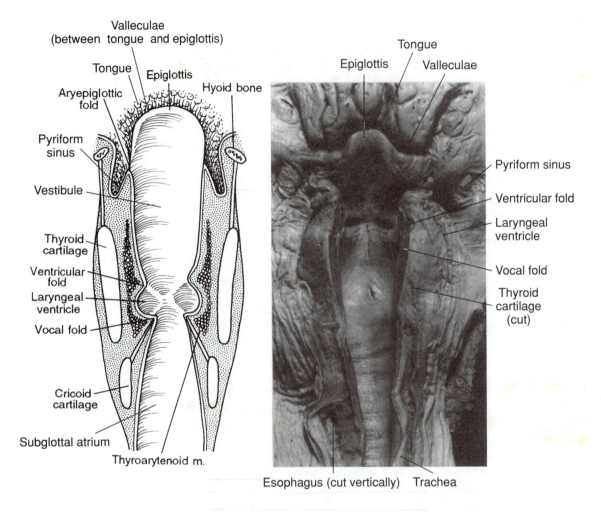

FIGURE 3–5. Cavity of the larynx with landmarks.

At the margins of the glottis are the vocal folds and the arytenoid cartilage. The anterior three fifths of the vocal margin is made up of the soft tissue of the vocal folds. (You might see this referred to as the membranous glottis because some anatomists define the glottis as the entire vocal mechanism.) In adult males the free margin of the vocal folds is approximately 15 mm long, and in females it is approximately 12 mm. This free margin of the vocal folds is the vibrating element that provides voice. The posterior two fifths of the vocal folds is the cartilage of the arytenoids. (This is often referred to as the cartilaginous glottis because *glottis* can refer also to the entire

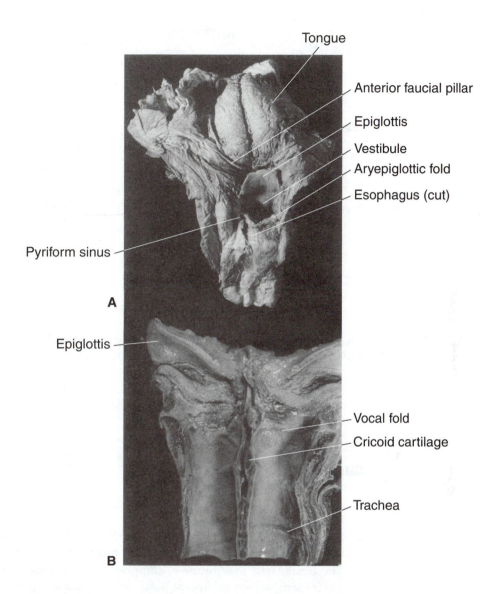

FIGURE 3–6. A. Larynx seen from behind and above. **B.** Larynx that has been cut sagittally and the sides reflected, revealing the two halves of larynx.

ANTERIOR

Valleculae

Epiglottis

Ventricular fold

Vocal fold

Pyriform sinus

Aryepiglottic fold

Prominence of cuneiform cartilage

Prominence of arytenoid cartilage

SUPERIOR VIEW

FIGURE 3-7. Vocal folds as seen from above.

vocal mechanism.) This portion of the vocal folds is between 4 mm and 8 mm long, depending on sex and body size.

The conus elasticus begins at the margins of the true vocal folds and extends to the inferior border of the cricoid cartilage, widening from the vocal folds to the base of the cricoid.

Summary

- The cavity of the larynx is a constricted tube with a smooth surface.
- Sheets and cords of ligaments connect the cartilages, and smooth mucous membrane covers the medial-most surface of the larynx.
- The fibroelastic membrane is composed of the upper quadrangular membranes and aryepiglottic folds, the lower conus elasticus, and the vocal ligament, which is actually the upward free extension of the conus elasticus.
- The aryepiglottic folds course from the side of the epiglottis to the arytenoid apex.
- The vocal ligament is made of elastin. The aditus is the entryway of the larynx, marking the entry to the vestibule.
- The ventricular and vocal folds are separated by the laryngeal ventricle.
- The glottis is the variable space between the vocal folds.

STRUCTURAL ELEMENTS OF THE LARYNX

Cricoid Cartilage

As the most inferior cartilage of the larynx, the cricoid cartilage is the approximate diameter of the trachea. It is higher in the back than in the front. There are several important landmarks on the cricoid. The low, anterior cricoid arch provides clearance for the vocal folds that will pass over that point, and the posterior elevation provides the point of articulation of the arytenoid cartilages. On the lateral surfaces of the cricoid are articular facets, or "faces," marking the point of articulation of the inferior horns of the thyroid cartilage (see Figure 3-8).

Thyroid Cartilage

The unpaired thyroid cartilage is the largest laryngeal cartilage. As you can see in Figure 3-9, the thyroid has a prominent anterior surface made up of two plates called the *thyroid laminae*, joined midline at the *thyroid angle*. At the superior-most point of that angle is the *thyroid notch*. On the lateral superficial aspect of the thyroid laminae you can see the *oblique line*. This marks the point of attachment for two of the muscles we will talk about shortly.

The posterior aspect of the thyroid is open, and it is characterized by two prominent sets of cornu, or horns. The *inferior cornua* project downward to articulate with the cricoid cartilage, and the *superior cornua* project upward to articulate with the hyoid. Some individuals have a small *triticial cartilage* (*cartilago triticea*) between the superior cornu of the thyroid cartilage and the hyoid bone.

Arytenoid and Corniculate Cartilages

The paired arytenoid cartilages are among the most important of the larynx. They reside on the superior surface of the cricoid cartilage and provide the mechanical structure that permits onset and offset of voicing. To aid visualization, the form of the arytenoid can be likened to a pyramid (see Figure 3-10). Each cartilage has two processes and four surfaces.

The apex is the superior portion of the arytenoid cartilage, and above it is the corniculate cartilage. The inferior surface of the arytenoid cartilage is termed the base, and its concave surface is the point of articulation with the convex arytenoid facet of the cricoid cartilage.

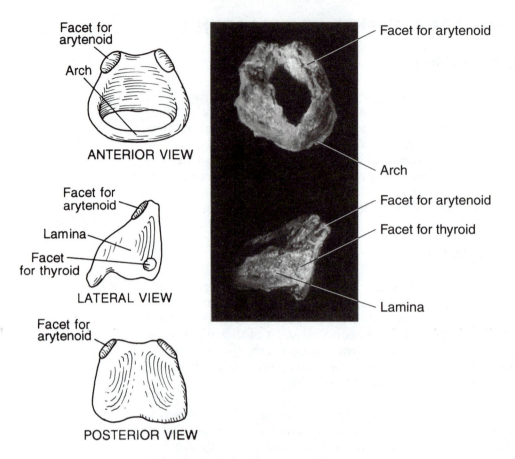

FIGURE 3-8. Cricoid cartilage and landmarks.

There are two processes on each arytenoid. The *vocal process* projects toward the thyroid notch, where the vocal folds attach in the anterior. The *muscular process* forms the lateral outcropping of the arytenoid pyramid and is the point of attachment for muscles that adduct and abduct the vocal folds.

Epiglottis

The unpaired epiglottis is a leaflike structure that arises from the inner surface of the angle of the thyroid cartilage just below the notch, attached there by the *thyroepiglottic ligament*. The sides of the epiglottis are joined with the arytenoid cartilages via the aryepiglottic folds, which are the product of the membranous lining draping over muscle and connective tissue.

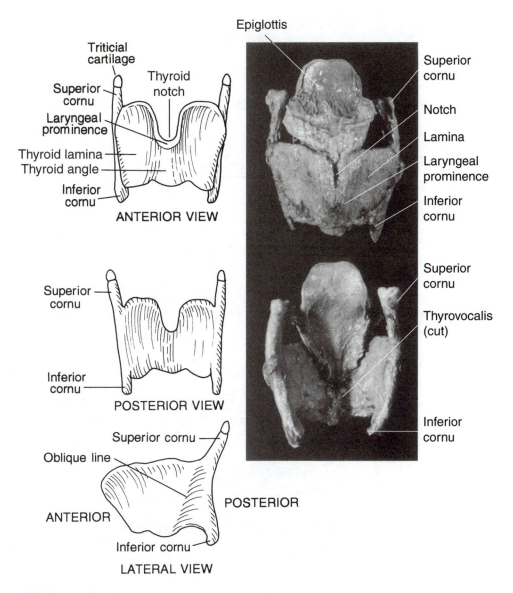

FIGURE 3-9. Thyroid cartilage and landmarks.

The epiglottis projects upward beyond the larynx and above the hyoid bone. It is attached to the root of the tongue by the median *glosso-epiglottic fold* and the paired lateral glosso-epiglottic folds. This juncture produces the **valleculae**, important landmarks in swallowing deficit. During swallowing, food passes over the epiglottis, and from there laterally to the *pyriform* (also piriform)

Valleculae: Pair of small indentations between the tongue and epiglottis.

FIGURE 3-10. Arytenoid cartilages articulated with cricoid cartilage.

Fossa: Indentation or cavity.

Pharyngeal recesses: Valleculae and pyriform sinuses.

sinuses, which are small **fossae,** or indentations, between the aryepiglottic folds medially and the mucous lining of the thyroid cartilage. Together the pyriform sinuses and valleculae are called the **pharyngeal recesses** (see Figure 3-7).

Cuneiform Cartilages

The cuneiform cartilages are small cartilages embedded in the aryepiglottic folds. They are situated above and anterior to the

Valleculae and Swallowing

The valleculae are "little valleys," formed by the membrane between the tongue and epiglottis. During normal swallowing the larynx elevates and the epiglottis folds down to protect the airway from food and liquid. The food and liquid pass over the back of the tongue, through the valleculae, on either side of the base of the epiglottis, into the pyriform sinuses lateral to the laryngeal aditus, and finally into the esophagus.

When swallowing is compromised, as in the deficit caused by cerebrovascular accident (CVA, or stroke), the larynx may not elevate properly, and food can accumulate in the valleculae. The resultant malodorous breath in a neurologically compromised individual may be a significant indicator of a dangerous swallowing dysfunction; if the epiglottis is not covering the airway, there is a good chance that the vocal folds are not doing their job in protecting the lungs.

corniculate cartilages, and they cause a small bulge on the surface of the membrane that looks white under illumination. These cartilages apparently provide support for the membranous laryngeal covering.

Hyoid Bone

The *hyoid bone* is the union between the tongue and the laryngeal structure. This unpaired small bone articulates loosely with the superior cornu of the thyroid cartilage, and it has the distinction of being the only bone of the body that is not attached to other bone (see Figure 3-11).

The front of the **corpus** of the hyoid bone is convex and the inner surface is concave. The corpus is the point of attachment for six muscles (mylohyoid, sternohyoid, omohyoid, stylohyoid, genioglossus, and geniohyoid). The greater **cornu** is on the lateral surface of the corpus, projecting posteriorly. At the junction of the corpus and greater cornu, you can see the *lesser cornu*. Three additional muscles (hypoglossus, middle constrictor, and thyrohyoid) are attached to these two structures.

Corpus: Body.

Cornu: Horn.

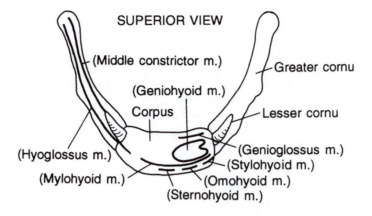

SUPERIOR VIEW

(Middle constrictor m.)　　Greater cornu

(Geniohyoid m.)

Corpus　　Lesser cornu

(Hyoglossus m.)　　(Genioglossus m.)

(Stylohyoid m.)

(Mylohyoid m.)　　(Omohyoid m.)

(Sternohyoid m.)

POSTERIOR VIEW

(Hyoepiglottic ligament)

Lesser cornu

(Thyrohyoid membrane)

(Thyrohyoid m.)

FIGURE 3-11. Hyoid bone seen from above and behind. Points of attachment of muscles and membranes are indicated in parentheses.

MOVEMENT OF THE CARTILAGES

The *cricothyroid* and *cricoarytenoid joints* are the only functionally mobile points of the larynx. The cricothyroid joint is the junction of the cricoid cartilage and inferior cornu of the thyroid cartilage. These joints permit the cricoid and thyroid to rotate and glide relative to each other. As seen in Figure 3-12, rotation at the cricothyroid joint permits the thyroid cartilage to rock down in front, and the joint also permits the thyroid to glide forward and backward slightly relative to the cricoid. This joint will provide the major adjustment for change in vocal pitch.

The cricoarytenoid joint is the articulation formed between the cricoid and arytenoid cartilages. These joints permit rocking, gliding, and minimal rotation. The arytenoid facet of the cricoid is a convex, oblong surface, and the axis of motion is around a line projecting

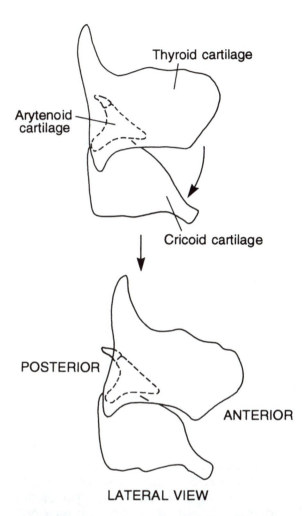

Thyroid cartilage

Arytenoid cartilage

Cricoid cartilage

POSTERIOR

ANTERIOR

LATERAL VIEW

FIGURE 3-12. Movement of the cricoid and thyroid cartilages about the cricothyroid joint. When the cricoid and thyroid move toward each other in front the arytenoid cartilage moves farther away from the thyroid cartilage, tensing the vocal folds.

back along the superior surface of the arytenoid and converging at a point above the arytenoid (see Figure 3-13). This rocking action folds the two vocal processes toward each other, permitting the vocal folds to make contact. The arytenoids are also capable of gliding on the long axis of the facet, facilitating changes in vocal fold length. The arytenoids may rotate upon a vertical axis drawn through the

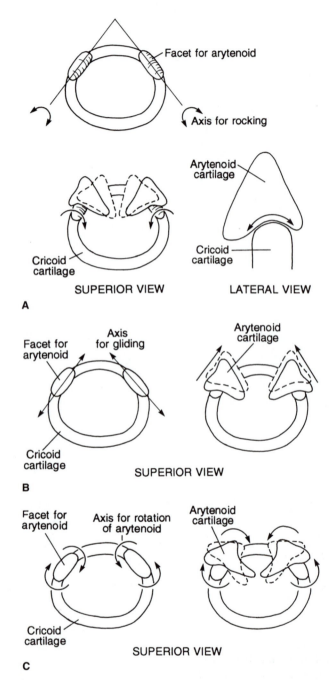

FIGURE 3–13. The articular facet for the arytenoid cartilage permits rocking, gliding and rotation. **A.** The shape of the articular facet of the arytenoid cartilage promotes inward rocking of the arytenoid cartilage and vocal folds (*arced arrows*). **B.** The long axis of the facet permits limited anterior-posterior gliding (bidirectional arrows). **C.** The arytenoids can also rotate, although this does not appear to be a functional gesture for adduction (circling arrows). (Based on data of Broad, 1973; Fink, 1978; Netter, 1989; Zemlin, 1998.)

Vocal Fold Hydration

The vocal folds are extremely sensitive to the internal and external environments. Although the effects of smoking and other pollutants are known to irritate the tissues of the vocal folds, the internal environment appears to have an impact as well.

When the vocal folds are subject to abuse, problems such as contact ulcers and vocal nodules may occur. Hydration therapy is a frequent prescription to counteract the problems of irritated tissue. Dry tissue does not heal as well as moist tissue, so the patient will be told to spray the throat, drink fluids, or even take medications to promote water retention. This type of therapy makes more than medical sense. Verdolini, Titze, and Fennell (1994) found that the effort of phonation increases as individuals become dehydrated and decreases when they are hydrated beyond normal levels. Indeed, the airflow required to produce the same phonation is greatly increased by a poorly lubricated larynx. In addition, the vocal folds vibrate much more periodically (that is, they have greatly reduced perturbation, or cycle-by-cycle variation) when lubricated (Fukida et al., 1988). When the relative periodicity of the vocal folds decreases, the voice is hoarse.

apex of the arytenoid, but this motion appears to be limited to extremes of abduction (Fink & Demarest, 1978). The combination of these gestures provides the mechanism for vocal fold approximation and abduction.

Your understanding of the movement of these cartilages in relation to each other will provide a valuable backdrop to understanding laryngeal physiology.

Summary

- The laryngeal cartilages have a number of important landmarks to which muscles are attached.
- The cricoid cartilage is shaped like a signet ring, higher in back.
- The arytenoid cartilages ride on the superior surface of the cricoid, with the cricoarytenoid joint permitting rotation, rocking, and gliding.
- The corniculate cartilages attach to the upper margin of the arytenoids.

Palpation of the Larynx

To palpate the larynx, first identify the prominent thyroid notch, or "Adam's apple." Once you have found it, place your index finger on the notch and your thumb and second finger on either side. Your thumb and second finger should feel a fairly flat surface, the thyroid lamina. Now bring your index finger straight down a little bit, and you will feel the prominent thyroid angle. Bring your finger back up to the top of the notch; the hard region contacting your fingernail is the corpus of the hyoid bone. In some people this is very hard to differentiate from the thyroid.

Palpate lateral to the notch on the superior surface and you will feel the superior cornu of thyroid. With a little discomfort you may feel the articulation of the hyoid and thyroid. If you draw your finger down the angle again, you can find the lower margin of the thyroid and feel the cricoid beneath. By carefully placing your thumb at the junction of the cricoid and thyroid, you can hum up and down the scale and feel the thyroid and cricoid moving closer together and farther apart as you do this. You will also feel the entire larynx elevate as you reach the upper end of your range. Finally, draw your finger down to find the lower margin of the cricoid, marking the beginning of the trachea. Palpate the tracheal rings.

- The thyroid cartilage has two prominent laminae, superior and inferior horns, and a prominent thyroid notch.
- The hyoid bone attaches to the superior cornu of thyroid, and the cricoid cartilage attaches to the inferior horn via the cricothyroid joint.
- The epiglottis attaches to the tongue and thyroid cartilage, dropping down to cover the larynx during swallowing.
- The cuneiform cartilages are embedded in the aryepiglottic folds.

LARYNGEAL MUSCULATURE

Intrinsic laryngeal muscles:
Muscles with both origin and insertion in the larynx.

Extrinsic laryngeal muscles:
Muscles with one attachment in the larynx and one attachment outside the larynx.

As summarized in Table 3-1, muscles of the larynx are categorized either as **intrinsic laryngeal muscles**, which have both origin and insertion on laryngeal cartilages, or **extrinsic laryngeal muscles**, which have one attachment on a laryngeal cartilage and the other attachment on a nonlaryngeal structure. The intrinsic muscles

Table 3-1. Muscles Associated with Laryngeal Function

Intrinsic Muscles of Larynx

Adductors
Lateral cricoarytenoid
Transverse arytenoid
Oblique arytenoid

Abductor
Posterior cricoarytenoid

Tensors
Thyrovocalis (medial thyroarytenoid)
Cricothyroid, pars recta and pars oblique

Relaxers
Thyromuscularis (lateral thyroarytenoid)

Suprahyoid and Infrahyoid Muscles

Hyoid and Laryngeal Elevators
Stylohyoid
Mylohyoid
Geniohyoid
Genioglossus
Hyoglossus
Inferior pharyngeal constrictor
Digastricus anterior and posterior

Hyoid and Laryngeal Depressors
Sternothyroid
Sternohyoid
Omohyoid
Thyrohyoid

assume responsibility for opening, closing, tensing, and relaxing the vocal folds, and the extrinsic muscles make major adjustments of the larynx.

Intrinsic Laryngeal Muscles

Adductors

The *lateral cricoarytenoid muscle* attaches to the cricoid and the muscular process of the arytenoid, causing the muscular process to move forward and medially (see Figure 3-14). The origin of the lateral cricoarytenoid muscle is the superior-lateral surface of the

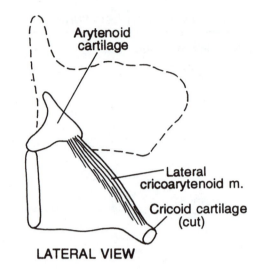

Arytenoid cartilage

Lateral cricoarytenoid m.

Cricoid cartilage (cut)

LATERAL VIEW

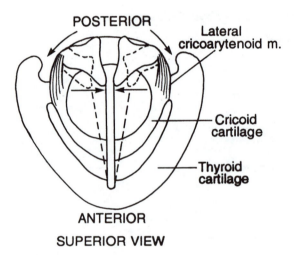

POSTERIOR

Lateral cricoarytenoid m.

Cricoid cartilage

Thyroid cartilage

ANTERIOR

SUPERIOR VIEW

FIGURE 3-14. Contraction of the lateral cricoarytenoid muscle pulls the muscular process forward, adducting the vocal folds.

cricoid cartilage. The muscle courses up and back to insert into the muscular process of the arytenoid cartilage. When it is contracted, the muscular process is drawn forward, which rocks the arytenoid inward and downward, adducting the vocal folds.

Innervation of all intrinsic muscles of the larynx is by means of the X *vagus nerve*. The *recurrent (inferior) laryngeal nerve (RLN)* is so named because of its course. The left RLN "re-courses" beneath the aorta, after which it ascends to innervate the larynx. The right RLN courses under the subclavian artery before ascending to the larynx.

The *transverse arytenoid muscle* also might be called the transverse interarytenoid muscle. This muscle spans the posterior surface of both arytenoid cartilages. Its function is to pull the two arytenoids closer together and to approximate the vocal folds. Motor innervation of the transverse arytenoid muscles is by means of the inferior branch of the recurrent laryngeal nerve arising from the X vagus nerve.

The *oblique arytenoid muscles* are immediately superficial to the transverse arytenoid muscles, and they perform a similar function. They take their origins at the posterior base of the muscular processes to course obliquely up to the apex of the opposite arytenoid. This course results in a characteristic X arrangement of the muscles as well as in the ability of these muscles to pull the apex medially. The result of this action is to promote adduction, enforce medial compression, and rock the arytenoid (and vocal folds) down and in. Innervation of the oblique arytenoid muscles is the same innervation of the transverse arytenoid muscles.

Abductor

The *posterior cricoarytenoid muscle* is the sole abductor of the vocal folds. As you can see in Figure 3-15, the posterior cricoarytenoid muscle originates on the posterior cricoid lamina. Fibers project up and out to insert into the posterior aspect of the muscular process of the arytenoid cartilage. The posterior cricoarytenoid muscles are direct antagonists to the lateral cricoarytenoids (see Figures 3-15 and 3-16).

Contraction of this muscle pulls the muscular process posteriorly, rocking the arytenoid cartilage out on its axis and abducting the vocal folds. The posterior cricoarytenoid is innervated by the recurrent laryngeal nerve, a branch of the X vagus nerve.

Glottal Tensors

The primary tensor of the vocal folds, the cricothyroid muscle, achieves its function by rocking the thyroid cartilage forward relative to the cricoid cartilage. The *cricothyroid muscle* is composed of two heads, the pars recta and pars oblique, as seen in Figure 3-17. The pars recta courses up and out to insert into the lower surface of

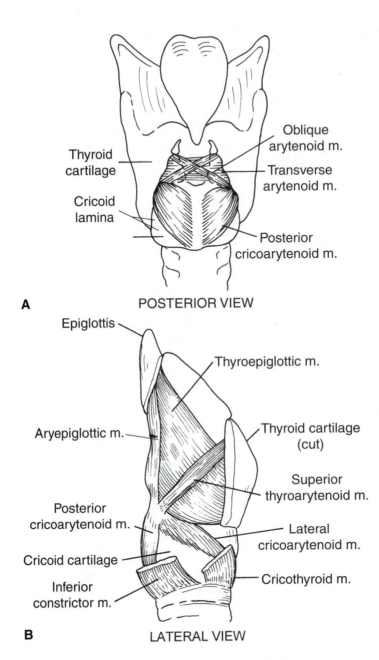

FIGURE 3-15. A. Schematic of posterior cricoarytenoid muscle and transverse and oblique arytenoid muscles. Contraction of the transverse and oblique arytenoid muscles pulls the arytenoids closer together, thereby supporting adduction. Contraction of the posterior cricoarytenoid muscle pulls the muscular process back, abducting the vocal folds. **B.** Schematic illustrating relationship among posterior cricoarytenoid, lateral cricoarytenoid, superior thyroarytenoid, and aryepiglottic muscles.

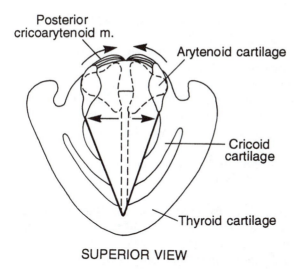

FIGURE 3-16. Superior view of action of the posterior cricoarytenoid muscle.

FIGURE 3-17. Cricothyroid muscle, pars recta and pars oblique.

the thyroid lamina. The pars oblique arises from the cricoid cartilage lateral to the pars recta, coursing obliquely up to insert at the juncture of the thyroid laminae and inferior horns.

Contraction of the pars recta rocks the thyroid cartilage downward, rotating on the cricothyroid joint. (Remember that the points of attachment of the vocal folds are the inner margin of the thyroid cartilage and arytenoid cartilages and that the arytenoid cartilages are well attached to the posterior cricoid cartilage). Rocking the thyroid cartilage forward stretches the vocal folds. That is, rocking the thyroid and cricoid closer together in front makes the posterior cricoid more distant from the thyroid. The cricothyroid is innervated by the external branch of the *superior laryngeal nerve* of the X vagus. This branch courses lateral to the inferior pharyngeal constrictor to terminate on the cricothyroid muscle.

The *thyrovocalis muscle* is actually the medial muscle of the vocal folds. Contraction of the thyrovocalis tenses the vocal folds, especially when contracted in concert with the cricothyroid (see Figure 3-18). The thyrovocalis (abbreviated *vocalis*) originates from the inner surface of thyroid cartilage near the thyroid notch and inserts into the lateral surface of the arytenoid vocal process. Contraction of this muscle will draw the thyroid and cricoid cartilages farther apart in front, making this muscle a functional antagonist of the cricothyroid muscle (which draws the anterior cricoid and anterior thyroid closer together). This antagonistic function has earned the thyrovocalis

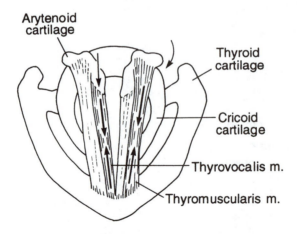

Arytenoid cartilage

Thyroid cartilage

Cricoid cartilage

Thyrovocalis m.

Thyromuscularis m.

SUPERIOR VIEW

FIGURE 3-18. The thyromuscularis muscle is the lateral muscular component of the vocal folds; the thyrovocalis is the medialmost muscle of the vocal folds. Together they are often referred to as thyroarytenoid muscle.

Referral in Voice Therapy

The phonatory mechanism is extremely sensitive, and vocal variations can indicate a broad range of problems. We must always refer an individual to a physician when we identify vocal dysfunction, even if we are fairly certain that the problem is behavioral. When a client comes to us with a hoarse voice, we may find that the person is abusing his or her phonatory mechanism by spending too much time in loud, smoky settings that require raising the voice to speak. What we don't know from this information is whether there is a vocal pathology, perhaps secondary to the same behavioral conditions, that is developing on the vocal folds. Although we suspect vocal nodules, the client could be showing early signs of laryngeal cancer.

In a similar vein, a client who comes to us with a voice that is progressively weaker during the day and for whom muscular effort of any sort is extremely difficult as the day wears on should be referred to a neurologist. *Myasthenia gravis* is a myoneural disease that results in a complex of speech disorders including progressive weakening of phonation, progressive degeneration of articulatory function, and progressive hypernasality, all arising from use of the speech mechanism over the course of a day or briefer time. The condition is quite treatable, but often the speech-language pathologist is the first to recognize the signs because the client sees it primarily as a speech problem. If you identify these signs in a patient, bring this to the attention to your supervising speech-language pathologist, who could assess further.

classification as a glottal tensor. The thyrovocalis is innervated by the recurrent laryngeal nerve, a branch of the X vagus.

Laryngeal Relaxer

The *thyromuscularis muscles* (or simply, *muscularis*) are immediately lateral to each thyrovocalis. The thyromuscularis originates on the inner surface of the thyroid cartilage, near the notch and lateral to the origin of the thyrovocalis. It runs back to insert into the arytenoid cartilage at the muscular process and base. Contraction of the medial fibers of the thyromuscularis relaxes the vocal folds. These fibers pull the arytenoids toward the thyroid cartilage without influencing medial rocking. The thyromuscularis is innervated by the recurrent laryngeal nerve, a branch of the X vagus.

Summary of Intrinsic Muscle Activity

The drawing in Figure 3-19 may help you to visualize the actions of phonation. Intrinsic muscles of the larynx include the thyrovocalis, thyromuscularis, cricothyroid, lateral and posterior cricoarytenoid,

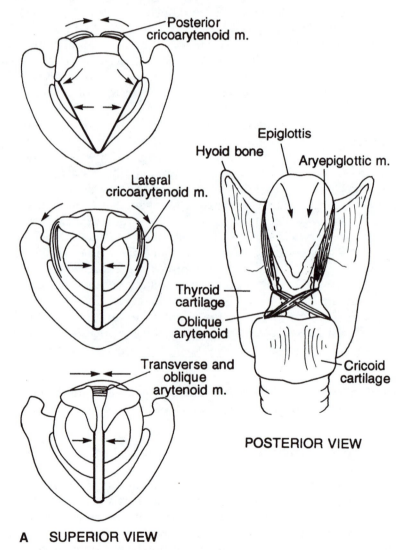

A   SUPERIOR VIEW

FIGURE 3-19. A. Thyrovocalis and thyromuscularis are tensed upon contraction of cricothyroid muscle (*continues*).

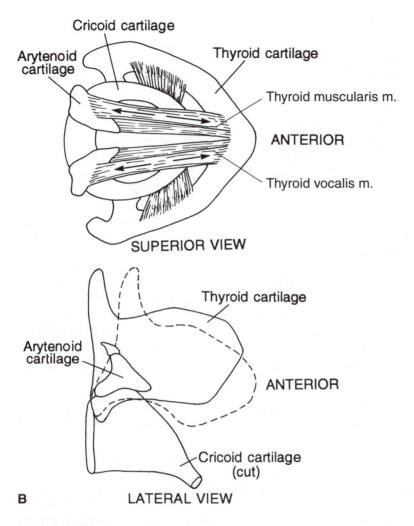

FIGURE 3-19. (*continued*) **B.** Contraction of muscle causes thyroid to rock forward and down as cricoid rocks up in front.

transverse arytenoid and oblique interarytenoid muscle, and superior thyroarytenoid muscles. The thyrovocalis and thyromuscularis muscles make up the muscular portion of the vocal folds. The cricothyroid pulls the anterior cricoid and anterior thyroid closer together, thereby stretching the vocal folds. The lateral cricoarytenoid adducts the vocal folds by rotating and rocking the arytenoids medially, while the posterior cricoarytenoid muscle abducts the vocal folds. The oblique and transverse arytenoid muscles pull the arytenoids closer together, assisting adduction. The superior

Vocal Hyperfunction

The range of phonatory "misbehavior" is broad and deep. The larynx is an exquisite structure of delicate tissues evolved for use as a protective mechanism. When we use it as a phonatory source, we capitalize on its flexibility. When we overuse the mechanism, we can get into trouble. Here are a few of the problems that occur from laryngeal misuse.

Vocal nodules arise from excessively loud phonation or excessively forceful adduction (shouting or screaming). Contact ulcers apparently develop from excessive force on the posterior aspect of the vocal folds, applied by attempting to force the vocal folds into a lower vocal range and higher vocal intensity.

The addition of toxins to your laryngeal environment can cause trouble as well. Alcohol consumption can irritate the vocal folds, as can cigarette and cigar smoke (primary or secondary smoke). Likewise, excessively dry air can irritate the vocal folds, leading to laryngitis. Esophageal reflux can also cause laryngeal irritation.

thyroarytenoid muscle is a variable muscle that may or may not be present. If present, it would be positioned to relax the vocal folds.

Adduction and abduction of the vocal folds is achieved by coordinated effort of many of the larynx's intrinsic muscles. The lateral cricoarytenoid muscle is responsible for rocking the arytenoid cartilage on its axis, causing the vocal folds to tip in and slightly down. This action is directly opposed by contraction of the posterior cricoarytenoid muscle, which will rock the arytenoid (and vocal folds) out on that same axis. Contraction of the transverse arytenoid muscle draws the posterior surfaces of the two arytenoids closer together, but it is most effective as an adductor if the lateral cricoarytenoid muscle is contracted as well. Contraction of the oblique arytenoid helps the vocal folds dip downward as they are adducted.

Changing vocal pitch is accomplished by altering the mass and tension of the vocal folds. Increasing the tension on the vocal folds stretches them and thereby reduces the mass per unit length. Stretching the vocal folds does not decrease the mass of the muscle, but it does spread them over the length of the muscle. Both increased tension and reduced mass per unit length increases frequency of vibration of the vocal folds, causing pitch to rise; relaxing the vocal folds causes the frequency and thus the pitch to drop. Note that when the cricothyroid is contracted, the thyrovocalis stretches. If you also contract the thyrovocalis, the vocal folds become more tense and the pitch increases.

Extrinsic Laryngeal Muscles

The extrinsic musculature consists of muscles with one attachment to a laryngeal cartilage. These include the sternothyroid, thyrohyoid, and thyropharyngeus muscles. A number of muscles attached to the hyoid also move the larynx: infrahyoid muscles run from the hyoid to a structure below and suprahyoid muscles attach to a structure above the hyoid. Infrahyoid muscles consist of the sternohyoid and omohyoid muscles; the suprahyoid muscles are digastricus, stylohyoid, mylohyoid, geniohyoid, genioglossus, and hyoglossus muscles. They are often called the strap muscles.

A more meaningful categorization is based on function relative to the larynx. Muscles that elevate the hyoid and larynx are laryngeal elevators (digastricus, stylohyoid, mylohyoid, geniohyoid muscles, genioglossus, hyoglossus, and thyropharyngeus muscles) and muscles that depress the larynx and hyoid are laryngeal depressors (sternohyoid, omohyoid, thyrohyoid, and sternothyroid muscles).

Hyoid and Laryngeal Elevators

Digastricus. As seen in Figure 3-20, the *digastricus muscle* is actually composed of two separate "bellies," or the central portion of a muscle. The anterior and posterior bellies of the digastricus muscle converge at the hyoid bone, and their paired contraction elevates the hyoid. The digastricus anterior muscle originates on the inner surface of the mandible at the digastricus fossa, courses medially and down to the level of the hyoid, and joins the posterior digastricus by means of an intermediate tendon. The posterior digastricus originates on the mastoid process of the temporal bone, behind and beneath the ear. The intermediate tendon passes through and separates the fibers of another muscle, the stylohyoid, as it inserts into the hyoid at the juncture of the hyoid corpus and greater cornu.

Contraction of the anterior component draws the hyoid up and forward, whereas contraction of the posterior belly draws the hyoid up and back. Simultaneous contraction results in hyoid elevation without anterior or posterior movement.

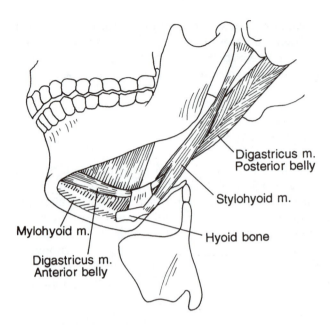

FIGURE 3-20. Schematic of digastricus, stylo-hyoid, and mylohyoid muscles. (After data and view of Netter, 1989.)

Muscles attached to the mandible, such as the digastricus, also may be depressors of the mandible. That is, the digastricus could help to pull the mandible down if the musculature below the hyoid were to fix it in place. The anterior belly is innervated by the mandibular branch of V trigeminal nerve via the mylohyoid branch of the inferior alveolar nerve. The posterior belly is supplied by the digastric branch of the VII facial nerve.

Stylohyoid Muscle. The *stylohyoid muscle* originates on the prominent styloid process of the temporal bone, a point medial to the mastoid process (see Figure 3-20). The course of this muscle is medially down, so that it crosses the path of the posterior digastricus and inserts into the corpus hyoid. Contraction of the stylohyoid elevates and retracts the hyoid bone. The stylohyoid is innervated by the motor branch of the VII facial nerves.

Mylohyoid Muscle. The *mylohyoid muscle* originates on the underside of the mandible and courses to the corpus hyoid. The mylohyoid is fanlike, originating along the lateral aspects of the inner mandible on a prominence known as the mylohyoid line. The anterior fibers converge at the *median fibrous raphe* (ridge), a structure that runs from the mandible to the hyoid. The posterior fibers course directly to the hyoid. The fibers of mylohyoid form the floor of the oral cavity. The relationship between digastricus and mylohyoid can be seen in Figure 3-21. The mylohyoid elevates the hyoid and projects it forward, or alternately depresses the mandible. Mylohyoid is innervated by the alveolar nerve, arising from the V trigeminal nerve, mandibular branch.

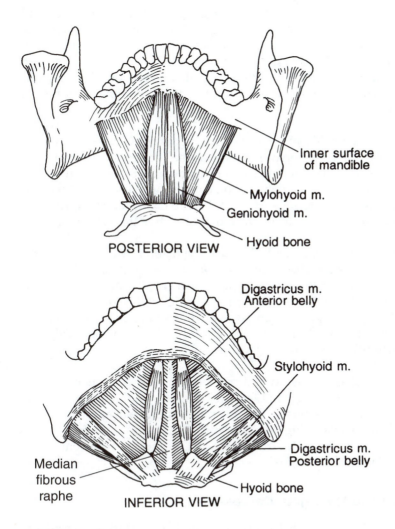

FIGURE 3-21. Schematic of the relationships among geniohyoid, mylohyoid, digastricus, and stylohyoid muscles.

Geniohyoid Muscle. The *geniohyoid muscle* is superior to the mylohyoid, originating at the mental spines projecting in a course parallel to the anterior belly of the digastricus from the inner mandibular surface (see Figure 3-21). Fibers of this narrow muscle course back and down to insert into the hyoid bone at the corpus. When contracted, the geniohyoid elevates the hyoid and draws it forward. It may depress the mandible also if the hyoid is fixed. The geniohyoid is innervated by the XII hypoglossal nerve.

Hyoglossus Muscle. The *hyoglossus* is a lateral muscle that arises from the entire superior surface of the greater cornu of hyoid and courses up into the side of the tongue. The point of insertion in the tongue is near that of the styloglossus, a muscle we will discuss in Chapter 4, which covers the articulators. The muscle takes on a quadrilateral appearance and is a lingual depressor or hyoid elevator. The hyoglossus muscle is innervated by the motor branch of the XII hypoglossal.

Genioglossus Muscle. Although the *genioglossus muscle* is more appropriately considered a muscle of the tongue, it definitely is a hyoid elevator. The genioglossus originates on the inner surface of the mandible at the symphysis and courses up, back, and down into the tongue and anterior surface of the hyoid corpus. The genioglossus muscle is innervated by the motor branch of the XII hypoglossal.

Thyropharyngeus and Cricopharyngeus Muscles of the Inferior Constrictor. The *thyropharyngeus* and *cricopharyngeus muscles* comprise the inferior pharyngeal constrictor. The cricopharyngeus is the sphincter muscle at the orifice of the esophagus, while the thyropharyngeus is involved in propelling food through the pharynx. Its attachment to the cricoid and thyroid provides an opportunity for laryngeal elevation.

The thyropharyngeus arises from the posterior pharyngeal raphe, coursing down fanlike and laterally to the thyroid lamina and inferior cornu. Contraction of this muscle promotes elevation of the larynx while constricting the pharynx. The inferior constrictors are innervated by branches from the X vagus and the recurrent laryngeal nerves off the vagus.

Hyoid and Laryngeal Depressors

Laryngeal depressors depress and stabilize the larynx via attachment to the hyoid, but also stabilize the tongue by serving as antagonists to the laryngeal elevators.

Sternohyoid Muscle. As the name implies, the *sternohyoid* runs from sternum to hyoid. It originates from the posterior-superior region of the manubrium sterni, as well as from the medial end of the clavicle (see Figure 3-22). It courses superiorly to insert into the inferior margin of the hyoid corpus. Contraction of the sternohyoid depresses the hyoid. The sternohyoid is innervated by the *ansa cervicalis* (*ansa* = loop; i.e., cervical loop), arising from spinal nerves C1 through C3.

Omohyoid Muscle. The *omohyoid* is a muscle with two bellies. The *superior belly* terminates on the side of the hyoid corpus, while the *inferior belly* has its origin on the upper border of the scapula. The bellies are joined at an intermediate tendon. As you can see from Figure 3-22, the omohyoid passes deep to the sternocleidomastoid that, along with the deep cervical fascia, restrains the muscle to retain that characteristic "dogleg" angle. When contracted, the omohyoid depresses the hyoid bone and larynx. The superior belly is

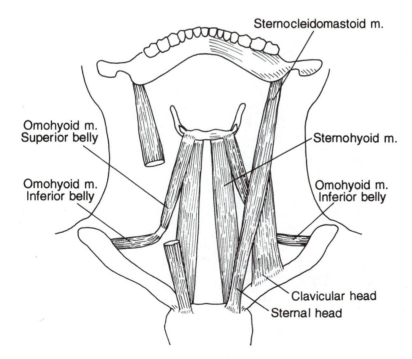

FIGURE 3-22. Schematic of the relationships among omohyoid, sternocleidomastoid, and sternohyoid muscles.

innervated by the superior ramus of the ansa cervicalis arising from spinal nerve C1, whereas the inferior belly is innervated by the main ansa cervicalis, arising from spinal nerves C2 and C3.

Sternothyroid Muscle. As shown in Figure 3-23, contraction of the *sternothyroid muscle* depresses the thyroid cartilage. It originates at the manubrium sterni and first costal cartilage, coursing up and out to insert into the oblique line of the thyroid cartilage. The sternothyroid is innervated by fibers from spinal nerves C1 and C2, which pass in the XII hypoglossal nerve.

Thyrohyoid Muscle. The *thyrohyoid muscle* courses from the oblique line of the thyroid cartilage to the inferior margin of the greater cornu of hyoid bone. The thyrohyoid muscle either depresses the hyoid or raises the larynx (see Figure 3-23). It is innervated by the fibers of spinal nerve C1, which course with the XII hypoglossal nerves.

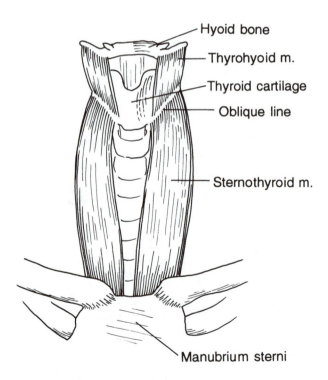

FIGURE 3-23. The sternothyroid and thyrohyoid muscles.

Summary

- The extrinsic muscles of the larynx are the sternothyroid, thyrohyoid, and thyropharyngeus muscles.
- The digastricus anterior and posterior together elevate the hyoid, whereas the stylohyoid retracts it.
- The mylohyoid and hyoglossus elevate the hyoid, and the geniohyoid elevates the hyoid and draws it forward.
- The thyropharyngeus and cricopharyngeus muscles elevate the larynx, and the sternohyoid, sternothyroid, thyrohyoid, and omohyoid muscles depress the larynx.

Interaction of Musculature

The larynx is virtually suspended from a broad sling of muscles that must work in concert to achieve the complex motions required for speech and nonspeech functions. Movement of the larynx and its cartilages requires both gross and fine adjustments. It appears that the gross movements associated with laryngeal elevation and depression provide stability for the fine adjustments of phonatory control. The suprahyoid and infrahyoid muscles raise and lower the larynx, changing the vocal tract length, but the intrinsic laryngeal muscles are responsible for the fine adjustments associated with phonation control.

The musculature works as a unit. The simple gesture of laryngeal elevation must be countered with the controlled antagonistic action of the laryngeal depressors. Elevation of the tongue tends to elevate the larynx and increase the tension of the cricothyroid, and this must be countered through intrinsic muscle adjustment to keep the articulatory system from driving the phonatory mechanism. It is time to move to physiology of phonation to see how these components work together.

PHYSIOLOGY OF PHONATION

Discussion of the function of the larynx and vocal folds revolves around the movable components and the results of that movement. We will concentrate on the nonspeech functions initially, which will help examine speech and vocal function. Speech-language pathologists and assistants use their knowledge of these nonspeech functions in the treatment of voice disorders, so you will need to be very familiar with these functions.

Laryngeal Stability

Laryngeal stability is the key to laryngeal control, and this stability is gained through development of the infrahyoid and suprahyoid musculature. You can think of the larynx as a box connected to a flexible tube on the lower end (trachea) and loosely attached above. This "box" has liberal movement in the vertical dimension and some horizontal movement as well, but there must be a great deal of control in contraction of all of this musculature for this arrangement to work.

The larynx is intimately linked, via the hyoid bone, to the tongue so that movement of the tongue is translated to the larynx. During development, the infant begins to gain control of neck musculature as early as 4 weeks, as seen in the ability to elevate the neck while prone. This ability to extend the previously flexed neck heralds the beginning of oral motor control because the ability to balance neck extension and flexion permits the child to control the gross movement of the head. During this stage, the larynx is quite elevated, so much so that you can easily see the superior tip of the epiglottis behind the tongue of a 2-year-old. In the early stages, the elevated larynx facilitates the anterior tongue protrusion required in infancy for nursing.

As the child develops, the larynx descends, starting a process of muscular differentiation between the tongue and the larynx. In the "nursing" position of the tongue, laryngeal stability is not very important. As the child begins to eat solid food, the ability to move food around in the oral cavity is quite important. Now the child will develop the ability to move the tongue and larynx independently, permitting a much wider set of oral gestures. With this differentiation comes the control needed for accurate speech production. For more information on head and neck control in children with motor dysfunction, you may wish to examine Jones-Owens (1991), and Bly (1994) provides more detail about the development of muscle control.

Nonspeech Laryngeal Function

Cough: Forceful expiration of air following tight adduction of the vocal folds, for the purpose of expelling foreign matter from the airway.

The protective function of the larynx is its most important role because failure to prohibit entry of foreign objects into the lungs is life-threatening. This function is fulfilled through the cough and other associated reflexive gestures. **Coughing** is a response by the

Vocal Fold Paralysis

Paralysis refers to loss of voluntary motor function, whereas **paresis** refers to weakness. Either occurs from damage to the neurons supplying the muscle.

Vocal fold paralysis takes several forms, depending on the nerve damage. If only one side of the recurrent laryngeal nerve is damaged, the result is unilateral vocal fold paralysis. Bilateral vocal fold paralysis results from bilateral lower motor neuron damage.

If the result of damage is adductor paralysis, the vocal folds remain in the abducted position. In unilateral paralysis, one vocal fold is still capable of motion. Phonation can still occur, but production will be markedly breathy. Bilateral adductor paralysis results in virtually complete loss of phonation. If the superior laryngeal nerve is involved, the individual loses the ability to alter vocal pitch because the cricothyroid is innervated by this nerve.

There are several causes of vocal fold paralysis but the most common is damage to the nerve during thyroid surgery and blunt trauma, often from the steering wheel of an automobile. Cerebrovascular accidents (CVA: hemorrhage or other condition causing loss of blood supply to the brain) may damage upper or lower motor neurons, resulting in paralysis, and a host of neurodegenerative diseases can weaken or paralyze the vocal folds. Paralysis may also occur as a result of aneurysm of the aortic arch. An aneurysm is a focal "ballooning" of a blood vessel caused by a weakness in the wall. When the aneurysm balloons out, it compresses the recurrent laryngeal nerve, causing paresis or paralysis. A phonatory **sign** (objective evidence of phonatory deficit) is not to be taken lightly.

Paralysis: Loss of voluntary motor function due to lesion in the nervous system.

Paresis: Weakness arising from lesion in the nervous system.

Sign: Measurable or objective component of illness or condition.

tissue of the respiratory passageway to an irritant or foreign object, mediated by the visceral afferent (sensory) portion of the X vagus innervating the bronchial mucosa. Coughing is a violent and broadly predictable behavior, which includes deep inhalation through widely abducted vocal folds, followed by tensing and tight adduction of the vocal folds and elevation of the larynx. The axis of movement of the arytenoids guarantees that, as they are rocked for adduction, they also are directed somewhat downward, providing more force in opposition to expiration. Significant positive subglottal pressure for the cough comes from tissue recoil and muscles of expiration. The high pressure of forced expiration blows the vocal folds apart.

The aerodynamic benefit of this is that the person coughing generates a maximal flow of air through the passageway to expel the irritating object. The negative side of the cough is the force required for its production. Chronic irritation of the respiratory system leads to vocal abuse in the form of repeated coughing. The "near cousin" of the cough is throat clearing. It is not as violent as the full cough, but is nonetheless stressful.

So far we have dealt primarily with laryngeal functions focused on tight adduction of the vocal folds, but abduction has its place as well. Abduction dilates the larynx, an important function for respiration during physical exertion. Oxygen use increases significantly during work and exertion. During normal quiet respiration, an adult's vocal folds are abducted to a width of about 8 mm. During forced respiration, the need for air causes you to dilate, or open, the respiratory tract as widely as possible, doubling that width.

Summary

- We use the larynx and associated structures for many nonspeech functions, including coughing, throat clearing, abdominal fixation, and increasing airflow.
- These functions serve important biological needs, and understanding them provides background for useful clinical intervention techniques.

Laryngeal Function for Speech

Phonation is an extremely important component of the speech signal. To accomplish phonation, we must adduct the vocal folds to begin phonation (attack), hold the vocal folds in a fixed position in the airstream to sustain phonation, and abduct the vocal folds to terminate phonation (see Figure 3-24).

Attack

Simultaneous vocal attack:
Phonation initiated through
simultaneous vocal folds
adduction and expiration.

Attack is the process of bringing vocal folds together to begin phonation. There are three basic types of attack. When we initiate phonation using **simultaneous vocal attack**, we coordinate adduction and onset of respiration so that they occur simultaneously. The vocal folds reach the critical degree of adduction at the same time

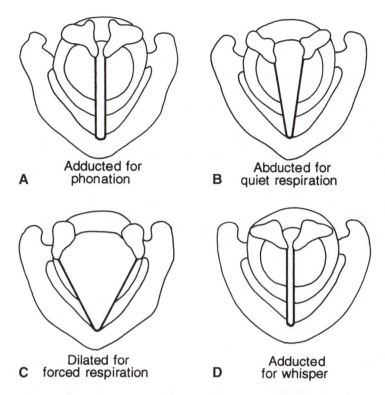

A Adducted for phonation

B Abducted for quiet respiration

C Dilated for forced respiration

D Adducted for whisper

FIGURE 3–24. Laryngeal postures for various functions. **A.** During adduction for phonation the vocal folds are approximated. **B.** For quiet respiration the folds are moderately abducted, but for forced respiration, **C**, they are widely separated. Adduction for whisper, **D**, involves bringing the folds close together but retaining an open space between the arytenoid cartilages.

that the respiratory flow is adequate to support phonation. You are using simultaneous attack when you say the word "zany," for example, because to start the flow of air before voicing would add the unvoiced /s/ to the beginning of the word.

Breathy vocal attack involves starting airflow before adducting the vocal folds. This occurs frequently during running speech, as in the sentence "Harry is my friend."

The third type of attack is **glottal attack**. In this attack, adduction of the vocal folds occurs prior to the airflow, much like a cough. Try this. Bring your vocal folds together (be gentle!) as if to cough, but instead of opening your vocal folds as you push air through the

Breathy vocal attack: Phonation by initiating expiration before adduction of the vocal folds.

Glottal attack: Phonatory onset that occurs with the adduction of the vocal folds before onset of expiration.

Ventricular Phonation

The false, or ventricular, vocal folds are technically unable to vibrate for voice, but in some instances clients may use them for this purpose. Boone (1999) cites instances in which clients use ventricular phonation as an adaptive response to severe vocal fold dysfunction, such as growths on the folds. Apparently the client forces the lateral superior walls closely together during the adductory gesture, permitting the folds to make contact and vibrate.

The ventricular folds are thick, and the phonation heard is deep and often raspy. The false folds may hypertrophy (increase in size), facilitating ventricular phonation.

---

folds, keep them adducted and say /a/. That was a glottal attack. You use a glottal attack when saying any word beginning with a vowel, such as "onion."

Termination

Termination of phonation requires that we abduct the vocal folds. We pull the vocal folds out of the airstream far enough to reduce the turbulence, and the vocal folds stop vibrating. As with attack, we terminate phonation many times during running speech to accommodate voiced and voiceless speech sounds.

Adduction is a constant in all types of attack. The arytenoid cartilages are capable of moving in three dimensions—*rotating, rocking,* and *gliding*. It appears that the primary arytenoid gesture for adduction is inward rocking. When the arytenoids are pulled medially on the convex arytenoid facet of the cricoid, the arytenoids will rock down. These motions are the product of the lateral cricoarytenoid muscle and the lateral portion of the thyromuscularis.

Sustained Phonation

Sustained phonation is the purpose of adduction and abduction for speech. Let us examine this closely. Vocal attack requires muscular action, as does termination of phonation. In contrast, sustaining phonation simply requires maintenance of a laryngeal posture through tonic (sustained tensing) contraction of musculature. This is a very important point. The vibration of the vocal folds is achieved by placing and holding the vocal folds in the airstream so

Vocal Fold Nodules

Vocal fold nodules are aggregates of tissue arising from abuse. This condition makes up a large share of the voice disorder cases seen by school clinicians. Common forms of vocal abuse are yelling, screaming, cheerleading, or "barking" commands (e.g., by a drill sergeant). The result of this abuse is a sequence of events that can lead to permanent change in the vocal fold tissue. You are probably familiar with laryngitis, which is hoarseness, often with loss of voice (**aphonia**). The laryngeal effect is swelling (edema) of the delicate vocal fold tissue so that it is difficult to make the folds vibrate. In fact, they are often bowed so badly that expiratory flow will pass between them, even as phonation occurs; we refer to this as a breathy voice.

Vocal abuse typically leads to soreness, which is a message from your body to stop doing what made the vocal folds hurt in the first place. Continued abuse results in growth of a protective layer of epithelium, which is callus-like and not a very effective oscillator. If the vocal hyperfunction continues, the hardened tissue will increase in size until a nodule may be found on one (unilateral) or both (bilateral) vocal folds. The site of abuse is usually at the juncture of the anterior and middle thirds of the vocal folds because this is the point of greatest impact during phonation. Although untreated vocal nodules may eventually have to be removed surgically, voice therapy to reverse the vocal behavior driving the phenomenon is always appropriate. If the vocal hyperfunction is not eliminated, the vocal nodules will return after surgery. Surgery may be avoided if therapy is initiated soon enough.

Aphonia: Loss of voicing.

their physical qualities interact with the airflow, causing vibration. The vocal folds are held in place during sustained phonation. Vibration of the vocal folds is *not* the product of repeated adduction and abduction of the vocal folds.

Vocal Register

The *mode of vibration* of the vocal folds during sustained phonation refers to the pattern of activity that the vocal folds undergo during a cycle of vibration. Moving from one point in the vibratory pattern to the same point again defines one cycle of vibration, and within one cycle, the vocal folds undergo some very significant changes, and these variations in vibratory pattern in large part differentiate vocal registers. A number of *modes* or *vocal registers* have been differentiated perceptually.

Sustained and Maximum Phonation

Physical systems, such as those encompassing the mechanisms of speech, are rarely employed at maximum output and stress. For instance, we generally don't breathe in maximally or speak using our entire vital capacity, although we are capable of doing so. When clinicians wish to examine whether there is a deficit in a system, one useful technique is to ask the client to perform a test of maximal output for a given parameter. In respiration, such tests would be examination of vital capacity, inspiratory reserve, and expiratory reserve.

This useful concept may be extended to voicing. If you ask a client to sustain a vowel for as long as he or she can, you are testing not only how well the vocal folds function but also the vital capacity and checking action of the person under examination. If the respiratory system is intact, an average adult female between the ages 17 and 41 years will be able to sustain the /a/ vowel for approximately 15 seconds, and the male will be able to sustain that vowel for 23 seconds. This function changes with age, increasing through the second decade of life. Generally you can expect the phonation time to increase from about 10 seconds at 6 years, but you may be interested in looking at the norms by age as summarized by Kent, Kent, and Rosenbek (1987). By the way, did you wonder why males are able to phonate a little longer than females? If you blamed it on larger vital capacity, you were right.

Another phonation-related task involves maximum duration of the sustained sibilants, /s/ and /z/. Boone (1999) states that individuals are able to sustain these phonemes for approximately the same durations, but that physical change to the vocal folds (such as vocal nodules) will cause a significant reduction in the duration of the voiced /z/. Males again produce longer fricatives (e.g., /s/), and the duration increases with age. Clinicians calculate the ratio of s:z duration to aid their decisions. If the two durations are the same, the value is 1.0, and as the /z/ duration drops, the ratio increases. Although the ratio undergoes continual examination for its clinical utility, many studies have substantiated the use of this clinical tool.

The three registers most commonly referred to are **modal register,** **glottal fry** or pulse register, and **falsetto**. We will be also interested in the variant **breathy** and **pressed phonatory** modes, as well as **whispered speech**.

Modal Register. The first register, known as the modal register, or modal phonation, refers to the pattern of phonation used most often. This pattern is the most important one for the speech-language pathologist and the speech-language pathology assistant, and it is the most efficient.

Figure 3-25 shows the vocal folds from the sides and from above. In the vertical mode of phonation, the vocal folds open from inferior to superior (bottom to top), and they also close from inferior to superior. The folds are an undulating wave of tissue, and it is more appropriate to think of air as "bubbling" through the adducted folds than of them opening and closing as if hinged.

The second mode of vibration of the vocal folds is in the anterior-posterior dimension. The vocal folds tend to open from posterior to anterior, but that closure at the end of a cycle is made by contact of the medial edge of the vocal fold, but with the posterior closing last.

The primary frequency of vibration of the vocal folds is the **fundamental frequency**. This is the number of cycles the vocal folds go through per second, and it is audible. The movement of the vocal folds in air produces an audible disturbance known as sound. That sound is transmitted through the air as a wave, with molecules compressed by movement of the vocal folds.

Besides the fundamental frequency, the vocal folds produce an extremely rich set of harmonics, which are whole-number multiples of the fundamental. These harmonics provide important acoustical information for identification of voiced phonemes.

Because the vocal folds offer resistance to airflow, the minimum driving pressure of the vocal folds in modal phonation is approximately 3 cm to 5 cm H_2O subglottal pressure. If pressure is lower than this, the folds will not be blown apart. This is clinically important because a client who cannot generate 3 cm to 5 cm H_2O and sustain it for 5 seconds cannot use the vocal folds for speech. (See Figure 3-26 for an illustration of a simple clinical manometer.)

Modal register: The mode of vibration used for daily speaking.

Glottal fry: A low-frequency mode of vibration characterized by syncopated rhythm and generated by low subglottal air pressure.

Falsetto: Phonation is high in frequency, which is produced by significant increase in laryngeal tension that results in thinned vocal fold margins.

Breathy phonation (pressed phonation): The mode of phonation produced with extra airflow through the partially adducted vocal folds.

Whispered speech: Speech produced without vocal fold vibration by causing air to pass along the edges of the tensed vocal folds, thus producing a friction sound source.

Fundamental frequency: The lowest component of a harmonic series. In phonation, the lowest frequency of the voiced source.

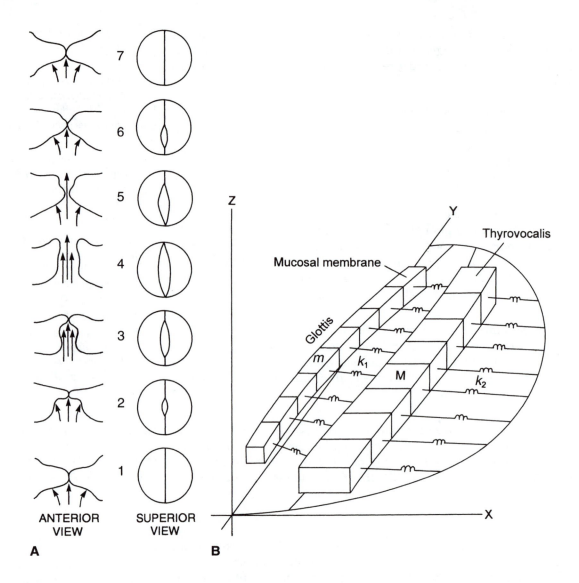

FIGURE 3-25. A. Graphic representation of vertical and transverse phase relationships during one glottal cycle. Notice that generally the vocal folds open from inferior to superior and also close from inferior to superior. Simultaneously, the glottis grows generally from posterior to anterior, but the vocal folds close from anterior to posterior. **B.** The mucoviscoaerodynamic theory of vocal fold vibration (Titze, 1973) holds that vocal fold vibration can be explained best if the mechanism is viewed as a series of masses (*m*) linked by spring elements (*k*). (Redrawn by permission, from Titze (1973). The human vocal cords: A mathematical model, Part I. *Phonetica, 28,* 129–170.)

Puberphonia

During normal development, children undergo a great deal of change during puberty, the time in a person's life when he or she becomes capable of reproduction. This occurs between 13 and 15 years for boys and between 9 and 16 years for girls and is characterized by rapid muscle development and significant gains in height and weight. The thyroid cartilage and thyroarytenoid are not left out of development. They grow rapidly during this time, although the larynges of boys grow considerably more than those of girls.

The result of this spurt of laryngeal growth is that the person (typically a boy) has periods of voice change (mutation) in which his voice "breaks down" in pitch as he is speaking. This is, of course, a normal result of the changing tissue and the young man's attempt to control it for phonation, but it is nonetheless disturbing. *Puberphonia* refers to the maintenance of the childhood pitch despite having passed through the developmental stage of puberty. It surely represents an attempt to hold something constant during the roller-coaster ride of puberty, but the result is a significant mismatch between the large body of the developing teenaged boy and the high-pitched voice of the prepubescent child. Typically, the young man is speaking in falsetto but is aware of the "lower" voice. To help the individual alter habitual pitch therapy performed over the summer vacation, in absence of peer pressures associated with school, is quite effective.

Glottal Fry. The second register is known as **glottal fry,** but is known also as pulse register. What "fry" and "pulse" allude to is the crackly, "popcorn" quality of this voice. Perceptually, this voice is extremely low in pitch and sounds rough, almost like eggs frying in a pan.

Glottal fry: Vocal register produced with low subglottal pressure, low vocal intensity, and low fundamental frequency.

Glottal fry is the product of a complex glottal configuration, and it occurs in frequencies ranging as low as 30 Hz, up to 80 or 90 Hz. This mode of vibration requires low subglottal pressure to sustain it (on the order of 2 cm H_2O), and tension of the vocalis is significantly reduced relative to modal vibration so that the vibrating margin is flaccid and thick. The lateral portion of the vocal folds is

c.m

H₂O

FIGURE 3-26. A useful clinical tool described by Hixon, Hawley, and Wilson (1982), this portable manometer gives the client feedback concerning respiratory ability and provides the clinician with a measure of function.

tensed, producing strong medial compression with short, thick vocal folds and low subglottal pressure. If either vocalis tension or subglottal pressure is increased, the popcorn-like perception of this mode of vibration is lost.

In glottal fry, the vocal folds take on a secondary, syncopated mode of vibration, with a secondary beat for every cycle of the fundamental frequency. In addition to this syncopation, the vocal folds spend up to 90% of the cycle in approximation.

Falsetto. The third and highest register of phonation, the **falsetto,** also is characterized by a vibratory pattern that varies from modal

Falsetto: Phonatory mode characterized by high fundamental frequency, and produced through reed-like vibration of vocal folds.

production. In falsetto, the vocal folds lengthen and become extremely thin and "reedlike." When set into vibration, they tend to vibrate along the tensed, bowed margins, in contrast to the complex pattern seen in other modes of phonation. Compared with modal phonation, the vocal folds make contact only briefly, and the degree of movement (amplitude of excursion) is reduced. The posterior portion of the vocal folds tends to be damped, so that the length of the vibrating surface is decreased to a narrow opening. Contrast this to elevated pitch in modal phonation, which involves lengthening the vocal folds.

The perception of falsetto is one of an extremely "thin," high-pitched vocal production. The difference between falsetto and modal vibration is not simply one of the frequencies of vibration (in the 300–600 Hz range). Although it is true that falsetto is the highest register, the modal and falsetto registers overlap.

Whispering. Whispering is not really a phonatory mode, because no voicing occurs. This does not mean that there are no laryngeal adjustments, but rather that they do not produce vibration in the vocal folds. Prove this to yourself. In respiration the vocal folds are abducted, but for whispering they must be partially adducted and tensed to develop turbulence in the airstream, and that turbulence is the noise you use to make speech.

The interplay of the elasticity and mass of the vocal folds leads them to vibrate in a periodic fashion. *Intensity* refers to the relative power or pressure of an acoustic signal, measured in decibels (abbreviated dB). In phonation, we may refer to the intensity of voice as vocal intensity. Intensity is a direct function of the amount of pressure exerted by the sound wave (as opposed to air pressure generated by the respiratory system). As molecules vibrate from movement of the vocal folds, the movement of molecules exerts an extremely small but measurable force over an area, and that is defined as pressure. The larger the excursion of the vibrating body, the greater the intensity of the signal produced because air will be displaced with greater force. The next two sections deal with frequency and intensity of vocal fold vibration.

Summary

- We must adduct the vocal folds to initiate phonation, and this may take several forms, including breathy, simultaneous, and glottal attacks.

- Termination of phonation requires abduction of the vocal folds, a process that must occur with the transition of voiced to voiceless speech sounds.
- Sustained phonation can take several forms, depending on the laryngeal configuration.
- Fundamental frequency is the measure of how fast the vocal folds vibrate.
- Falsetto occupies the upper range of laryngeal function, while glottal fry is found in the lower range.
- Vocal fold vibration varies among phonatory modes, and the differences are governed by laryngeal tension, medial compression, and subglottal pressure.

FREQUENCY, PITCH, AND PITCH CHANGE

Prosody: Combination of changes in fundamental frequency and vocal intensity that provides linguistically relevant information.

Hypertonus: Abnormal increase in muscle tone.

Prosody and Neuromuscular Disorder

The prosodic element of speech can be a window on speech physiology in neuropathology. **Prosody** is the combination of changes in fundamental frequency and vocal intensity that produces linguistically relevant intonation and stress characteristics, such as emphasizing the word *he* in the sentence "He went to town." When the neuromuscular system is compromised, prosody may be affected. When muscle tone increases (**hypertonus**) due to spasticity, the individual may demonstrate prosody characterized by even and equal stress with inappropriately high vocal intensity on each syllable or word. It is as if each syllable is forced out, the uttered sentence has an essentially flat intonation contour.

When an individual has ataxic signs from cerebellar damage, she will have disrupted prosody from the discoordination of respiratory, phonatory, and articulatory systems. Speech syllable timing will be defective, and control of phonatory elements will be seriously deficient.

In many of the hyperkinetic dysarthrias the element of speech control is over-ridden by movements of speech structures that are involuntary and uncontrollable. In these cases, prosody will be seriously affected as the articulatory or phonatory gesture is interrupted by the spontaneous movements.

Pitch is the perceptual correlate of frequency and is closely related to frequency: As frequency increases, pitch increases, and as frequency decreases, so does pitch.

The vocal folds are made up of mass and elastic elements that promote **oscillation,** or repeated vibration, at the same frequency, and as long as mass and elasticity are constant the vocal folds vibrate at the same frequency. Alteration of mass and elasticity changes the frequency of vibration.

Several important terms describe aspects of perceived pitch. Unfortunately, most of these terms refer to perceived pitch when they really describe physical frequency! Let us take a look at optimal and habitual pitch, average fundamental frequency, and range of fundamental frequency.

Pitch: The perceptual correlate of frequency of vibration.

Oscillation: Repeated vibration of a body at the same frequency.

Optimal Pitch

The term **optimal pitch** is used to refer to the pitch (actually, the frequency) of vocal fold vibration that is optimal or most appropriate for an individual. This frequency of vibration is the most efficient for a given pair of vocal folds and is a function of the mass and elasticity of the vocal folds. Some voice scientists and clinicians estimate optimal pitch directly from the individual's range of phonation because it is considered to be approximately $\frac{1}{4}$ octave above an individual's lowest frequency of vibration. Others estimate it from a cough or throat-clearing because frequency of the vibrating vocal folds during throat-clearing approximates conditions associated with conversational frequency but without social conditions associated with use of phonation for communication.

Optimal pitch: The frequency of vibration of the vocal folds that is most efficient for the vocal folds.

Optimal pitch varies as a function of sex and age. You can expect an adult female to have a fundamental frequency of approximately 212 Hz during a reading task, whereas the optimal fundamental frequency for adult males is be much lower, around 132 Hz for the same task.

The reason for the difference in fundamental frequency between males and females has to do with tissue mass and length of vocal folds. Children of both sexes have fundamental frequency in the range of 300 Hz, but that changes during puberty. During puberty, males undergo a significant growth of muscle and cartilage, resulting in greater muscle mass even in the vocal mechanism. This results in the prominent "Adam's apple" and a drop in fundamental frequency arising from the increased mass of the folds (see Figure 3-27).

Laryngeal stridor: Harsh sound produced upon inhalation or exhalation.

Laryngeal Stridor

Laryngeal stridor refers to a harsh sound produced during respiration. The sound is associated with some obstruction in the respiratory passageway and is always a sign of dysfunction. Stridor may arise from a growth in the larynx or trachea, causing turbulence during respiration, or it may arise from the dysfunction of vocal folds. If the vocal folds are paralyzed in the adducted position (abductor paralysis), they not only obstruct the airway but also vibrate as the air of inspiration passes by them. In this case, the harsh sound is referred to as inhalatory stridor. You may want to imitate this yourself so that you can learn to recognize this sign of obstruction. Phonate while breathing out, and then, without abducting your vocal folds, force your inspiration through the closed vocal folds. You will notice not only a harsh sound but also the extreme difficulty of inhaling through an obstruction.

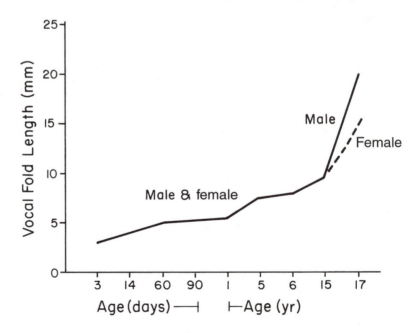

FIGURE 3–27. Changes in vocal fold length for males and females as a function of age. Note that males and females have essentially the same length of vocal folds until puberty, at which time both sexes undergo marked physical development. (Data of Kaplan, 1971.)

Habitual Pitch

We use the term **habitual pitch** to refer to the frequency of vibration of vocal folds that is habitually used during speech. In the ideal condition, this would be the same as optimal pitch. Some individuals alter their everyday pitch in speech beyond the range expected for their age, size, or gender. Although the choice to use an abnormally higher or lower fundamental frequency is often not a conscious decision, it has an effect on phonatory efficiency and effort. When the vocal folds are forced into the extremes of their range of ability, greater effort is required to sustain phonation, and this results in vocal and physical fatigue.

Habitual pitch: The frequency of vibration of the vocal folds habitually used by an individual during speech.

Average Fundamental Frequency

The **average fundamental frequency** of vibration of the vocal folds during phonation can be measured during a variety of tasks (e.g., reading aloud, conversational speech, counting aloud, etc.). Different tasks result in variations of average fundamental frequency, but they all provide measures of habitual pitch.

Average fundamental frequency: The average frequency of vibration taken over a given time period of phonation.

Pitch Range

Pitch range refers to the range of fundamental frequency for an individual and is calculated as the difference between the highest and lowest frequencies. The vocal mechanism is capable of approximately two octaves of change in fundamental frequency from the lowest possible to the highest frequency. An individual with a lowest-possible fundamental frequency of 90 Hz can reach a high of about 360 Hz (octave 1 = 90 Hz to 180 Hz; octave 2 = 180 Hz to 360 Hz).

Pitch range: The range of phonation possible, calculated as the highest frequency of vibration minus the lowest frequency of vibration.

Pitch Changing Mechanism

Fundamental frequency increase comes from stretching and tensing the vocal folds using the cricothyroid and thyrovocalis muscles. Here is the mechanism of this change.

Tension, Length, and Mass

The changeable elements of the vocal folds are tension, length, and mass. We can change the *mass per unit length* by spreading the muscle, mucosa, and ligament out over more distance. We can change the *tension* of the vocal folds by stretching them tighter or relaxing them. Both of these changes arise from elongation.

When the cricothyroid muscle is contracted, the thyroid tilts down, lengthening the vocal folds and increasing the fundamental frequency. When the tension on the vocal folds is increased, the natural frequency of vibration increases.

The thyrovocalis is also a tenser of the vocal folds. Contraction of this muscle pulls both cricoid and thyroid closer together, an action opposed by the simultaneously contracted cricothyroid.

Lowering fundamental frequency requires the opposite manipulation. Contraction of the thyromuscularis shortens the vocal folds so they become more massive and less tense.

Subglottal Pressure and Frequency Change

Increasing pitch requires increasing the tension of the system, thereby increasing the glottal resistance to airflow. If airflow is to remain constant through the glottis, air pressure must increase. It appears, however, that increases in subglottal pressure are a response to, rather than a cause of, the increased tension required for frequency change. Subglottal pressure does increase, but by itself has little effect on frequency change.

Summary

- Pitch is the perceptual correlate of frequency of vibration, although the term has come to refer in common usage to phenomena associated with the physical vibration of the vocal folds.
- Optimal pitch is the frequency of vibration that is most efficient for a given pair of vocal folds, and habitual pitch is the frequency of vibration habitually used by an individual.
- Fundamental frequency is the lowest component of a harmonic series. In phonation, it is the lowest frequency of the voiced source.
- The pitch range of an individual spans approximately two octaves.
- Changes in vocal fundamental frequency are governed by the tension of the vocal folds and their mass per unit length.
- Increasing the length of the vocal folds increases vocal fold tension and decreases the mass per unit area, which increases the fundamental frequency.

- The respiratory system responds to increased vocal fold tension with increased subglottal pressure, so that pitch and subglottal pressure tend to covary.
- Increased subglottal pressure is a response to increased vocal fold tension.

INTENSITY AND INTENSITY CHANGE

Just as pitch is the perceptual correlate of frequency, **loudness** is the perceptual correlate of intensity. Intensity (or its correlate, sound pressure level) is the physical measure of power (or pressure) ratios, but loudness is how we perceive power or pressure differences. As with pitch and frequency, there is a close relationship between loudness and intensity.

Loudness: The perceptual correlate of intensity.

To increase the vocal intensity of vibrating vocal folds, one must somehow increase the vigor with which the vocal folds are forced open by air pressure. In sustained phonation, the vocal folds move only as a result of the air pressure beneath them and the flow between them. Subglottal pressure and flow provide the energy for this vocal engine, so to increase the intensity or strength of the phonatory product we will have to increase the energy that drives it. We increase subglottal pressure to increase vocal intensity. To prove this to yourself, do the following. You need to feel what you do to produce loud speech. You may be in a quiet setting right now and you really may not want to yell, but that is fine. Pay attention to your lungs and larynx as you prepare to yell as loudly as you can to someone across the room. Without even yelling, you should have been able to feel your lungs take in a large charge of air, and you also should have felt your vocal folds tighten. These are the two gestures of significance for increasing vocal intensity: increased subglottal pressure and medial compression.

To explain the effect that medial compression has on vocal intensity requires a return to discussion of a cycle of vocal fold vibration. We can break a cycle of vibration into stages. There is an opening stage, in which the vocal folds are opening, a closing stage, in which the vocal folds are returning to the point of approximation, and a closed stage, in which there is no air escaping between the vocal folds (see Figures 3-28 and 3-29). In modal phonation at conversational intensities, it has been found that the vocal folds spend about 50% of their time in the opening phase, 37% of the time in the closing phase, and 13% of the cycle completely closed. When the vocal folds are tightly adducted for increased vocal intensity, they tend to return to the closed position more quickly and to stay closed for a longer time. The opening phase reduces to approximately 33%, while the closed

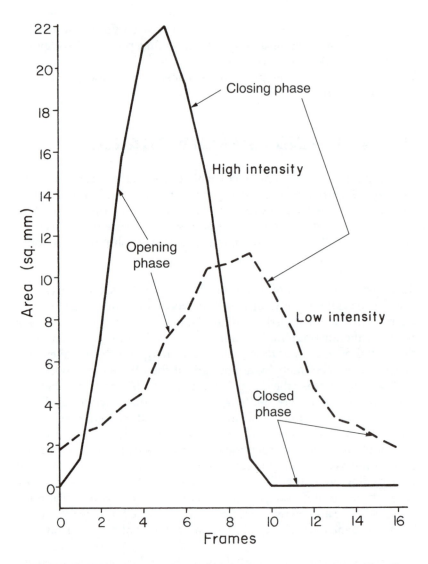

FIGURE 3–28. Effect of vocal intensity on vocal fold vibration. During low-intensity speech the opening and closing phases occupy most of the vibratory cycle, as revealed in the area of the glottis. During high-Intensity speech the opening phase is greatly compressed, as is the closing phase, while the time spent in the closed phase is greatly increased. (Data from Fletcher, 1950.)

FIGURE 3-29. Effect of vocal intensity shown on electroglotto-graphic trace. The electroglottograph measures impedance across the vocal folds; the peak represents the closed phase of the glottal cycle. **A.** Conversational-level sustained vowel. **B.** High-level sustained vowel.

phase increases to more than 30%, depending on the intensity increase (Fletcher, 1950).

The concept you should retain is this: To increase vocal intensity, the vocal folds are tightly compressed, it takes more force to blow them open, they close more rapidly, and they tend to stay closed because they are tightly compressed. This is the cause side of the equation. The effect portion is that because so much energy is required to hold the folds in compression, the release of the folds from this condition is going to be markedly stronger. Each time the folds open, they do so with vigor, producing an explosive compression of the air medium. The harder that eruption of the vocal folds is, the greater is the amplitude of the cycle of vibration. If you remember that as the amplitude of the signal increases so does the intensity, you will recognize the difference of intensity in Figure 3-29A and 3-29B.

The two waveforms in Figure 3-30 are different in intensity, but not in frequency. The time between the cycles is exactly the same, so the

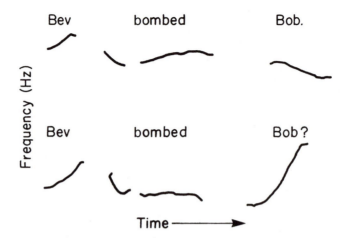

FIGURE 3-30. Fundamental frequency fluctuation for declarative statement and question form. Note the difference in falling and rising intonation between these two sentence forms.

frequency must be the same. From this situation comes a very important point: Intensity and frequency are controlled independently, and you can increase intensity without increasing frequency. Here is the paradox. Increases in intensity and fundamental frequency depend on the same basic mechanism (tension/compression and subglottal pressure), so it is difficult to increase intensity without increasing pitch, but trained or well-controlled speakers can do this. The tendency is for frequency and intensity to increase together, which is a natural phenomenon that you can demonstrate for yourself. Find a place where you can shout, and then say a word before shouting it. Your pitch will most certainly go up when you shout, unless you try very hard to avoid it.

The relationship between subglottal pressure and the actual sound pressure output of the vocal folds depends on the speaker. However, it appears that for every doubling of subglottal pressure there is an increase of between 8 and 12 decibels in vocal intensity.

Summary

- Vocal intensity is to the increase in sound pressure of the speech signal.
- To increase vocal intensity of phonation, the speaker must increase medial compression through the muscles of adduction.

- This increased adductory force requires greater subglottal pressure to produce phonation and forces the vocal folds to remain closed for a longer time.
- The increased laryngeal tension required for increasing intensity also increases the vocal fundamental frequency, although the trained voice is capable of controlling fundamental frequency and vocal intensity independently.

LINGUISTIC ASPECTS OF PITCH AND INTENSITY

Pitch and intensity are elements of suprasegmental aspects of communication. **Suprasegmental** elements are the parameters of speech above the segment (phonetic) level. The phonetic level of speech refers to the *phonemes*, or unique sounds, of speech (although some speech scientists consider segments to be the components of phonemes, such as aspiration, frequency transitions, etc.). The term *segment* arises from the need to parse out the independent and unique sounds that represent meaning in speech (phonemes), but we would be remiss if we did not note that the subsegmental elements, such as the specific frequency transition of a stop phoneme, are critical to the accurate identification of the segment. The term *suprasegmental* generally refers to elements of **prosody**, the system of phoneme, syllable, and word stress (emphasis) used to vary meaning in speech. The prosodic elements include pitch, intonation, loudness, stress, duration, and rhythm. These elements convey much of the emotion, intent, and meaning of speech. Even though it is beyond the scope of this text to deeply examine these suprasegmental elements, pitch and intensity play such a large role in speech that we will discuss them here.

Suprasegmental elements are largely a product of phonation. **Intonation** refers to the changes in pitch in speech, and **stress** refers to syllable or word emphasis relative to an entire utterance. For example, say the following sentence out loud: "My cat's name is Mary." You end it with a falling intonation and put more stress on "cat's" than on "name" or "Mary." To a large extent, these elements both arise out of variation in vocal intensity and fundamental frequency. Intonation can be considered the melodic envelope that contains the sentence and serves to mark sentence type. Generally, statements have falling intonation at the end and questions have rising intonation. For example, Figure 3-30 shows traces of the fundamental frequency for the productions of "Bev bombed Bob." and "Bev bombed Bob?" If you say these two sentences, you can hear the

Suprasegmental: Information within the speech signal that spans two or more phonemes, generally called prosodic elements.

Prosody: The suprasegmental elements governing allocation of stress to speech, including vocal pitch, intonation, loudness, duration, and rhythm.

Stress: The emphasis on a word produced in continuous speech, relative to the emphasis of the entire utterance.

Intonation: The changes in pitch in continuous speech.

changes that are so strong in the second sentence. Hirano, Ohala, and Vennard (1969) used this sentence contrast to show that the lateral cricoarytenoid, thyrovocalis, and cricothyroid are all quite active in these rapid laryngeal adjustments.

Stress helps punctuate speech, providing emphasis to syllables or words through both intensity and frequency changes. To increase stress, we increase fundamental frequency and intensity through increasing subglottal pressure, medial compression, and glottal tension. Remember from our earlier discussion that both frequency and intensity involve adjustments of these variables. We capitalize on the fact that both intensity and fundamental frequency vary together, so that stressed syllables or words show changes in both.

The musculature involved in stress is similar to that of intonation, with an increase in subglottal pressure. The changes in fundamental frequency are on the order of 50 Hz (Netsell, 1973), governed by the lateral cricoarytenoid, thyrovocalis, and cricothyroid. The changes in subglottal pressure will be small but rapid, or pulsatile (Hixon, 1973). Because they require bursts of increased expiratory force, they are driven by expiratory muscles.

Monopitch: Speech with little or no perceived variation in pitch.

Monoloud: Of unvarying vocal loudness.

Although stress and intonation are not essential for communication, they are essential for natural sounding speech. Clearly you can speak in a **monopitch** (unvarying vocal pitch) or **monoloud** voice (unvarying vocal loudness), but the effect is so distracting that it interferes with communication. You may find individuals with neurological impairments who show both of these characteristics. Treatment directed toward increased muscular effort at points requiring stress will greatly enhance the naturalness of speech because increasing vocal effort at the points inevitably increases both fundamental frequency and vocal intensity.

THEORIES OF PHONATION

The myoelastic-aerodynamic theory of phonation states that vibration of the vocal folds depends on the elements embodied in the name of the theory. The *myoelastic element* is the elastic component of muscle (*myo* = muscle) and associated soft tissues of the larynx, and the aerodynamic component is that of the airflow and pressure through this constricted tube. Van den Berg (1958) recognized that the combination of tissue elasticity, which causes the vocal folds to return to their original position after being distended, and the Bernoulli effect, which helped promote this return by dropping the pressure at the constriction, could account for the sustained vibration shown in even a cadaverous specimen provided with an artificial source of expiratory charge.

Titze (1994) has sought to explain how complex acoustic output can come from a seemingly simple oscillator such as the vocal folds. We have long recognized that the vocal folds undulate in the modes discussed earlier. Titze recognized that this complex vibration arises from the loosely bound masses associated with the membranous cover of the vocal folds (the epithelium and superficial layer of the lamina propria) and the body of the vocal folds (the intermediate and deep layers of lamina propria and thyrovocalis muscle). The loosely bound elastic tissue supports oscillation, and viewing the soft tissue as an infinite (or at least uncountable) number of masses reveals that a very large number of modes of vibration is possible. This discussion in no way gives justice to the elegance of this theory, and we recommend that you take time for the exceptionally readable work of Titze.

The phonatory mechanism is an important component of the speaking mechanism, providing the voiced source for speech. In the next chapter, we explore what happens to the voice source after it leaves the larynx.

CHAPTER SUMMARY

Phonation is the product of vibrating vocal folds in the larynx. The vocal folds vibrate as air flows past them, capitalizing on the Bernoulli principle and tissue elasticity to maintain phonation. The interaction of subglottal pressure, tissue elasticity, and constriction of the airflow caused by the vocal folds produces sustained phonation as long as pressure, flow, and vocal fold approximation are maintained.

The larynx comprises the cricoid, thyroid, and epiglottis cartilages, as well as the paired arytenoid, corniculate, and cuneiform cartilages. The thyroid and cricoid cartilages articulate by means of the cricothyroid joint, which lets the two cartilages come closer together in front. The arytenoid and cricoid cartilages also articulate with a joint, which permits a wide range of arytenoid motion. The epiglottis is attached to the thyroid cartilage and base of the tongue. The corniculate cartilages rest on the upper surface of the arytenoids, and the cuneiform cartilages reside in the aryepiglottic folds.

The cavity of the larynx is a constricted tube with a smooth surface. Sheets and cords of ligaments connect the cartilages, and smooth mucous membrane covers the medial-most surface of the larynx. The valleculae are found between the tongue and the epiglottis, in folds formed by the lateral and median glossoepiglottic ligaments. The fibroelastic membrane is composed of the upper quadrangular membranes and aryepiglottic folds, the lower conus elasticus, and the vocal ligament, which is actually the upward free extension of the conus elasticus.

The vocal folds are five layers of tissue, the deepest being muscle. The aditus is the entryway of the larynx.

Intrinsic muscles of the larynx include the thyrovocalis, thyromuscularis, cricothyroid, lateral and posterior cricoarytenoid, transverse arytenoid and oblique interarytenoid, and superior thyroarytenoid muscles. Extrinsic muscles of the larynx include infrahyoid and suprahyoid muscles. The digastricus anterior and posterior elevate the hyoid, and the stylohyoid retracts it. The mylohyoid and hyoglossus elevate the hyoid, and the geniohyoid elevates the hyoid and draws it forward. The thyropharyngeus and cricopharyngeus muscles elevate the larynx, and the sternohyoid, sternothyroid, and omohyoid muscles depress the larynx.

Movement of the vocal folds into and out of approximation requires coordinated effort of the intrinsic muscles of the larynx. The lateral cricoarytenoid muscle rocks the arytenoid cartilage on its axis, tipping the vocal folds in and slightly down. The posterior cricoarytenoid muscle rocks the arytenoid out. The transverse arytenoid muscle draws the posterior surfaces of the arytenoids closer together. The oblique arytenoid assists the vocal folds to dip downward when they are adducted. Vocal fundamental frequency is increased by increasing tension, a function of the thyrovocalis and cricothyroid muscles.

We must adduct the vocal folds to initiate phonation, and this may take several forms, including breathy, simultaneous, and glottal attacks. Termination of phonation requires abduction of the vocal folds, a process that must occur with the transition of voiced to voiceless speech sounds. Sustained phonation can take several forms, depending on the laryngeal configuration. Falsetto occupies the upper range of laryngeal function, and glottal fry is found in the lower range. Vocal fold vibration among phonatory modes, and the differences are governed by laryngeal tension, medial compression, and subglottal pressure.

Pitch is the perceptual correlate of frequency of vibration, although the term has come into common usage when referring to phenomena associated with the physical vibration of the vocal folds. Optimal pitch refers to the frequency of vibration that is most efficient for a given pair of vocal folds, and habitual pitch is the frequency of vibration habitually used by an individual. Fundamental frequency is the lowest component of a harmonic series. In phonation, it is the lowest frequency of the voiced source. The pitch range of an individual spans approximately two octaves. Changes in vocal fundamental frequency are governed by the tension of the vocal folds and their mass per unit length. Increasing the length of the vocal folds increases vocal fold tension and decreases the mass per unit area, which increases the fundamental frequency. The respiratory system responds to increased vocal fold tension with increased subglottal pressure, so that pitch and subglottal pressure tend to covary.

Increased subglottal pressure is a response to increased vocal fold tension. Vocal intensity refers to the increase in sound pressure of the speech signal. To increase vocal intensity of phonation, the speaker must increase medial compression through the muscles of adduction. This increased adductory force requires greater subglottal pressure to produce phonation and forces the vocal folds to remain in the closed portion of the phonatory cycle for a longer time. The increased laryngeal tension required for increasing intensity also increases the vocal fundamental frequency, although the trained voice is capable of controlling fundamental frequency and vocal intensity independently.

Suprasegmental elements are the parameters of speech above the segment (phonetic) level, generally referring to elements of prosody (pitch, intonation, loudness, stress, duration, and rhythm). Intonation refers to the changes in pitch in speech, and stress refers to syllable or word emphasis relative to an entire utterance. Intonation can be considered the melodic envelope that contains the sentence and can mark sentence type. Stress provides emphasis to syllables or words through both intensity and frequency changes.

The myoelastic-aerodynamic theory of phonation states that vibration of the vocal folds depends on the elements embodied in the name of the theory. Titze (1994) enlarged this theory to encompass the complex vibratory modes responsible for the rich acoustics of speech.

Endnote: Mechanics of Vibration

You may be familiar with the notion that things are capable of vibrating perhaps by plucking a guitar string. When a physical body is set into vibration, it tends to continue vibrating (that is, oscillating), and that vibration tends to continue at the same rate.

Let us examine why a body tends to oscillate. If you have a guitar or other stringed instrument, pluck one of the strings. As you listen to the twang of the string, you will notice that it continues vibrating for quite a while before finally quieting down. The tone remains about the same pitch throughout the audible portion of its vibration.

The process of vibration is determined by a lawful interplay among the elastic restoring forces of a material; the stiffness of the material; and inertia, a quality of its mass. Elasticity is the property of a material that causes it to return to its original shape after being displaced. Stiffness refers to the strength of the forces held within a given material that restore it to its original shape on being distended. Inertia is the property of mass that dictates that a body in motion tends to stay in motion. If we discuss the vibration of the guitar string in detail, the interaction of these elements may become clearer. Look at Figure 3-31 as we discuss this.

In Figure 3-31A, the guitar string is at its resting point; all forces are balanced. Next, the string is being displaced by someone's finger; a displacing force is distending the string. In part C, the string has been released and is moving toward its starting point. This is a direct result of the restoring forces of the elastic material. The elastic qualities of the material from which the string is made and the stiffness of that material determine the efficiency with which the string returns. (If you tried this with a very inelastic material, such as a bar of lead or a slab of roast beef, would it return?)

In part D, when the string reaches it original position, it is moving too fast to stop and sails on by it, even though it is the point of equilibrium. Just as when you push someone in a swing, the swing does not simply return to the point of rest and stop, but rather overshoots that point. The reason the string travels past the point of rest is that it has mass. It takes energy to move mass and it takes energy to stop it once it has started moving. The string will not only return to its original resting position due to elastic restoring forces, but it will fly past that position due to the inertia associated with moving the mass of the object. In part E, the string eventually stops moving because it is now being distended in the opposite direction. The energy you expended in the first distension has now been translated into an opposite distortion as a result of inertia. In the final panel, the string can now begin its return trip toward the starting point, but it will once again overshoot that point because of inertia.

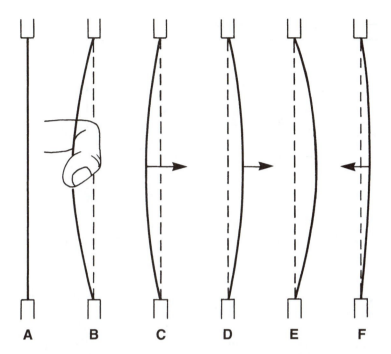

FIGURE 3-31. A guitar string illustrates oscillation. **A.** The string is at rest. **B.** A finger forces the string into displacement. **C.** The string is released and its elastic elements cause it to return toward the rest position. **D.** The string overshoots the rest position because of its inertia. **E.** The string reaches the extreme point of its excursion past the rest position. **F.** Elastic forces in the string cause the string to return toward the rest position.

If you had set a pencil into vibration instead of a string and we had moved a sheet of paper in front of it as it vibrated, it might have drawn a picture something like Figure 3-32, which depicts the periodic motion of a vibrating body. This picture is a graphic representation of the vibration of that object. The drawing represents a waveform, which is the representation of displacement of a body over time, and displays what the pencil or string was doing as it vibrated.

This waveform is periodic. When we say that vibration is periodic, we mean that it repeats itself in a predictable fashion. If it took the ruler 1/100 of a second to move from the first point of distension back to that point again, it will take 1/100 of a second to repeat that cycle if it is vibrating periodically.

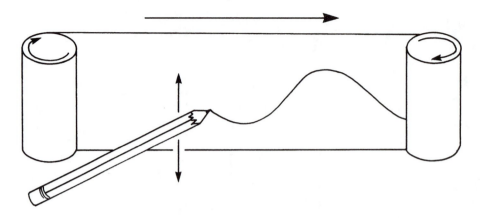

FIGURE 3–32. Periodic motion of a vibrating body graphically recorded.

Moving from one point in the vibratory pattern to the same point again defines one cycle of vibration, and the time it takes to pass through one cycle of vibration is referred to as the period. In our example, the period of vibration was 1/100 second, or 0.01 second. Frequency refers to how often something occurs, as in the frequency with which you shop for groceries (e.g., two times per month). The frequency of vibration is how often a cycle of vibration repeats itself, which in our example is 100 times per second. Frequency and period are the inverse of each other, and that relationship may be stated as $f = 1/T$ or $T = 1/f$. That is, frequency (f) equals 1 divided by period (T for "Time"). For our example, frequency = 1/0.01 second. If you take a moment with your calculator, you will find that this calculation gives a result of 100.

Because frequency refers to the repetition rate of vibration, we speak of it in terms of number of cycles per second. The pencil vibrated with a frequency of 100 cycles per second, but shorthand notation for cycles per second is Hertz (Hz), after Heinrich Hertz. When we set the pencil into vibration, it vibrated with a period of .01 seconds and a frequency of 100 Hz.

We said that a body's frequency of vibration is governed by its elasticity, stiffness, and mass. If you had added a large weight to the guitar string, it would have vibrated slower. As mass increases, frequency of vibration decreases.

If you were to make the string stiffer, it would vibrate more rapidly. Increased stiffness would drive the string to return to its point of equilibrium faster, increasing the frequency of vibration.

Study Questions

1. Identify the structures indicated on the figure.

A. _____ cartilage

B. _____ cartilage

C. _____ cartilage

D. _____ cartilage

E. _____ cartilage

F. _____ bone

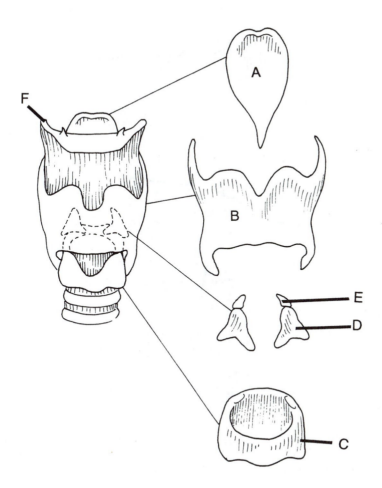

2. Identify the landmarks indicated on the figure.

A. _____

B. _____

C. _____

D. _____

E. _____

F. _____

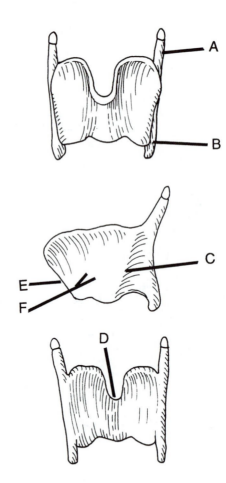

3. Identify the landmarks indicated on the figure.

A. _____ process

B. _____ process

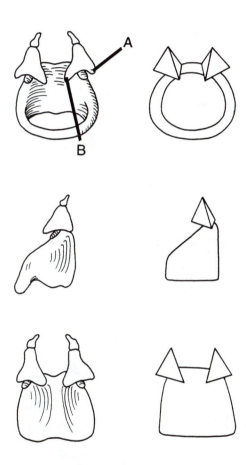

4. Identify the muscles indicated in the following figure.

    A. _____

    B. _____

    C. _____

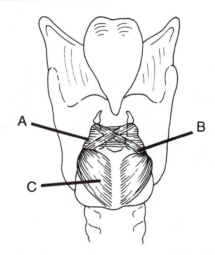

5. Identify the muscles indicated in the following.

    A. _____

    B. _____

    C. _____

    D. _____

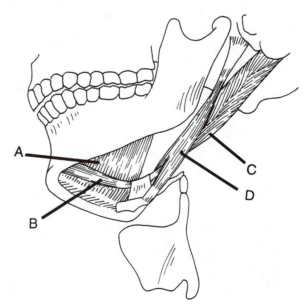

6. Identify the muscles indicated in the following figure.

    A. _____

    B. _____

    C. _____

    D. _____

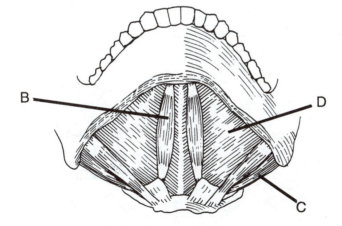

7. This is a view of the laryngeal opening from above. Identify the indicated structures.

A. _____

B. _____

C. _____

D. _____

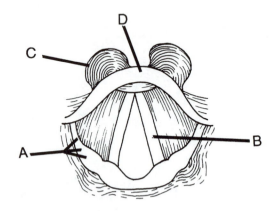

8. Identify the two muscles in the following figure.

A. _____

B. _____

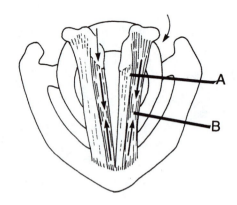

9. The _____ muscle is the primary muscle responsible for change of vocal fundamental frequency.

10. The space between the vocal folds is the _____ .

11. The _____ effect states that given a constant volume flow of air or fluid, at a point of constriction there will be a decrease in air pressure perpendicular to the flow and an increase in velocity of the flow.

12. Laryngeal cancer sometimes necessitates complete removal of the larynx. Because the respiratory and digestive systems share the pharynx, removal of this protective mechanism poses a problem for the needs of breathing and swallowing. What surgical changes would permit both processes?

13. _____ is the process of capturing air in the thorax to provide the muscles with a structure upon which to push or pull.

14. In _____ attack, the vocal folds are adducted before initiation of expiratory flow.

15. In _____ attack, the vocal folds are adducted after the initiation of expiratory flow.

16. In _____ attack, the vocal folds are adducted simultaneous with initiation of expiratory flow.

17. During modal phonation, the vocal folds open from _____ (inferior/superior) to _____ (inferior/superior). The folds close from _____ (inferior/superior) to _____ (inferior/superior).

18. The minimum subglottal driving pressure for speech is _____ cm H_2O.

19. In the mode of vibration known as _____ , the vocal folds vibrate at a much lower rate than in modal phonation, and the folds exhibit a syncopated vibratory pattern.

20. In the mode of vibration known as _____ , the vocal folds lengthen and become extremely thin and reedlike.

21. Presence of vocal nodules or other space-occupying laryngeal pathology may result in _____ phonation.

22. To increase vocal intensity, one must _____ (increase/decrease) subglottal pressure and _____ (increase/decrease) medial compression.

23. To increase vocal fundamental frequency, one must _____ vocal fold tension by _____ (lengthening/shortening) the vocal folds.

24. _____ is the pitch of phonation that is optimal or most appropriate for an individual.

25. _____ is the vocal pitch habitually used during speech.

26. As vocal intensity increases, the closed phase of the vibratory cycle _____ (increases/decreases).

27. We had occasion to record the speech of an individual with a maxillary fistula secondary to squamous cell carcinoma. The cancerous condition had required removal of part of her maxilla, which meant that the oral cavity was continuous with the nasal cavity. While working with the physician who was fitting her for an oral prosthesis, we recorded her speech, only to find that when speech was produced with the open fistula, the fundamental frequency was highly irregular but became regular again when the oral prosthesis was in place. What could be the link between the vocal folds and the oral–nasal communication?

REFERENCES

Abrahams, P. H., McMinn, R. M. H., Hutchings, R. T., Sandy, C., Mark, S. (2003). *McMinn's color atlas of human anatomy* (5th ed.). Philadelphia: Mosby.

Adair, R. K. (1990). *The physics of baseball* (3rd ed.). New York: HarperCollins.

Adair, R. K. (1995). The physics of baseball. *Physics Today, 48*(5), 26–31.

Aronson, E. A. (1985). *Clinical voice disorders.* New York: Thieme.

Baer, T., Sasaki, C., & Harris, K. (1985). *Laryngeal function in phonation and respiration.* Boston: College-Hill Press.

Baken, R. J., & Orlikoff, R. F. (1999). *Clinical measurement of speech and voice,* (2nd ed.). San Diego: Singular Publishing Group.

Bateman, H. E. (1977). *A clinical approach to speech anatomy and physiology.* Springfield, IL: Charles C. Thomas.

Beck, E. W., Monson, H., & Groer, M. (1982). *Mosby's atlas of functional human anatomy.* St. Louis: Mosby.

Berkovitz, B. K. B., & Moxham, B. J. (2002). *Head and neck anatomy: A clinical reference.* London: Martin Dunitz.

Bless, D. M., & Abbs, J. H. (1983). *Vocal fold physiology.* San Diego: College-Hill Press.

Bly, L. (1994). *Motor skills acquisition in the first year.* Tucson, AZ: Therapy Skill Builders.

Boone, D. R. (1999). *The voice and voice therapy.* Englewood Cliffs, NJ: Prentice-Hall.

Broad, D. J. (1973). Phonation. In F. D. Minifie, T. J. Hixon, & F. Williams, (Eds.), *Normal aspects of speech, hearing, and language.* Englewood Cliffs, NJ: Prentice-Hall.

Carrau, R. L., & Murry, T. (1999). *Comprehensive management of swallowing disorders.* San Diego: Singular Publishing Group.

Childers, D. G., Hicks, D. M., Moore, G. P., Eskenazi, L., & Lalwani, A. L. (1990). Electroglottography and vocal fold physiology. *Journal of Speech and Hearing Research, 33,* 245–254.

Chusid, J. G. (1985). *Correlative neuroanatomy and functional neurology* (17th ed.). Los Altos, CA: Lange Medical Publications.

Daniloff, R. G. (1989). *Speech science.* San Diego: College-Hill Press.

Doyle, P. C., Grantmyre, A., & Myers, C. (1989). Clinical modification of the tracheostoma breathing valve for voice restoration. *Journal of Speech and Hearing Disorders, 54,* 189–192.

Durrant, J. D., & Lovrinic, J. H. (1995). *Bases of hearing science.* Baltimore: Williams & Wilkins.

Eckel, F., & Boone, D. (1981). The s/z ratio as an indicator of laryngeal pathology. *Journal of Speech and Hearing Disorders, 46,* 147–149.

Fink, B. R. (1975). *The human larynx.* New York: Raven Press.

Fink, B. R., & Demarest, R. J. (1978). *Laryngeal biomechanics.* Cambridge, MA: Harvard University Press.

Fletcher, W. W. (1950). *A study of internal laryngeal activity in relation to vocal intensity.* Doctoral dissertation, Northwestern University, Evanston, IL.

Fucci, D. J., & Lass, N. J. (1999). *Fundamentals of speech science.* Boston: Allyn & Bacon.

Frable, M. A. (1961). Computation of motion of the cricoarytenoid joint. *Archives of Otolaryngology, 73,* 551–556.

Fujimura, O. (1988). *Vocal fold physiology. Vol. 2. Vocal physiology.* New York: Raven Press.

Fukida, H., Kawaida, M., Tatehara, T., Ling, E., Kita, K., Ohki, K., Kawasaki, Y., & Saito, S. (1988). A new concept of lubricating mechanisms of the larynx. In Fujimura, O. (Ed.), *Vocal physiology: Voice production, mechanisms and functions* (pp. 83–92). New York: Raven Press.

Ganong, W. F. (2003). *Review of medical physiology,* (2nd ed.). New York: McGraw-Hill/Appleton & Lange.

Gosling, J. A., Harris, P. F., Humpherson, J. R., Whitmore, I., & Willan, P. L. T. (1985). *Atlas of human anatomy.* Philadelphia: J. B. Lippincott.

Gray, H., Bannister, L. H., Berry, M. M., & Williams, P. L. (Eds.). (1995). *Gray's anatomy.* London: Churchill Livingstone.

Grobler, N. J. (1977). *Textbook of clinical anatomy (Vol. 1).* Amsterdam: Elsevier Scientific.

Hirano, M. (1974). Morphological structure of the vocal cord as a vibrator and its variations. *Folia Phoniatrica, 26,* 89–94.

Hirano, M., Kirchner, J. A., & Bless, D. M. (1987). *Neurolaryngology.* Boston: College-Hill Press.

Hirano, M., Kiyokawa, K., & Kurita, S. (1988). Laryngeal muscles and glottic shaping. In O. Fujimura (Ed.), *Vocal physiology: Voice production, mechanisms and functions* (pp. 49–65). New York: Raven Press.

Hirano, M., Ohala, J., & Vennard, W. (1969). The function of laryngeal muscles in regulation of fundamental frequency and intensity of phonation. *Journal of Speech and Hearing Research, 12,* 616–628.

Hixon, T. J. (1973). Respiratory function in speech. In F. D. Minifie, T. J. Hixon, & F. Williams (Eds.), *Normal aspects of speech, hearing, and language* (pp. 73–126). Englewood Cliffs, NJ: Prentice-Hall.

Hixon, T. J. (1982). Speech breathing kinematics and mechanism inferences therefrom. In S. Grillner, A. Persson, B. Lindblom, & J. Lubker (Eds.), *Speech motor control* (pp. 75–94). New York: Pergamon.

Hixon, T. J., Hawley, J. L., & Wilson, K. J. (1982). An around-the-house device for the clinical determination of respiratory driving pressure: A note on making simple even simpler. *Journal of Speech and Hearing Disorders, 47,* 413–415.

Hollien, H., & Moore, G. P. (1968). Stroboscopic laminography of the larynx during phonation. *Acta Otolaryngologica, 65,* 209–215.

Hufnagle, J., & Hufnagle, K. K. (1988). S/Z ratio in dysphonic children with and without vocal cord nodules. *Language, Speech, and Hearing Services in Schools, 19,* 418–422.

Husson, R. (1953). Sur la physiologie vocale. *Annals of Otolaryngology, 69,* 124–137.

Isshiki, N. (1964). Regulatory mechanisms of voice intensity variation. *Journal of Speech and Hearing Research, 7,* 17–29.

Jones-Owens, J. L. (1991). Prespeech assessment and treatment strategies. In M. B. Langley, & L. J. Lombardino (Eds.), *Neurodevelopmental strategies for managing communication disorders in children with severe motor dysfunction.* Austin: Pro-Ed.

Kaplan, H. M. (1971). *Anatomy and physiology of speech.* New York: McGraw-Hill.

Kent, R. D. (1997). *The speech sciences.* San Diego: Singular Publishing Group.

Kent, R. D., Kent, J. F., & Rosenbek, J. C. (1987). Maximum performance tests of speech production. *Journal of Speech and Hearing Disorders, 52,* 367–387.

Kirchner, J. A., & Suzuki, M. (1968). Laryngeal reflexes and voice production. In M. Krauss (Ed.), *Sound production in man. Annals of the New York Academy of Sciences, 155,* 98–109.

Kuehn, D. P., Lemme, M. L., & Baumgartner, J. M. (1989). *Neural bases of speech, hearing, and language.* Boston: Little, Brown.

Langley, M. B., & Lombardino, L. J. (1991). *Neurodevelopmental strategies for managing communication disorders in children with severe motor dysfunction.* Austin: Pro-Ed.

Lieberman, P. (1968a). *Intonation, perception, and language.* Research monograph No. 38. Cambridge, MA: M.I.T. Press.

Lieberman, P. (1968b). Vocal cord motion in man. *Annals of the New York Academy of Sciences, 155,* 28–38.

Lieberman, P. (1977). *Speech science and acoustic phonetics: An introduction.* New York: Macmillan.

Liebgott, B. (2001). The anatomical basis of dentistry. St. Louis, MO: Mosby.

Logemann, J. (1998). *Evaluation and treatment of swallowing disorders* (2nd ed.). Austin: Pro-Ed

McMinn, R. M. H., Hutchings, R. T., & Logan, B. M. (1994). *Color atlas of head and neck anatomy.* London: Mosby-Wolfe.

Netsell, R. (1973). Speech physiology. In F. D. Minifie, T. J. Hixon, & F. Williams (Eds.), *Normal aspects of speech, hearing, and language* (pp. 134–211). Englewood Cliffs, NJ: Prentice-Hall.

Netsell, R., & Hixon, T. J. (1978). A noninvasive method for clinically estimating subglottal air pressure. *Journal of Speech and Hearing Disorders, 43,* 326–330.

Netter, F. H. (1983a). *The CIBA collection of medical illustrations. Vol. 1. Nervous System. Part I. Anatomy and physiology.* West Caldwell, NJ: CIBA Pharmaceutical Company.

Netter, F. H. (1983b). *The CIBA collection of medical illustrations. Vol. 1. Nervous system. Part II. Neurologic and neuromuscular disorders.* West Caldwell, NJ: CIBA Pharmaceutical Company.

Netter, F. H. (1989). *Atlas of human anatomy.* West Caldwell, NJ: CIBA Pharmaceutical Company.

Netter, F. H. (1997). *Atlas of human anatomy.* Los Angeles: Icon Learning Systems.

Nishizawa, N., Sawashima, M., & Yonemoto, K. (1988). Vocal fold length in vocal pitch change. In O. Fujimua (Ed.), *Vocal physiology: Voice production, mechanisms and functions* (pp. 49–65). New York: Raven Press.

Proctor, D. F. (1968). The physiologic basis of voice training. In M. Krauss (Ed.), *Sound production in man. Annals of the New York Academy of Sciences, 155,* 208–228.

Ptacek, P. H., & Sander, E. K. (1963). Maximum duration of phonation. *Journal of Speech and Hearing Disorders, 28*(2), 171–182.

Ramig, L. A., & Ringel, R. L. (1983). Effects of physiological aging on selected acoustic characteristics of voice. *Journal of Speech and Hearing Research, 26,* 22–30.

Rastatter, M. P., & Hyman, M. (1982). Maximum phoneme duration of /s/ and /z/ by children with vocal nodules. *Language, Speech, and Hearing Services in Schools, 13,* 197–199.

Rohen, J. W., Yokochi, C., Lutjen-Drecoll, E. L., & Romrell, L. J. (2002). *Color atlas of anatomy: A photographic study of the human body* (5th ed.). Philadelphia: Lippincott, Williams & Wilkins.

Rosse, C., Gaddum-Rosse, P., & Rosse, G. (1997). *Hollinshead's textbook of anatomy.* Philadelphia: Lippincott-Raven.

Sapienza, C. M., & Stathopoulos, E. T. (1994). Respiratory and laryngeal measures of children and women with bilateral vocal fold nodules. *Journal of Speech and Hearing Research, 37,* 1229–1243.

Shepard, T. H. (1998). *Catalog of teratogenic agents* (9th ed.). Baltimore: Johns Hopkins University Press.

Sonninen, A. (1968). The external frame function in the control of pitch in the human voice. In M. Krauss (Ed.), *Sound production in man. Annals of the New York Academy of Sciences, 155,* 68–89.

Sorensen, D. N., & Parker, P. A. (1992). The voiced/voiceless phonation time in children with and without laryngeal pathology. *Language, Speech, and Hearing Services in Schools, 23,* 163–168.

Tait, N. A., Michel, J. F., & Carpenter, M. A. (1980). Maximum duration of sustained /s/ and /z/ in children. *Journal of Speech and Hearing Disorders, 15,* 239–246.

Timcke, R., Von Leden, H., & Moore, G. P. (1958). Laryngeal vibrations: Measurements of the glottic wave I: The normal vibratory cycle. *Archives of Otolaryngology, 68,* 1–19.

Titze, I. R. (1973). The human vocal cords: A mathematical model, Part I. *Phonetica, 28,* 129–170.

Titze, I. R. (1988). The physics of small amplitude oscillation of the vocal folds. *Journal of the Acoustical Society of America, 83*(4), 1536–1552.

Titze, I. R. (1994). *Principles of voice production.* Englewood Cliffs, NJ: Prentice-Hall.

Van den Berg, J. W. (1958). Myoelastic-aerodynamic theory of voice production. *Journal of Speech and Hearing Research, 1,* 227–244.

Van den Berg, J. W. (1968). Sound production in isolated human larynges. In M. Krauss (Ed.), *Sound production in man. Annals of the New York Academy of Sciences, 155,* 18–27.

Van den Berg, J. W., & Tan, T. S. (1959). Results of experiments with human larynxes. *Practica Oto-rhino-laryngologica, 21,* 425–450.

Verdolini, K., Titze, I. R., & Fennell, A. (1994). Dependence of phonatory effort on hydration level. *Journal of Speech and Hearing Research, 37,* 1001–1007.

Whillis, J. (1946). Movements of the tongue in swallowing. *Journal of Anatomy, 80,* 115–116.

Zemlin, W. R. (1998). *Speech and hearing science. Anatomy and physiology* (4th ed.). Needham Heights, MA: Allyn & Bacon.

CHAPTER

4

Anatomy and Physiology of Articulation and Resonation

OUTLINE

I. Anatomy of Articulation and Resonance

A. Articulation: Bringing mobile and immobile articulators into contact to shape the sounds of speech

B. Source-filter theory of vowel production

C. Articulators
    1. Mobile articulators
        a. Tongue
        b. Mandible
        c. Soft palate (velum)
        d. Lips
        e. Cheeks
        f. Fauces
        g. Pharynx
    2. Immobile articulators
        a. Alveolar ridge of maxillae
        b. Hard palate
        c. Teeth

D. Bones of the face and cranial skeleton
    1. Bones of the face
        a. Mandible
        b. Maxillae
        c. Nasal
        d. Palatine processes
        e. Nasal conchae
        f. Vomer
        g. Zygomatic
        h. Hyoid
    2. Bones of the cranial skeleton
        a. Ethmoid
        b. Sphenoid
        c. Frontal
        d. Parietal
        e. Occipital
        f. Temporal

E. Dentition
    1. Alveoli
    2. Categorized as incisors, cuspids, bicuspids, and molars
    3. Each tooth has a root and crown, the crown's surface composed of enamel overlying dentin
    4. Each tooth has medial, distal, lingual, buccal (or labial), and occlusal surfaces
    5. Clinical eruption
    6. The permanent arch
    7. Types of occlusion
        a. Class I occlusion
        b. Class II malocclusion
        c. Class III malocclusion

8. Aberrant orientation
    a. Torsiversion
    b. Labioversion
    c. Linguaversion
    d. Distoversion
    e. Mesioversion
    f. Infraversion
    g. Supraversion

F. Cavities of the vocal tract
  1. Pharynx
    a. Oropharynx
    b. Nasopharynx
    c. Laryngopharynx
  2. Oral cavity
  3. Buccal cavity
  4. Nasal cavities

G. Muscles of the face and mouth
  1. Muscles of the face
    a. Orbicularis oris
    b. Risorius
    c. Buccinator
    d. Levator labii superioris
    e. Zygomatic minor
    f. Levator labii superioris alaeque nasi
    g. Levator anguli oris
    h. Zygomatic major, Zygomatic minor,
    i. Depressor labii inferioris
    j. Depressor anguli oris
    k. Mentalis
    l. Platysma
  2. Tongue
    a. Intrinsic tongue muscles
    b. Extrinsic tongue muscles
  3. Muscles of mastication
    a. Mandibular elevators
    b. Mandibular depressors
  4. Muscles of the soft palate
    a. Palatal elevators
    b. Palatal depressors
  5. Muscles of the pharynx
    a. Superior pharyngeal constrictor
    b. Middle pharyngeal constrictor
    c. Inferior pharyngeal constrictor
    d. Cricopharyngeal muscle
    e. Stylopharyngeus

II. Physiology of Articulation and Resonation

    A. Biological functions
        1. Mastication and deglutition
            a. Oral preparatory stage
            b. Oral stage
            c. Pharyngeal stage
            d. Esophageal stage
    B. Speech function
        1. Extralabial force of mentalis muscle
        2. Mandible adjustments
        3. Tongue function
    C. Development of articulatory ability
        1. Reflexive responses
        2. Voluntary control

If you asked most people what is involved in the process of speaking, they would probably mention the elements of articulation. You now know, of course, that there is much more to speech than moving the lips, tongue, and mandible. Still, the articulatory system is an extremely important element in our communication system.

Articulation: The process of bringing the mobile and immobile articulators into contact for the purpose of shaping the sounds of speech.

Articulation is the process of bringing the mobile and immobile articulators into contact for the purpose of shaping the sounds of speech produced by laryngeal vibration. Laryngeal vibration produces the sound required for voicing in speech.

SOURCE-FILTER THEORY OF VOWEL PRODUCTION

A widely accepted description of how the oral cavity creates some speech sounds is the *source-filter theory* of vowel production. The theory states that a voicing source is generated by the vocal folds and routed through the vocal tract where it is shaped into the sounds of speech. Changes in the shape and configuration of the tongue, mandible, soft palate, and other articulators govern the resonance characteristics of the vocal tract, and the resonances of the tract determine the sound of a vowel.

Vocal tract: The oral cavity, the pharynx, and the nasal cavity.

The **vocal tract**, consisting of the mouth (oral cavity), the region behind the mouth (pharynx), and the nasal cavity, can be thought of as a series of linked tubes (see Figure 4-1). You probably know that if you blow carefully across the top of a glass or plastic bottle, you will hear a tone. If you decrease the volume of the air in the bottle by adding fluid to it, the frequency of vibration of the tone increases. Likewise, if you blow across the top of a bottle with larger air volume, the tone

FIGURE 4–1. Visualization of the oral, nasal, and pharyngeal cavities as a series of linked tubes. This linkage provides the variable resonating cavity that produces speech.

decreases in frequency. As the volume of the air in the bottle increases, the frequency of the tone decreases. As the volume decreases, the frequency increases. You are experimenting with the resonant frequency of a cavity, which is the frequency of sound to which the cavity most effectively responds. You might think of the bottle as a filter that lets only one frequency of sound through and rejects the other frequencies, much as a coffee filter lets the liquid through but traps the grounds. The airstream blowing across the top of the bottle is actually producing a very broad-spectrum signal, but the bottle selects the frequency components that are at its resonant frequency. The resonant frequency of a cavity is largely governed by its volume and length.

When you move your tongue around in your mouth, you are changing the shape of your oral cavity. This, then, is the source-filter theory of speech production. The vocal folds produce a tone that is passed through the filter of your vocal tract. Because the vocal tract filter is changeable, you are able to reconfigure its shape and therefore change the sound.

Summary

- The source-filter theory states that speech is the product of sending an acoustic source, such as the sound produced by the vibrating vocal folds, through the filter of the vocal tract, which shapes the output.
- The ever-changing speech signal is the product of moving articulators.

Let us now examine the structures of the articulatory system. As with the phonatory system, we must examine the support structure (the skull and bones of the face) and the muscles that move the articulators. Before we begin, we will define the articulators used in speech production.

THE ARTICULATORS

Articulators can be mobile or immobile. In speech we often move one articulator to make contact with another, thus positioning a mobile articulator in relation to an immobile articulator. The largest mobile articulator is the tongue, with the lower jaw (mandible) a close second (see Figure 4-2). The velum, or soft palate, is another mobile articulator, used to differentiate nasal sounds such as /m/ and /n/ from non-nasal sounds. The lips are moved to produce different speech sounds, and the cheeks play a role in changes of resonance of the cavity. The region behind the oral cavity (the *fauces*, shown in a later figure, and the pharynx) can be moved through muscular action, and the larynx and hyoid bone both change to accommodate different articulatory postures.

There are three immobile articulators. The alveolar ridge of the upper jaw (maxilla, pl. maxillae) and the hard palate are both significant articulatory surfaces. The teeth are used to produce a variety of speech sounds.

Of these mobile and immobile articulators, the tongue, mandible, teeth, hard palate, and velum are the major players, although all surfaces and cavities in the articulatory-resonatory system contribute to the production of speech. You may wish to refer to Figures 4-3 through 4-7 as we begin our discussion of the bones of the facial and cranial skeleton. In addition, Table 4-1 may help you to organize this body of material.

BONES OF THE FACE AND CRANIAL SKELETON

Bones of the Face

The face has numerous bones, with which you should become familiar (see Table 4-1).

A   SAGITTAL VIEW

FIGURE 4-2. A. Relationships among the articulators. **B.** Photograph of articulators seen through sagittal section.

A.

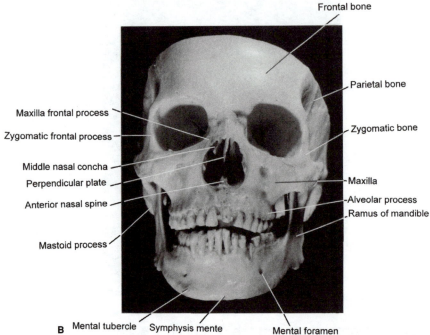

B.

FIGURE 4–3. A. Anterior view of the skull. **B.** Photograph of anterior skull.

The *mandible* is the massive bone making up the lower jaw of the face. It begins as a paired bone but fuses at the midline by the child's first birthday. As you can see in Figure 4-8, there are several landmarks of interest on both outer and inner surfaces. The point of fusion of the two halves of the mandible is the *symphysis mente,* or mental symphysis. Lateral to this on either side is the *mental foramen,* the hole through which the mental nerve of V trigeminal passes in life. On the side is the corpus, or body, and the point at which the mandible bends upward is the *angle.* The plate rising up from the mandible is

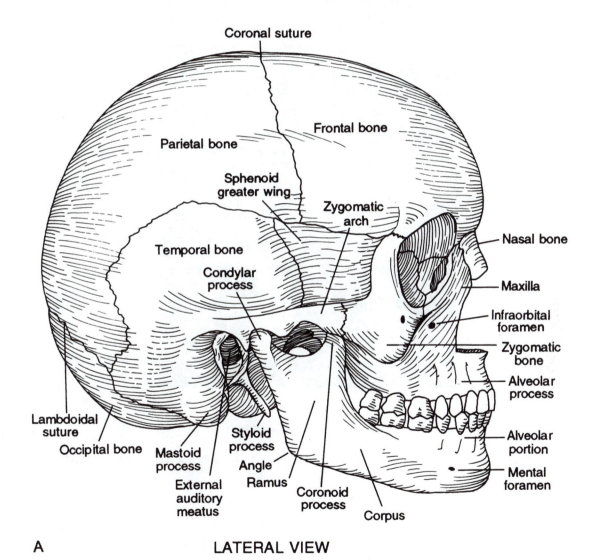

A   LATERAL VIEW

FIGURE 4-4. A. Lateral view of the skull. (*continues*)

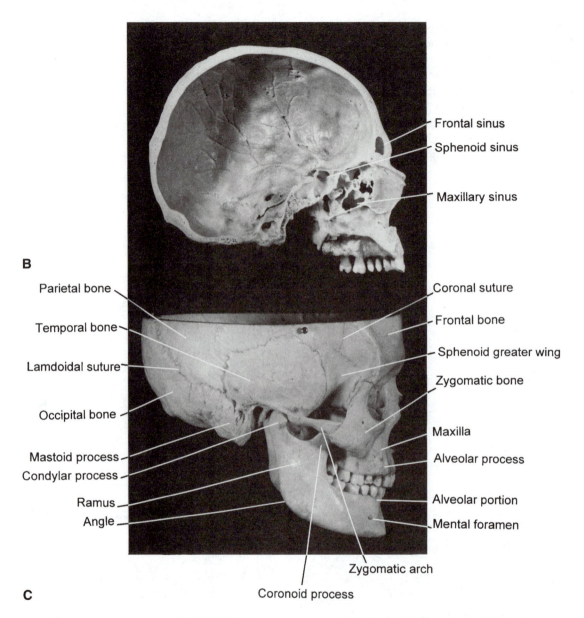

FIGURE 4–4. *(continued)* **B.** Medial surface of the skull. **C.** Photo of lateral skull.

the *ramus,* and the *condylar process* is an important landmark because the head of the condylar process articulates with the skull, permitting rotation of the mandible. Teeth in small *dental alveoli* (sacs, not shown) on the upper surface of the *alveolar part* of the mandible.

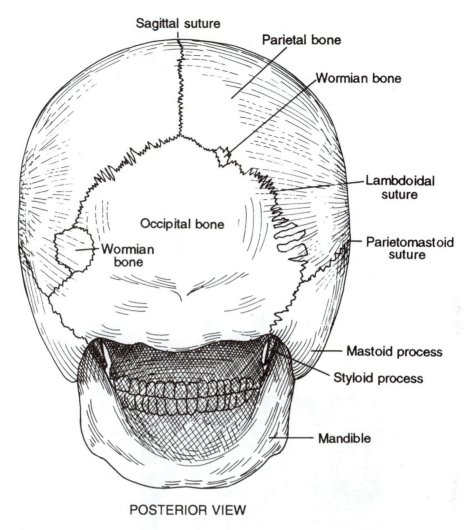

FIGURE 4-5. Posterior view of the skull.

On the inner surface of the mandible is the *mandibular foramen*, which houses the inferior alveolar nerve that provides sensory innervation for the teeth and gums.

The left and right maxillae are the bones of the upper jaw, most of the roof of the mouth (hard palate), nose, and upper dental ridge (see Figure 4-9). Supporting the eye is the *orbital process*, the lower portion of the orbital surface. The *zygomatic process* of the maxilla bone articulates with the zygomatic bone. At the midline, you can see the *anterior nasal spine* and *nasal crest*, and lateral to this is the *nasal notch*. The alveolar process contains alveoli that hold teeth in

A   SUPERIOR VIEW

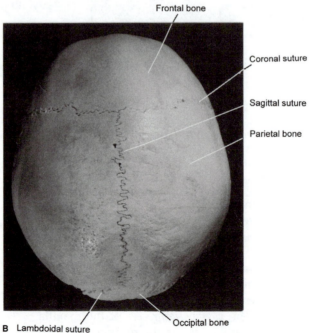

FIGURE 4-6. A. Superior view of the skull. **B.** Superior view photo of the skull.

FIGURE 4–7. A. Inferior view of the skull. **B.** Photo of inferior view of the skull.

Table 4-1. Bones of the Face and Cranial Skeleton

Bones of the Face	Bones of the Cranial Skeleton
Mandible	Ethmoid bone
Maxillae	Sphenoid bone
Nasal bone	Frontal bone
Palatine bone and	Parietal bone
nasal conchae	Occipital bone
Vomer	Temporal bone
Zygomatic bone	
Lacrimal bone	
Hyoid bone	

the intact adult maxilla. A medial view reveals the *maxillary sinus,* the *palatine process,* and the inner margin of the *alveolar process.*

Figure 4-10 shows an inferior view of the maxillae. As you can see, the two *palatine processes* of the maxillae articulate at the *intermaxillary suture.* This suture marks the point of a cleft of the hard palate. The palatine process makes up three fourths of the hard palate; the other one fourth is the *horizontal plate of the palatine bone.*

The *incisive foramen* in the anterior aspect of the hard palate is a conduit for the nasopalatine nerve serving the nasal mucosa. Trace the *premaxillary suture* forward from the incisive foramen to the alveolar process and you have identified the borders of the *premaxilla.* The premaxilla is difficult to see on the adult skull, but it is an important landmark. Note that the premaxillary suture neatly separates the lateral incisors from the cuspids.

The *nasal bones* are small, making up the superior nasal surface. Recall that the posterior one fourth of the hard palate is made up of the horizontal plate of the palatine bone (see Figure 4-11). When viewed from the front, you can see that the articulated palatine bones echo the nasal cavity defined by the maxillae.

The *inferior nasal conchae* (inferior *turbinates*) are small, scroll-like bones on the lateral surface of the nasal cavity. These small bones articulate with the maxilla, palatine, and ethmoid bones. The middle and superior nasal conchae, processes of the ethmoid bone (to be discussed), are above the inferior conchae. The mucosal lining covering the nasal conchae is the thickest of the nose and is richly endowed with vascular supply. Air passing over the nasal conchae is warmed and humidified before reaching the delicate tissues of the

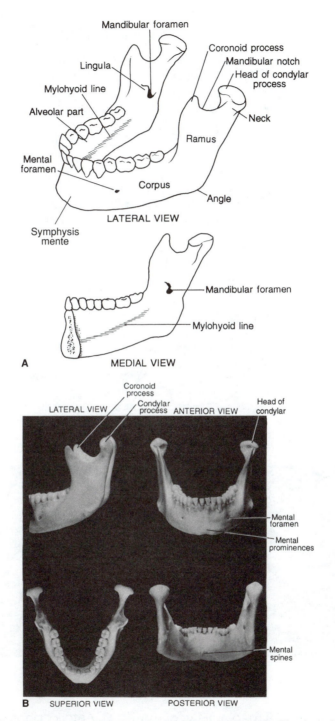

FIGURE 4-8. A. Lateral and medial views of the mandible. **B.** Photo of the mandible from lateral, anterior, superior, and posterior aspects.

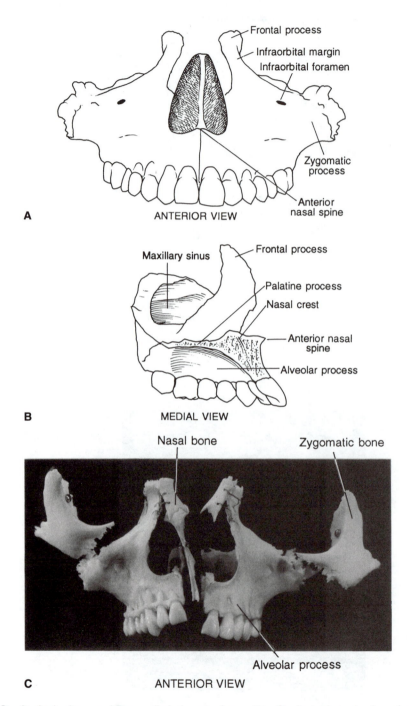

FIGURE 4–9. A. Anterior and **B** medial views of maxilla. **C.** Anterior photo of maxillae showing relationship with nasal and zygomatic bones.

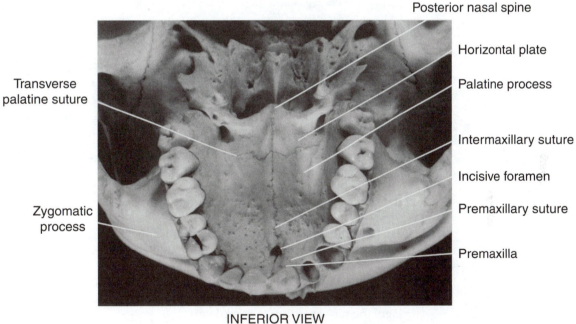

INFERIOR VIEW

FIGURE 4-10. Schematic and photograph of inferior view of the hard palate.

On Use of the Bite Block

A bite block is a device used to stabilize the mandible so that other articulators can be evaluated or exercised. Bite blocks come in many shapes, sizes, and textures, ranging from acrylic blocks about 1 cm square to bite blocks that are created of dental-impression material. The softer, more pliable dental-impression bite block provides a better surface for sustained use and is particularly good for clients who have limited motor control.

A bite block is used when a client cannot differentiate the contribution of the mandible from the lips or tongue during articulation. For instance, if you say /la la la la la/ repeatedly while lightly holding your mandible, you will feel the mandible move, even though the dominant articulator is the tongue. If you wanted to strengthen the tongue, by having it push toward the roof of the mouth against a resistance, you could place a bite block between the molars and have your client push up against a tongue depressor.

Needless to say, having your client perform oral motor activities such as the one just mentioned requires that you have a firm understanding of the anatomy and physiology of articulation, as well as a deep knowledge of motor development. Oral motor therapy focuses on remediating muscle imbalance, and inappropriate application of oral motor activities can create even greater problems! For an excellent discussion, see Langley and Lombardino, 1991.

lower respiratory system. The shape of the conchae greatly increases the surface area, which promotes rapid heat exchange.

There is only one *vomer* because it is a midline bone. It makes up the inferior and posterior nasal septum, which is the dividing plate between the two nasal cavities (see Figure 4-12). The bony nasal septum is made of two elements: the vomer and the perpendicular plate of the ethmoid bone. With the addition of the midline septal cartilage, the nasal septum is complete.

The *zygomatic bone* makes up the prominent structure we identify as the cheekbone. As you can see from Figure 4-13, the zygomatic bone articulates with the maxillae, frontal bone, and temporal bone (you cannot see the articulation with the sphenoid bone) and makes up the lateral orbit. The *zygomatic arch* consists of the temporal process of the zygomatic bone and the zygomatic process of the temporal bone.

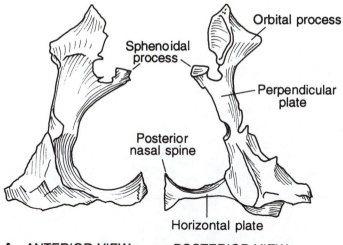

FIGURE 4–11. A. Anterior and posterior views of palatine bones. (*continues*)

These small bones are almost hidden in the intact skull. They articulate with the maxillae, frontal bone, nasal bone, and inferior conchae. They constitute a small portion of the lateral nasal wall and form a small portion of the medial orbit as well.

The *hyoid bone* is discussed in Chapter 3, but it rightfully belongs in this chapter as well. Its presence in this listing should remind you of the interconnectedness of the phonatory and articulatory systems.

Bones of the Cranial Skeleton

The bones of the cranium include those that define the cranial cavity. The *ethmoid bone* is a complex, delicate structure with a presence in the cranial, nasal, and orbital spaces (Figure 4-14). If the cranium and facial skeleton were an apple, the ethmoid would be the core. When the ethmoid is viewed from the front, it is easy to identify the *crista galli*, which protrudes into the cranial space. The *perpendicular plate* makes up the *superior nasal septum*. The *cribriform plates* separate the nasal and cranial cavities and provide the conduit for the *olfactory nerves* as they enter the cranial space.

Figure 4-15 shows that the *sphenoid* consists of a corpus and three pairs of processes, the *greater wings of sphenoid, lesser wings of sphenoid,* and *pterygoid processes.* When the sphenoid is viewed from above, you can see the *hypophyseal fossa*, the indentation that holds the pituitary gland (hypophysis).

Projecting downward from the greater wing and corpus are the *lateral* and *medial pterygoid plates*. These plates and the fossa between

Perpendicular plate
Orbital process / Posterior nasal spine

ANTERIOR VIEW

Horizontal plate

B INFERIOR VIEW

FIGURE 4-11. (*continued*) **B.** Articulated palatine bones from front and beneath. Note that the left perpendicular plate is incomplete.

Mandibular Hypoplasia and Micrognathia

Congenital mandibular hypoplasia is a condition of inadequate development of the mandible. Although some specific genetic syndromes have this as a trait (e.g., Pierre Robin syndrome), micrognathia (small jaw) may occur without a known mediating condition. The misalignment of the mandibular and maxillary arches can be corrected through surgery to extend the mandible. It is hypothesized that during development, micrognathia leads to cleft palate: The mandible may not develop adequately to accommodate the tongue, which in turn blocks the extension of the palatine processes of the maxillae.

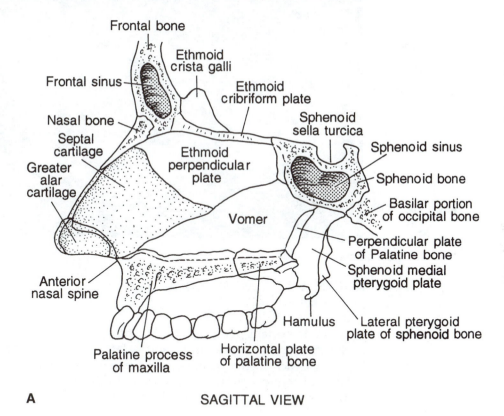

A   SAGITTAL VIEW

FIGURE 4–12. A. Medial view of the nasal septum. Notice that the septum is composed of the perpendicular plate of ethmoid, the vomer, and the septal cartilage. (*continues*)

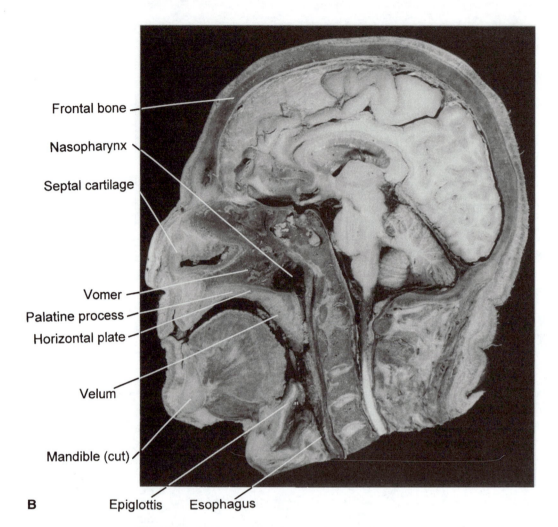

Frontal bone —

Nasopharynx

Septal cartilage

Vomer —

Palatine process —

Horizontal plate —

Velum

Mandible (cut) —

B   Epiglottis   Esophagus

FIGURE 4-12. (*continued*) **B.** Sagittal section through the nasal septum.

them are important points of attachment for one of the muscles of mastication and a muscle of the soft palate. A *hamulus* (hook) projects from each medial lamina, and the tendon of the tensor veli palatini of the soft palate passes around this on its course to the velum, as will be discussed.

The frontal bone shown in Figure 4-16 makes up the bony forehead, anterior cranial case, and supraorbital region. The *coronal suture* (see Figure 4B) is where the frontal and parietal bones articulate.

The *parietal bones* form the upper middle portion of the braincase (see Figure 4-17). These bones are joined at the *sagittal suture*, and join the

Cleft Lip and Cleft Palate

Cleft lip and cleft palate occur during early fetal development. Cleft lip is either unilateral or bilateral, occurring along the premaxillary suture. Cleft lip is rarely midline, but it can involve soft tissue alone or include a cleft of the maxilla up to the incisive foramen. Cleft palate can involve both hard and soft palates.

Cleft lip results from a failure of embryonic facial and labial tissue to fuse during development. It is assumed that tissues migrate and develop normally, but for some reason either fail to fuse or the fusion of the migrating medial nasal, maxillary, and lateral nasal processes breaks down. Cleft palate apparently results from some mechanical intervention in development. Prior to the seventh embryonic week, the palatine processes of the maxillae have been resting alongside the tongue so the tongue separates the processes. As the oral cavity and mandible grow, the tongue drops away from the processes, and the processes can extend, make midline contact, and fuse. If something blocks the movement of the tongue (such as micrognathia), the palatine processes will not move in time to make contact. The head grows rapidly, and the plates will have missed their chance to become an intact palate.

occipital bones by means of the *lambdoidal suture*. The temporal bone articulates with the parietal bone by means of the *squamosal suture*.

The *occipital bone* (see Figure 4-18) makes up the posterior braincase. It articulates with the temporal, parietal, and sphenoid bones. From beneath you can see that the occipital bone forms the base of the skull, wrapping beneath the brain. The *foramen magnum* provides the conduit for the spinal cord and beginning of the medulla oblongata, and the *condyles* mark the resting point for the first cervical vertebra.

The *temporal bone* is an important structure for students of speech pathology and audiology. The temporal bone is extremely dense and is remarkably rich in important landmarks (see Figure 4-19). This complex bone is divided into four segments: the squamous, tympanic, mastoid, and petrous portions. The *squamous portion* is fan-shaped and thin. The lower margin includes the roof of the *external auditory meatus*, the conduit for sound energy to the middle ear. The *zygomatic process* also arises from the squamous portion, forming part of the *zygomatic arch* (not shown). Beneath the base of the zygomatic

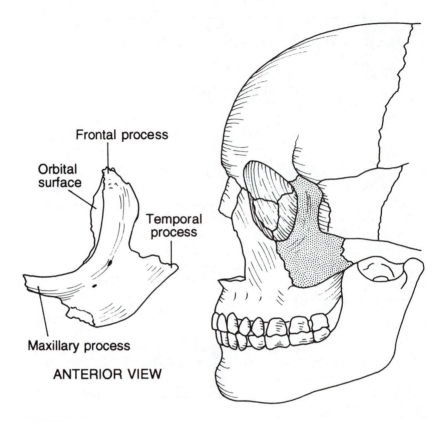

Frontal process

Orbital surface

Temporal process

Maxillary process

ANTERIOR VIEW

FIGURE 4-13. Anterior view of the zygomatic bone.

process is the *mandibular fossa* of the temporal bone with which the condyloid process of the mandible articulates.

The *mastoid portion* is the posterior part of the temporal bone. Air cells deep within in the mastoid portion communicate with the *tympanic antrum*. Above the antrum is the *tegmen tympani*, a thin plate of bone, and medial to it is the *lateral semicircular canal*. On the anterior surface of the temporal bone is the *mastoid process*, which arises from the *mastoid portion*. The *tympanic portion* of the temporal bone includes the anterior and inferior walls of the external auditory meatus (or ear canal). The *styloid process* protrudes beneath the external auditory meatus and medial to the mastoid process. The *petrous portion* includes the *cochlea* and *semicircular canals*.

The *temporal fossa* is a region that includes a portion of the temporal, parietal, and occipital bones, and is the point of origin of the fan-shaped temporalis muscle used for mastication (chewing). The medial surface

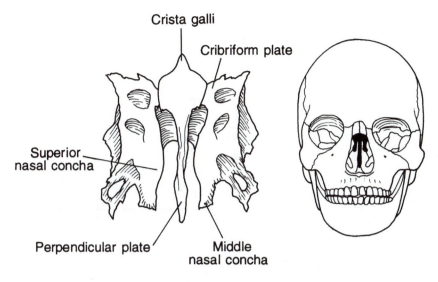

ANTERIOR VIEW

FIGURE 4-14. Anterior view of the ethmoid bone.

of the temporal bone reveals the *internal auditory meatus* through which the VIII cranial nerve passes on its way to the brainstem.

Summary

- The mandible provides the lower dental arch, alveolar region, and the resting location for the tongue.
- The maxillae provide the hard palate, point of attachment for the soft palate, alveolar ridge, upper dental arch, and dominant structures of the nasal cavities.
- The midline vomer articulates with the perpendicular plate of ethmoid and the cartilaginous septum to form the nasal septum.
- The zygomatic bone articulates with the frontal bone and maxillae to form the cheekbone. The small nasal bones provide the upper margin of the nasal cavity.
- The ethmoid bone serves as the core of the skull and face, with the prominent crista galli protruding into the cranium and the perpendicular plate dividing the nasal cavities.
- The frontal, parietal, temporal, and occipital bones of the skull overlie the lobes of the brain of the same names.
- The sphenoid bone has a marked presence in the braincase, with the prominent greater and lesser wings of sphenoid lateral to the corpus.
- The hypophyseal fossa houses the pituitary gland.

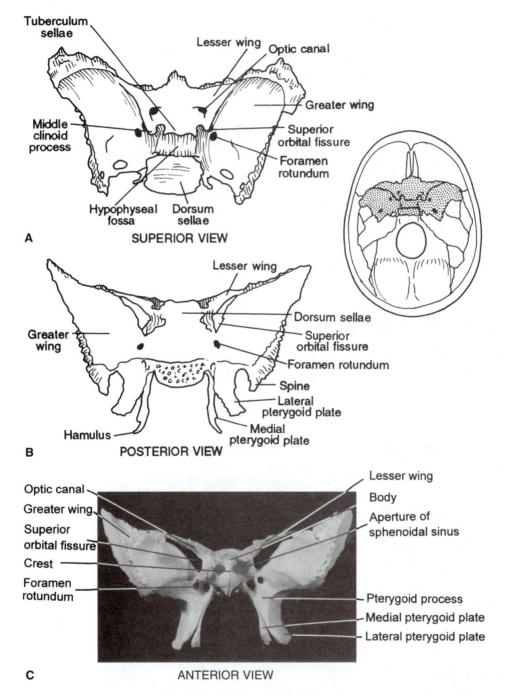

FIGURE 4-15. Schematics of superior and posterior sphenoid, and photograph of anterior view of sphenoid.

Table 4–2. Terms Related to Dentition

Surfaces

Medial/mesial	Surface of individual tooth closest to midline point on arch between central incisors.
Distal	Surface of individual tooth most distant from midline point on arch between central incisors.
Buccal	Surface of a tooth that could come in contact with the buccal wall.
Lingual	Surface of a tooth that could come in contact with the tongue.
Occlusal	The contact surface between teeth of the upper and lower arches.

Development

Intraosseous eruption	Eruption of teeth through the alveolar process.
Clinical eruption	Eruption of teeth into the oral cavity.
Successional teeth	Teeth that replace deciduous teeth.
Superadded teeth	Teeth in the adult arch not present within the deciduous arch.
Supernumerary	Teeth in excess of the normal number for an arch.

Dental Occlusion

Overjet	Normal projection of upper incisors beyond lower incisors.
Overbite	Normal overlap of upper incisors relative to lower incisors.
Class I occlusal relationship	Relationship between upper and lower teeth in which the first molar of the mandibular arch is one-half tooth advanced of the maxillary molar.
Class I malocclusion	Occlusal relationship in which there is normal orientation of the molars but an abnormal orientation of the incisors.
Class II malocclusion	Relationship of upper and lower arches in which the first mandibular molars are retracted at least one tooth from the first maxillary molars.
Class III malocclusion	Relationship of upper and lower arches in which the first mandibular molar is advanced greater than one tooth beyond the first maxillary molar.
Relative micrognathia	Condition in which mandible is small in relation to the maxillae.

Axial Orientation

Torsiversion	An individual tooth is rotated or twisted on its long axis.
Labioverted	An individual tooth tilts toward the lips.
Linguaverted	An individual tooth tilts toward the tongue.
Buccoversion	An individual tooth tilts toward cheek.
Distoverted	An individual tooth tilts away from midline of dental arch.
Mesioverted	An individual tooth tilts toward the midline of the dental arch.
Infraverted	A tooth is inadequately erupted.
Supraverted	A tooth protrudes excessively into the oral cavity, causing inadequate occlusion of other dentition.
Persistent open bite	Front teeth do not occlude because of excessive eruption of posterior teeth.
Persistent closed bite	Posterior teeth do not occlude because of excessive eruption of anterior dentition.

Supraorbital
margin

Zygomatic
process

ANTERIOR VIEW

FIGURE 4-16. Anterior view of frontal bone.

DENTITION

The teeth are vital components of the speech mechanism. Housed in the alveoli of the maxillae and mandible, teeth provide the mechanism for mastication, as well as articulatory surfaces for several speech sounds. Before we discuss the specific teeth, let us begin with an orientation to the dental arch. The upper and lower dental arches contain equal numbers of teeth of four types: incisors, cuspids, bicuspids, and molars (Figure 4-20 and Table 4-2).

Generally, teeth in the upper arch are larger than those in the lower arch, and the upper arch typically overlaps the lower arch in front. Each tooth has a *root*, hidden beneath the protective gingival, or gum, line (see Figure 4-21). The *crown* is the visible one third of the tooth, and the juncture of the crown and root is the *neck*. The surface of the crown is composed of the *dental enamel*, an extremely hard surface that overlies the *dentin*, or ivory, of the tooth. At the heart of the tooth is the *pulp*, in which the nerve supplying the tooth resides. The tooth is held in its socket by *cementum*, which is a thin layer of bone. As teeth shift from pressures (such as the forces accompanying tongue thrust), the cementum develops to ensure that the tooth remains firmly in its socket.

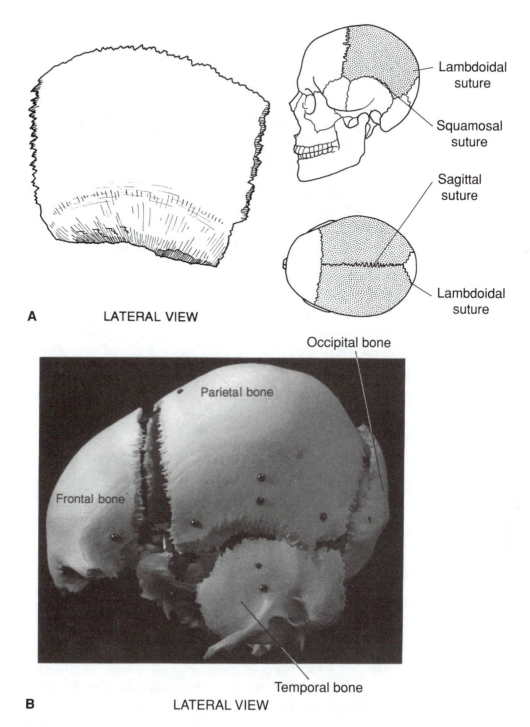

FIGURE 4-17. A. Lateral view of parietal bone. **B.** Photo of disarticulated parietal, frontal, temporal, and occipital bones.

Craniosynostosis

As an infant develops, the sutures of the skull become ossified, a process called synostosis. Complete synostosis normally occurs well into childhood, but in some instances synostosis occurs prenatally. Continued normal growth of the brain, especially during the first postnatal year, places pressure on the skull. The effects of premature synostosis on skull development, or craniosynostosis, are profound. With premature sagittal synostosis, the child's head becomes peaked along the suture and elongated in back. In Apert syndrome, a genetic condition, the affected child's stereotypic "peaked head" is the result of premature closure of the coronal suture, resulting in pronounced bulging along that articulation.

Five surfaces are important to remember when discussing teeth. To understand the terminology you need to alter your thinking about the dental arch a bit. Examine Figure 4-22 and you will see that the center of the dental arch is the point between the two central incisors, in front. Follow the arch around toward the molars in back and you have traced a path distal to those incisors. That is, *medial* refers to movement along the arch toward the midline between the central incisors, and *distal* refers to movement along the arch away from that midpoint. From this you can see that the *medial*, or *mesial*, *surface* of any tooth is the surface "looking" along the arch toward the midpoint between the central incisors. The *distal surface* is the surface of any tooth that is farthest from that midline point. Every tooth has a medial and a distal surface.

The *buccal surface* of a tooth is that which could come in contact with the buccal wall (cheek), and the *lingual surface* is the surface facing the tongue. The *occlusal surface* is the contact surface between teeth of the upper and lower arches. Not surprisingly, the thickest enamel overlays the occlusal surface because it receives the most abrasion.

Incisors clearly are designed for cutting, as their name implies (see Figure 4-23). The *central incisors* of the upper dental arch present a large, spadelike tooth with a thin cutting surface. The *lateral incisors* present a smaller but similar surface.

The *cuspid* (also canine; eyetooth) is well named. It has a single *cusp*, or point, that is used for tearing. In carnivores this tooth is particularly

FIGURE 4-18. A. Posterior and lateral views of the occipital bone (shaded areas). **B.** Occipital bone seen from inferior and superior aspects. **C.** Photo of occipital bone, inferior view.

FIGURE 4-19. Schematic and photo of lateral view of the temporal bone.

well suited for separating the fibers of muscle to permit meat eating. Lateral to the cuspids are the *first* and *second bicuspids*, or *premolars*. These teeth have two cusps on the occlusal surface, and they are absent from the deciduous dental arch.

Molars are large teeth with great occlusal surfaces designed to grind material, and their placement in the posterior arch capitalizes on the significant force available in the muscles of mastication. This mix of cutting teeth (incisors, cuspids, bicuspids) and grinding

MAXILLARY DENTAL ARCH

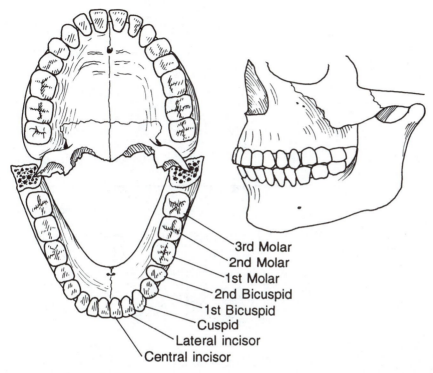

3rd Molar
2nd Molar
1st Molar
2nd Bicuspid
1st Bicuspid
Cuspid
Lateral incisor
Central incisor

MANDIBULAR DENTAL ARCH

FIGURE 4–20. Permanent dental arches.

teeth (molars) is just right for *omnivorous* humans: We will eat virtually anything! There are three molars in each half of the adult dental arch.

Dental Development

Dental development clearly parallels that of the individual. Infants develop **deciduous**, or *shedding, teeth* (also known as milk teeth) that give way to the *permanent teeth* that must last a lifetime. Deciduous teeth actually begin to grow early in prenatal development and start erupting through the bone (**intraosseous eruption**) and the gum (**clinical eruption**) between 6 and 9 months of age.

Deciduous (shedding) teeth:
The primary set of teeth.

Intraosseous eruption:
Eruption of dentition through the bone.

Clinical eruption: Eruption of dentition through the gum.

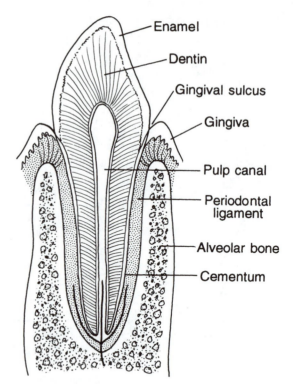

FIGURE 4-21. Components of a tooth.

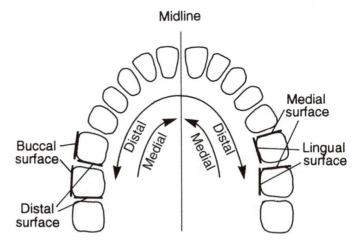

FIGURE 4-22. Surface referents of teeth and the dental arch.

Dental Anomalies

There are numerous developmental dental anomalies. Children may be born with supernumerary teeth (teeth in addition to the normal number), or teeth may be smaller than appropriate for the dental arch (microdontia). Teeth may fuse together at the root or crown. In addition, enamel may be extremely thin or even missing from the surface of the tooth (amelogenesis imperfecta), or the enamel may be stained from excessive use of the antibiotic tetracycline or fluoride.

Supernumerary teeth arise from a developmental anomaly in which the embryonic dental lamina produces excessive numbers of tooth buds. When this occurs, the individual is born with more teeth than predicted, often resulting in "twinning" of incisors. Below is a report from J. M. Harris, D.D.S., of a child he saw in his dental practice in Idaho Falls, Idaho.

An 8-year-old girl was brought to Dr. Harris's clinic with the complaint that one of her deciduous teeth needed to be extracted due to the patient's age. Dr. Harris performed pan-elipse radiography to verify that the permanent teeth were present prior to the extraction, but the X ray revealed supernumerary teeth in the left mandibular arch in the bicuspid region.

Extraction of the decayed deciduous tooth revealed a pocket of 15 supernumerary teeth: Some were simply tooth buds, but some had developed small roots and looked like fully formed molars. In an arch built ultimately for 16 teeth, that would be a significant addition!

The cluster was removed, Gelfoam was placed in the cavity, and sutures closed the space. There were no complications.

Tooth buds form when the developing mandible and maxillae are only 1 mm long, but by birth the buds have spread out to match the jaw, which is 40 times longer. These teeth are not only much smaller than adult teeth, matching the size of the arch, but there are fewer of them. Generally, central incisors emerge first (lower, then upper), followed by lateral incisors (upper, then lower). The first molars emerge at approximately the same time as the cuspids

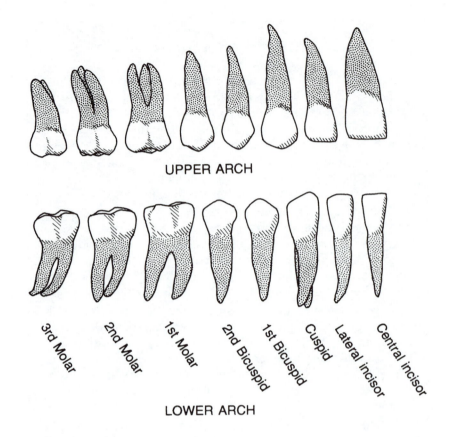

UPPER ARCH

3rd Molar 2nd Molar 1st Molar 2nd Bicuspid 1st Bicuspid Cuspid Lateral incisor Central incisor

LOWER ARCH

FIGURE 4–23. Types of teeth.

(between 15 and 20 months), and the second molars will have erupted by the second birthday. You will notice that there is no third molar or first or second bicuspids. These teeth are reserved for the adult arch. Each deciduous arch has 10 teeth, whereas the adult arch has 16 (see Figure 4-24).

Your first-grade school photograph will remind you of the period during which *shedding* begins. That gap-toothed grin of the 6-year-old child comes from shedding of the deciduous arch, beginning with the incisors (6 through 9 years), followed by first molars and cuspids (9 to 12 years), and finally second molars (beginning around 10 years of age).

FIGURE 4-24. Age of eruption of teeth in the permanent and deciduous arches.

The permanent teeth that replace deciduous teeth are called **successional teeth**. The third molar and bicuspids erupt in addition to the original constellation, and thus are referred to as *superadded*.

Successional teeth: Teeth in the mature dental arch that replace corresponding teeth of the deciduous arch.

Dental Occlusion

Occlusion is the process of bringing the upper and lower teeth into contact, and proper occlusion is essential for successful mastication. We will discuss orientation of the upper and lower dental arches, as well as orientation that the individual teeth can take within the

Occlusion: Closing.

Class I occlusal relationship (neutroclusion): The normal occlusal relationship characterized by the maxillary and mandibular molar relationship in which the maxillary first molar is retracted one-half tooth relative to the mandibular first molar.

Overjet: Condition of normal dentition in which the upper incisors project beyond the lower incisors.

Neutroclusion: The normal occlusal relationship characterized by the maxillary and mandibular molar relationship in which the maxillary first molar is retracted one-half tooth relative to the mandibular first molar.

Class II malocclusion: The occlusal relationship characterized by the maxillary and mandibular molar relationship in which the maxillary first molar is retracted at least one tooth relative to the mandibular first molar.

Micrognathia: Small mandible relative to the maxillae.

Class III malocclusion: The occlusal relationship characterized by the maxillary and mandibular molar relationship in which the maxillary first molar is advanced at least one tooth relative to the mandibular first molar.

Torsiversion: Twisted on the long axis.

Labioversion: Tilted toward the lip.

Linguaversion: Tilted toward the tongue.

Buccoversion: Tilted toward the cheek.

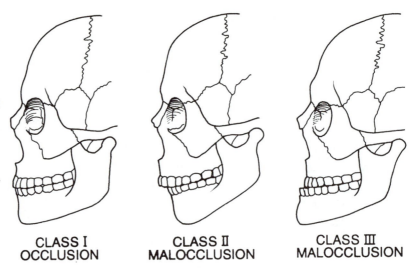

CLASS I OCCLUSION   CLASS II MALOCCLUSION   CLASS III MALOCCLUSION

FIGURE 4–25. Types of malocclusion.

arches. A **Class I occlusal relationship** between your upper and lower teeth is that in which the first molar of the mandibular arch is one-half tooth advanced of the first maxillary molar. The upper incisors project beyond the lower incisors vertically by a few millimeters (**overjet**), and the upper incisors naturally hide the lower incisors (overbite) so that only a little of the lower teeth will show. This Class I occlusion (also known as **neutroclusion**) (see Figure 4-25) is the normal relationship between the molars of the dental arches. Extreme overbite, however, can be clinically significant.

In **Class II malocclusion**, the first mandibular molars are retracted at least one tooth behind the first maxillary molars. This is sometimes the product of relative **micrognathia**, a condition in which the mandible is small in relation to the maxillae.

A **Class III malocclusion** is identified if the first mandibular molar is advanced farther than one tooth ahead of the first maxillary molar. Thus, in Class II malocclusion the mandible is retracted, whereas in Class III the mandible is protruded.

Individual teeth can be misaligned as well. If a tooth is rotated or twisted on its long axis, it has undergone **torsiversion**. If it tilts toward the lips, it is as **labioverted**, whereas tilting toward the tongue is **linguaverted** (see Figure 4-26). When molars tilt toward the cheeks, it is called **buccoversion**. A tooth that tilts away from the

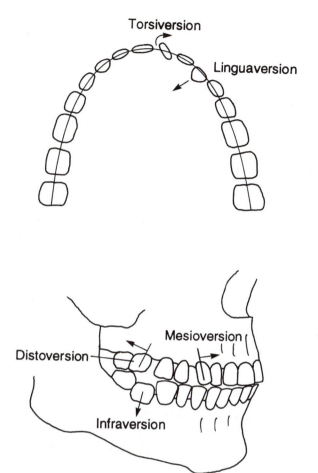

FIGURE 4-26. Graphic representation of torsiversion, linguaversion, infraversion, distoversion, and mesioversion.

Distoversion: Tilted away from the midline of the dental arch.
Mesioversion: Tilted toward the midline of the dental arch.
Infraversion: Inadequate eruption relative to the other teeth in the arch.
Supraversion: Excessive eruption relative to the majority of teeth in the arch.
Persistent open bite: Anterior dentition fails to occlude properly as a result of supraversion of the posterior teeth.
Persistent closed bite: Posterior dentition fails to occlude properly as a result of supraversion of the anterior teeth.

midline along the arch is **distoverted**, whereas one tilting toward that midline between the two central incisors is **mesioverted**. When a tooth does not erupt sufficiently to make occlusal contact with its pair in the opposite arch it is **infraverted**, whereas the tooth that erupts too far is **supraverted**. In some cases the front teeth do not demonstrate the proper occlusion because teeth in the posterior arch prohibit anterior contact, which is termed **persistent open bite**. If supraversion prohibits the posterior teeth from occlusion, it is called **persistent closed bite**.

Summary

- The teeth are housed in the alveoli of the maxillae and mandible and they consist of incisors, cuspids, bicuspids, and molars.
- Each tooth has a root and crown, with the surface of the crown composed of enamel overlying dentin.
- Each tooth has a medial, distal, lingual, buccal (or labial), and occlusal surface, and the occlusal surface reflects the function of the teeth in the omnivorous human dental arch.
- Clinical eruption of the deciduous arch begins between 6 and 9 months of age, and the permanent arch emerges between 6 and 9 years.
- Class I occlusion refers to normal orientation of mandible and maxillae; Class II malocclusion refers to a relatively retracted mandible; and Class III malocclusion refers to a relatively protruded mandible.
- Individual teeth may have aberrant orientation in the alveolus, including torsiversion, labioversion, linguaversion, distoversion, and mesioversion.
- Inadequately erupted or hypererupted teeth are referred to as infraverted and supraverted.

CAVITIES OF THE VOCAL TRACT

We mentioned that the source-filter theory depends on cavities to shape the acoustic output. Before we show you the muscles associated with articulation, let us discuss the cavities that are shaped by moving those muscles. These are the oral, buccal, nasal, and pharyngeal cavities (see Figure 4-27).

The *oral cavity* extends from the oral opening, or mouth, in front to the *faucial pillars* (also *fauces, faucial arches*) in back. The oral opening is strongly involved in articulation, being the point of exit of sound for all orally emitted phonemes (i.e., all sounds except those emitted nasally: see Figure 4-28).

This is a good opportunity to take a guided tour of your own mouth. Palpate the roof of your mouth (you can use your tongue to feel this if you wish). The hard roof of your mouth is the *hard palate*. The prominent ridges running laterally are the *rugae*, potentially useful structures in formation of the **bolus** of food during deglutition (swallowing) and serving as a landmark in articulation. The *median raphe* divides the hard palate into halves.

Bolus: *A mass of masticated food ready to be swallowed.*

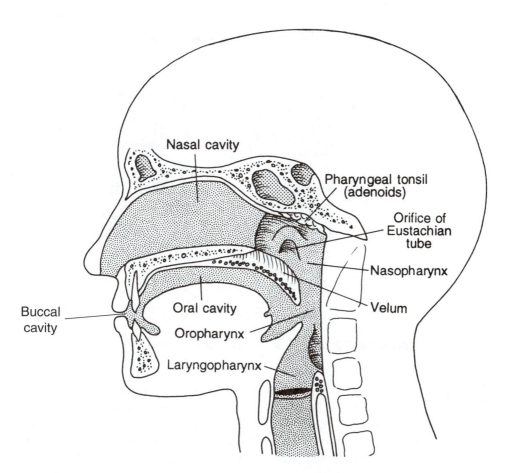

FIGURE 4–27. Oral, nasal, and pharyngeal cavities.

As you run your tongue or finger back along the roof of your mouth, you can feel the point at which the hard palate suddenly becomes soft. This is the juncture of the hard and soft palate. The soft portion is the *soft palate*, or *velum*, with the *uvula* marking the terminus of the velum. The velum is the movable muscle mass that separates the oral and nasal cavities (or more technically, the oropharynx and nasopharynx). The velum is attached in front to the palatine bone and is thus a muscular extension of the hard palate.

On each side of the soft palate and continuous with it are prominent bands of tissue. These are the *anterior* and *posterior faucial pillars* (also *posterior faucial arches*), and they mark the posterior margin of the oral cavity. The teeth and alveolar ridge of the maxillae make up the lateral margins of the oral cavity. The tongue occupies most of the lower mouth.

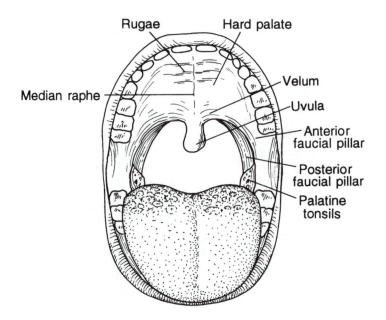

FIGURE 4–28. Anterior view of oral cavity.

Between the anterior and posterior faucial pillars you may see the *palatine tonsils*. These masses of lymphoid tissue are situated between the pillars on each side and even invade the lateral under-surface of the soft palate. Medial to these tonsils, on the surface of the tongue, are the *lingual tonsils*.

The *buccal cavity* lies lateral to the oral cavity, composed of the space between the posterior teeth and the cheeks of the face. It is bounded by the cheeks laterally, the lips in front, and the teeth medially. The posterior margin is at the third molar.

Although the oral cavity is fairly easy to view and palpate, only a small portion of the pharyngeal cavity is. The *pharyngeal cavity*, or pharynx, is broken into the oropharynx, laryngopharyx, and nasopharynx. The *oropharynx* is the portion of the pharynx immediately posterior to the fauces and bounded above by the velum. The lower boundary of the oropharynx is the hyoid bone. The *laryngopharynx* is bounded anteriorly by the epiglottis and inferiorly by the esophagus. The third pharyngeal space is the *nasopharynx*, the space above the soft palate. It is bounded in back by the pharyngeal protuberance of the occipital bone and in front by the nasal *choanae*. The lateral nasopharyngeal wall contains the orifice of the *eustachian*, or *auditory, tube*.

Although minute, the eustachian tube serves an extremely important function in that it provides a means of aerating the middle ear cavity. Recognize that the nasopharynx is on level with the ears, so that the tube connecting the nasopharynx with the middle ear space must course slightly up, back, and out to reach that cavity. The eustachian tube is actively opened through contraction of the tensor veli palatini muscle, as will be discussed.

Also in the nasopharynx is the pharyngeal tonsil (also known as adenoids). This mass of lymphoid tissue typically is found to arise from the base of the posterior nasopharynx. Removal of the adenoids from children with short or hypotrophied soft palates may result in persistent hypernasality.

Eustachian Tube Development

The eustachian tube is the communicative port between the nasopharynx and the middle ear cavity. It is opened during deglutition and yawning and provides a means of aeration of the middle ear cavity. In the adult, the eustachian courses down at an angle of about 45°. In the infant, the tube is more horizontal, with the shift in angle of descent brought about by head growth. It is thought that this horizontal course in the infant contributes to middle ear disease, the assumption being that liquids and bacteria have a low-resistance path to the middle ear from the nasopharynx of an infant being bottle-fed in the supine position.

The final cavities of concern to articulation are the nasal cavities (see Figure 4-29). The nasal cavities are produced by the paired maxillae, palatine, and nasal bones, and are divided by the nasal septum (made up of the singular vomer bone, the perpendicular plate of ethmoid, and the cartilaginous septum). The nasal cavities and turbinates are covered with mucous membrane endowed with beating and secreting epithelia, as well as a rich vascular supply. Air entering the nasal cavities is quickly warmed and humidified to protect the lungs, and fine nasal hairs help prevent particulate matter from entering the lower respiratory passageway. Beating epithelia propel encapsulated pollutants toward the nasopharynx, from which point they slowly work their way toward the esophagus, to be swallowed (a much better fate than to be deposited in the lungs).

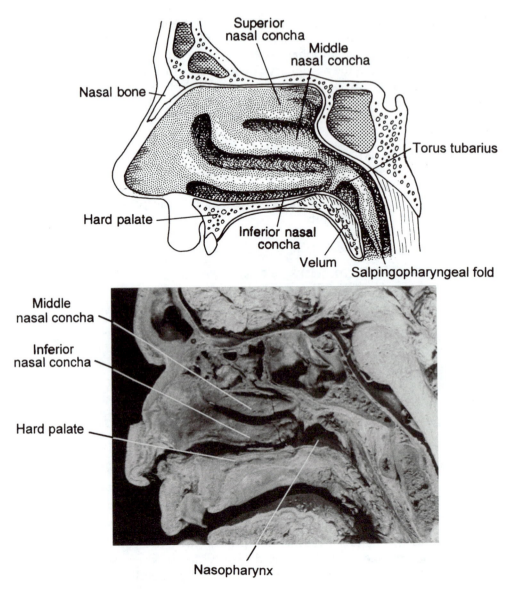

FIGURE 4-29. Nasal cavity and nasopharynx.

Nares: Nostrils.

The **nares**, or nostrils, mark the anterior boundaries of the nasal cavities and the nasal choanae are the posterior portals connecting the nasopharynx and nasal cavities. The floor of the nasal cavity is the hard palate of the oral cavity, specifically the palatine processes of maxillae and horizontal plates of the palatine bones.

Summary

- The most posterior of the tubes is the vertically directed pharynx, made up of the laryngopharynx, oropharynx, and nasopharynx.
- The horizontally coursing tube representing the nasal cavities arises from the nasopharynx, with the nasal and nasopharyngeal regions entirely separated from the oral cavity by elevation of the soft palate.
- The large tube representing the oral cavity is flanked by the small buccal cavities.
- The shape and size of the oral cavity is altered through movement of the tongue and mandible, and the nasal cavity may be coupled with the oral/pharyngeal cavities by means of the velum.
- The shape of the pharyngeal cavity is altered primarily by use of the pharyngeal constrictor muscles and by elevation or depression of the larynx.

Let us now examine the muscles involved in the articulatory system.

MUSCLES OF THE ARTICULATORY SYSTEM

The articulatory system is dominated by three significant structures: the lips, the tongue, and the velum. Movement of the lips for speech is a product of the muscles of the face. The tongue capitalizes on its own musculature and that of the mandible and hyoid for its movement. The muscles of the velum elevate that structure to separate the oral and nasal regions. Table 4-3 may assist you in organizing the muscles of the face and mouth, while Figure 4-30 will help you recognize their functions.

Table 4-3. Muscles of Articulation

Muscles of the Face

Orbicularis oris
Risorius
Buccinator
Levator labil superioris muscle
Zygomatic minor muscle
Levator labil superioris alaeque nasi muscle
Levator anguli oris muscle
Zygomatic major muscle
Depressor labil inferioris muscle
Depressor anguli oris muscle
Mentalis
Platysma

(continues)

Table 4-3. (*continued*)

Intrinsic Tongue Muscles

Superior longitudinal muscle of tongue
Inferior longitudinal muscle of tongue
Transverse muscle of tongue
Vertical muscle of tongue

Extrinsic Tongue Muscles

Genioglossus muscle
Hyoglossus muscle
Styloglossus muscle
Chondroglossus muscle
Palatoglossus muscle

Mandibular Elevators and Depressors

Masseter
Temporalis muscle
Medial pterygold muscle
Lateral pterygold muscle
Digastricus muscle
Mylohyoid muscle
Geniohyold
Platysma

Muscles of the Velum

Levator veli palatini muscle
Musculus uvulae
Tensor veli palatini muscle
Palatoglossus muscle
Palatopharyngeus muscle

Pharyngeal Musculature

Superior pharyngeal constrictor
Middle pharyngeal constrictor
Inferior pharyngeal constrictor
Cricopharyngeal muscle
Thyropharyngeus muscle
Salpingopharyngeus
Stylopharyngeus muscle

Muscles of the Face

The lips form the focus of the facial muscles; their movement largely determines their function in both facial expression and speech (see Figure 4-31). The lips comprise muscle and mucous membrane that

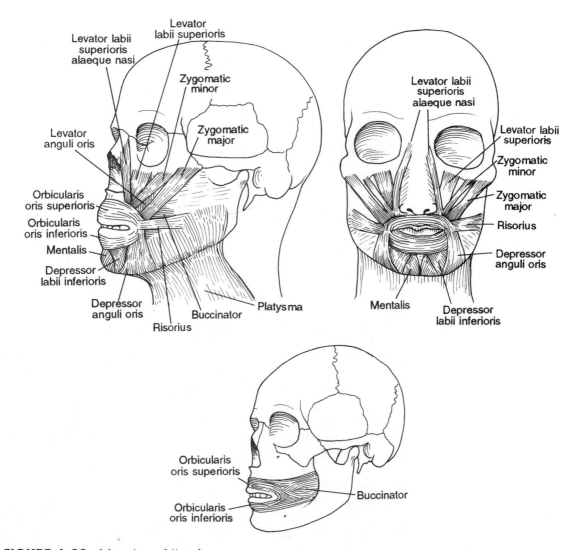

FIGURE 4–30. Muscles of the face.

is richly invested with vascular supply, a trait made apparent by the translucent superficial epithelia.

The *orbicularis oris* is really two muscles, the upper orbicularis oris and the lower orbicularis oris. The upper and lower orbicularis oris act much like a drawstring to pull the lips together and effect a labial seal. Both upper and lower orbicularis oris muscles are innervated by the VII facial nerve.

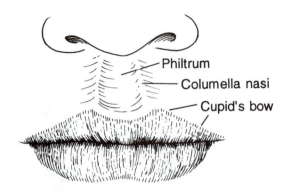

Philtrum
Columella nasi
Cupid's bow

FIGURE 4-31. Landmarks of the lips.

The upper and lower orbicularis oris serves as the point of insertion for many other muscles and interacts with the muscles of the face to produce the wide variety of facial gestures of which we are capable. The muscles inserting into the orbicularis oris have different effects, based on their course and point of insertion into the lips. The *risorius* and *buccinator* muscles insert into the corners of the mouth and retract the lips. The *depressor labii inferioris* depresses the lower lip, and the *levator labii superioris, zygomatic minor*, and *levator labii superioris alaeque nasi* muscles elevate the upper lip. The *zygomatic major* muscle elevates and retracts the lips, whereas the *depressor anguli oris* depresses the corner of the mouth. The *levator anguli oris* pulls the corner of the mouth up and medially.

The *buccinator muscle* ("bugler's muscle") lies deep to the risorius, following a parallel course. It originates on the *pterygomandibular ligament*, a tendinous slip running from the hamulus of the internal pterygoid plate of the sphenoid to the posterior mylohyoid line of the inner mandible. The posterior fibers are continuous with those of the superior pharyngeal constrictor. The buccinator courses forward to insert into the upper and lower orbicularis oris.

The buccinator, like the risorius, is involved primarily in mastication. The buccinator is used to move food onto the grinding surfaces of the molars, and contraction of this muscle tends to constrict the oropharynx. The risorius and buccinator are innervated by the VII facial nerve. The risorius muscle is superficial to the buccinator, originating from the posterior region of the face along the fascia of the masseter muscle. Besides assisting in mastication, the risorius muscles retract the lips at the corners, facilitating smiling.

The *levator labii superioris, zygomatic minor*, and *levator labii superioris alaeque nasi* share a point of insertion into the mid-lateral region of the upper lip. The three hold the major responsibility for elevation of the upper lip. The levator labii superioris alaeque nasi arises from the frontal process of maxilla, the levator labii superioris arises from the infraorbital margin of the maxilla, and the zygomatic minor arises from the zygomatic bone. Working together, these muscles dilate the oral opening, and fibers from the levator labii superioris alaeque nasi that insert into the wing of the nostril can flare the nasal opening. The levator labii superioris, zygomatic minor, and levator labii superioris alaeque nasi are innervated by the VII facial nerve.

The *levator anguli oris* arises from the canine fossa of the maxilla, coursing to insert into the upper and lower lips. This muscle is hidden by the levator labii superioris. The levator anguli oris draws the corner of the mouth up and medial. The levator anguli oris is innervated by the VII facial nerve.

The *zygomatic major* muscle arises lateral to the *zygomatic minor* on the zygomatic bone and inserts into the corner of the orbicularis oris. The zygomatic major elevates and retracts the angle of the mouth, as in smiling. The zygomatic major muscle is innervated by the buccal branches of the VII facial nerve.

The *depressor labii inferioris* originates from the mandible at the oblique line, coursing up and into the lower lip. Contraction of the depressor labii inferioris dilates the orifice of the mouth by pulling the lips down and out. The depressor labii inferioris is innervated by the VII facial nerve.

The *depressor anguli oris* originates along the lateral margins of the mandible on the oblique line. Its fanlike fibers converge on the orbicularis oris and upper lip at the corner. Contraction of the depressor anguli oris depresses the corners of the mouth and helps compress the upper lip against the lower lip. The depressor anguli oris is innervated by the VII facial nerve.

The *mentalis muscle* arises from the region of the incisive fossa of the mandible, inserting into the skin of the chin below. Contraction of the mentalis elevates and wrinkles the chin and pulls the lower lip out. The mentalis receives its innervation by means of VII facial nerve.

The *platysma* is more typically considered a muscle of the neck, but it is discussed here because of its function as a mandibular depressor.

The platysma arises from the fascia overlying the pectoralis major and deltoid, coursing up and into the corner of the mouth, the region below the symphysis mente, and the lower margin of the mandible, fanning as well to insert into the skin near the masseter. The platysma is highly variable but appears to assist in depression of the mandible. The platysma is innervated by the VII facial nerve.

Summary

- Numerous muscles insert into the orbicularis oris inferior and superior muscles, providing a flexible system for lip protrusion, closure, retraction, elevation, and depression.
- The risorius and buccinator muscles assist in retraction of the lips.
- Contraction of the levator labii superioris, zygomatic minor, and levator labii superioris alaeque nasi elevate the upper lip, and contraction of the depressor labii inferioris depresses the lower lip.
- Contraction of the zygomatic major muscle elevates and retracts the corner of the mouth, and the depressor labii inferioris pulls the lips down and out.
- The depressor anguli oris muscle depresses the corner of the mouth, the mentalis muscle pulls the lower lip out, and the platysma depresses the mandible.

Muscles of the Mouth

Musculature of the mouth is dominated by intrinsic and extrinsic muscles of the tongue, as well as those responsible for elevation of the soft palate.

The Tongue

The *tongue* is a massive structure that occupies the floor of the mouth (see Figure 4-32). We divide the muscles of the tongue into intrinsic and extrinsic musculature. The extrinsic muscles move the tongue into the general region desired and the intrinsic muscles tend to provide the fine, graded control of the articulatory gesture. Aside from its role in speech, the tongue is involved primarily in mastication and deglutition, being responsible for movement of food within the oral cavity to position it for chewing and to propel it backward for swallowing.

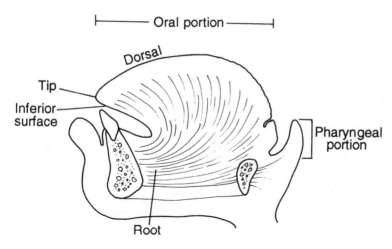

FIGURE 4-32. Demarcation of regions of the tongue.

The tongue is divided longitudinally by the *median fibrous septum*, a wall between right and left halves that serves as the point of origin for the transverse muscle of the tongue. The septum originates on the body of the hyoid bone via the *hyoglossal membrane*, forming the tongue attachment with the hyoid. The septum courses the length of the tongue.

It is useful to divide the tongue into regions as we discuss its characteristics (see Figure 4-33). The superior surface is the *dorsum*, and the anterior-most portion is the *tip*, or *apex*. The base of the tongue is the portion of the tongue that resides in the oropharynx. The portion of the tongue surface in the oral cavity is the *oral*, or *palatine, surface*, which makes up about two thirds of the surface of the tongue. The other third of the tongue surface, the *pharyngeal surface*, lies in the oropharynx.

Beneath the membranous lining of the pharyngeal surface of the tongue are *lingual tonsils*, groups of lymphoid tissue. Taken in conjunction with the pharyngeal and palatine tonsils, the lingual tonsils form the final portion of the ring of lymph tissue in the oral and pharyngeal cavities. Tonsils tend to *atrophy* (lose mass) over time. Although the pharyngeal and palatine tonsils may be quite prominent during childhood, they are markedly diminished by puberty.

The tongue is invested with sensors, or "taste buds." The tip of the tongue is sensitive to both sweet and sour tastes, and the sides of the tongue are sensitive only to sour tastes. Bitter tastes are sensed in the posterior tongue.

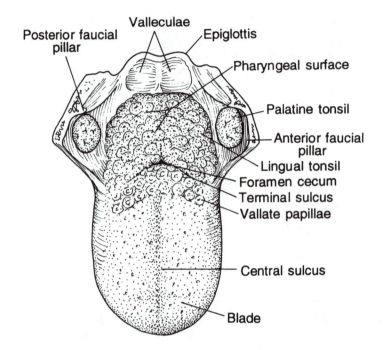

FIGURE 4-33. Landmarks of the tongue.

If you examine the inferior surface of your tongue in a mirror, you will see three important landmarks (see Figure 4-34). Notice the rich vascular supply on the under-surface. Medications administered under the tongue (sublingually) are absorbed very quickly into the bloodstream. The band of tissue running from the inner mandibular mucosa to the underside of the tongue is the *lingual frenulum,* or *lingual frenum.* Notice also the transverse band of tissue on the sides of the tongue (the *sublingual fold*). At this point reside the ducts for the sublingual salivary glands. Lateral to the lingual frenulum are the ducts for the *submandibular salivary glands* that are hidden under the mucosa on the inner surface of the mandible.

Intrinsic Tongue Muscles. The intrinsic muscles of the tongue include two pairs of muscles running longitudinally, as well as muscles coursing transversely and vertically. The intrinsic muscles interact in a complex fashion to produce the rapid, delicate articulations for speech and nonspeech activities. As we discuss each muscle, we

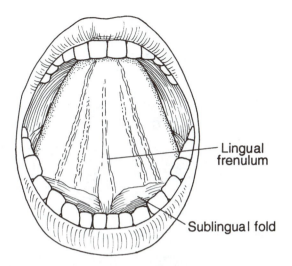

FIGURE 4-34. Inferior surface of tongue.

"Tongue Tie"

The lingual frenulum is a band of tissue that connects the tongue to the floor of the mouth. It appears to assist in stabilizing the tongue during movement, but occasionally it is too short for proper lingual function. This condition, colloquially referred to as "tongue tie," results in difficulty elevating the tongue for phonemes that require palatal or alveolar contact. The tongue may appear heart-shaped when protruded, resulting from the excessive tension on the midline by the short frenulum. A surgical procedure to correct the condition might be useful, although the surgery is not minor.

will tell you its basic function. Examination of Figure 4-35 will assist you in our discussion of these very important lingual muscles.

The paired *superior longitudinal muscles* course the length of the tongue, comprising the upper layer of the tongue. These muscles originate from the fibrous submucous layer near the epiglottis, the hyoid, and from the median fibrous septum. The fibers fan forward and outward to insert into the lateral margins of the tongue and region of the apex. The superior longitudinal muscles elevate the tip of the tongue. If one superior longitudinal muscle is contracted without the other, it pulls the tongue toward the side of contraction.

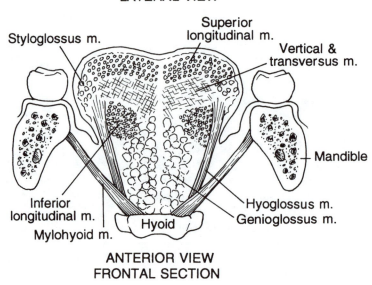

FIGURE 4–35. Intrinsic muscles of the tongue. (From data of Netter, 1997.)

The *inferior longitudinal muscle* originates at the root of the tongue and corpus hyoid, with fibers coursing to the apex of the tongue. This muscle occupies the lower sides of the tongue but is absent in the medial tongue base. The inferior longitudinal muscle pulls the tip of the tongue downward and assists in retraction of the tongue if cocontracted with the superior longitudinal. As with the superior

Tongue Thrust

As with other motor functions, swallowing changes and matures as the organism develops. The immature swallow capitalizes on the needs of the moment. An infant needs to compress his or her mother's nipple to stimulate release of milk, so the tongue moves forward naturally during this process. As the infant develops teeth, anterior movement of the tongue is blocked even as the need for it diminishes. The child begins eating semisolid and solid food, and chewing becomes more important than sucking. The mature swallow propels a bolus back toward the oropharynx, a maneuver that requires posterior direction of the tongue.

If the child fails to develop the mature swallow, he or she has a condition known as tongue thrust. The anterior direction of the tongue causes labioversion of the incisors. This child may have flaccid oral musculature, weak masseter action during swallow, and a disorganized approach to generation of the bolus. Considering that we swallow between 400 and 600 times per day, the immature swallow is difficult (but far from impossible) to reorganize into a mature swallow. Many speech-language pathologists specialize in oral myofunctional therapy directed toward remediation of such problems, a rewarding practice that results in (literally) smiling clients (see Ziekefoose, 1989).

longitudinal, unilateral contraction of the inferior longitudinal causes the tongue to turn toward the contracted side and downward.

The *transverse muscles of the tongue* provide a mechanism for narrowing the tongue. Fibers of these muscles originate at the median fibrous septum and course laterally to insert into the side of the tongue in the submucous tissue. The transverse muscle of the tongue pulls the edges of the tongue toward midline, effectively narrowing the tongue.

The *vertical muscles of the tongue* run at right angles to the transverse muscles and flatten the tongue. Fibers of the vertical muscle course from the base of the tongue and insert into the membranous cover. The fibers of the transverse and vertical muscles interweave. Contraction of the vertical muscles of the tongue pulls the tongue down into the floor of the mouth. Innervation of all intrinsic muscles of the tongue is by means of the XII hypoglossal nerve.

Extrinsic Tongue Muscles. The extrinsic muscles of the tongue tend to move the tongue as a unit. It appears that they set the general posture for articulation, with the intrinsic muscles performing the refined perfection of that gesture.

The *genioglossus* is the prime mover of the tongue, making up most of its bulk. The genioglossus (see Figure 4-36) arises from the inner mandibular surface at the symphysis and fans to insert into the tip and dorsum of the tongue, as well as to the corpus of the hyoid bone.

The genioglossus muscle occupies a medial position in the tongue, with the inferior longitudinal muscle, hyoglossus, and the styloglossus lateral to it. Fibers of the genioglossus insert into the entire surface of the tongue but are sparse to absent in the tip. Contraction of the anterior fibers of the genioglossus muscle retracts the tongue, whereas contraction of the posterior fibers draws the tongue forward to aid protrusion of the apex. If both anterior and posterior portions are contracted, the middle portion of the tongue will be drawn down into the floor of the mouth, functionally cupping the tongue along its length. The genioglossus is innervated by the XII hypoglossal nerve.

As the name implies, the *hyoglossus* arises from the length of the greater cornu and lateral body of the hyoid bone, coursing upward to insert into the sides of the tongue between the styloglossus and the inferior longitudinal muscles. The hyoglossus pulls the sides of the tongue down, in direct antagonism to the palatoglossus. The hyoglossus is innervated by the XII hypoglossal nerve.

If you examine Figure 4-36 again, you will see that the *styloglossus* originates from the anterolateral margin of styloid process of the temporal bone, coursing forward and down to insert into the inferior sides of the tongue. It divides into two portions, with one interdigitating with the inferior longitudinal muscle and the other with the fibers of the hyoglossus. Contraction of the styloglossus draws the tongue back and up. The styloglossus is innervated by the XII hypoglossal nerve.

The *chondroglossus muscle* is often considered part of the hyoglossus muscle. As with the hyoglossus, the chondroglossus arises from the hyoid (lesser cornu), coursing up to interdigitate with the intrinsic muscles of the tongue medial to the point of insertion of the hyoglossus. The chondroglossus is a depressor of the tongue. The chondroglossus is innervated by the XII hypoglossal nerve.

FIGURE 4-36. Genioglossus and related muscles of the tongue.

The *palatoglossus* can be functionally defined as a muscle of the tongue or of the velum, although it is more closely allied with palatal architecture and origin. It is described in a later section, but you should realize that it serves the dual purpose of depressing the soft palate or elevating the back of the tongue.

Summary

- The tongue is a massive structure that occupies the floor of the mouth. It is divided by a median fibrous septum that provides the origination for the transverse intrinsic muscle of the tongue.
- The tongue is divided into dorsum, apex (tip), and base.
- Fine movements are produced by contraction of the intrinsic musculature (transverse, vertical, inferior longitudinal, and superior longitudinal muscles of the tongue).
- Larger adjustments of lingual movement are completed through use of extrinsic muscles. The genioglossus retracts, protrudes, or depresses the tongue. The hyoglossus and chondroglossus depress the tongue, and the styloglossus and palatoglossus elevate the posterior tongue.

Muscles of Mastication: Mandibular Elevators and Depressors

The process of chewing food, or *mastication*, requires movement of the mandible so the molars can make a solid, grinding contact. The muscles of mastication are among the body's strongest, and the coordinated contraction of these muscles is required for proper preparation of food for swallowing. The muscles of mastication include the mandibular elevators (masseter, temporalis, medial pterygoid), muscles of protrusion (lateral pterygoid), and depressors (digastricus, mylohyoid, geniohyoid, platysma).

The *masseter* (see Figure 4-37) is the most superficial of the muscles of mastication. This massive muscle originates on the lateral, inferior, and medial surfaces of the zygomatic arch, coursing down to insert primarily into the ramus of the mandible, but some of the deeper fibers terminate on the coronoid process. The course and attachments of the masseter make it ideally suited for placing maximum force on the molars. Contraction of this muscle elevates the mandible. The masseter is innervated by the anterior trunk of the mandibular nerve arising from the V trigeminal.

The *temporalis muscle* is deep to the masseter, arising from a region of the temporal and parietal bones known as the temporal fossa (see

Palpation of the Oral Cavity

This palpation exercise would be well performed with one of your friends, and requires aseptic procedures. You will want to perform it under the guidance of your instructor, because this is a procedure that will carry into the oral peripheral examination in your clinical practice. A flashlight will help you identify structures.

Have your friend open her mouth as you look inside. Ensure that your nondominant hand (e.g., left hand if you are right-handed) is the only hand that holds or touches the flashlight; the other hand is gloved and must not touch anything but your friend. Ask your friend to say "ah" and watch the velum in back elevate. Look for presence or absence of the palatine tonsils between the faucial pillars. Shine the light on the hard palate and note the median raphe and rugae. Now palpate both of these structures, running your finger back along both sides of the median raphe of the hard palate. Palpate the margin of the hard and soft palates, being sensitive to the fact that this may elicit a gag reflex in some people. As you palpate the hard palate, be sensitive to the possible presence of occult (hidden; submucous) clefts of the hard palate.

Have your friend bite lightly on her molars and hold her teeth closed but lips open for an /i/ vowel. With the gloved finger, palpate the lateral margins of the teeth and gums. With a tongue depressor, move the cheeks away from the teeth and examine the relationship between the upper and lower teeth for occlusion.

Pull the lower lip down gently and examine the labial frenulum. Ask your friend to open her mouth and elevate her tongue, and examine the lingual frenulum.

Figure 4-38). The terminal tendon of the temporalis passes through the zygomatic arch and inserts in the coronoid process and ramus of the mandible. The temporalis elevates the mandible and draws it back if protruded. The temporalis is innervated by the temporal branches arising from the mandibular nerve of V trigeminal.

The *medial,* or *internal, pterygoid muscle* originates from the medial pterygoid plate and lateral fossa of the sphenoid. Fibers from the muscle course down and back to insert into the mandibular ramus. The medial pterygoid muscle elevates the mandible.

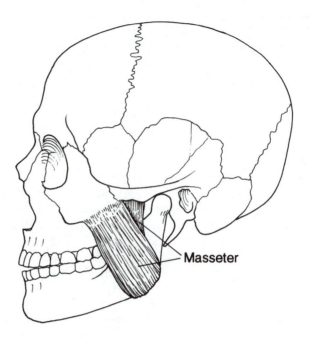

FIGURE 4-37. Graphic representation of the masseter muscle.

The *lateral*, or *external, pterygoid muscle* arises from the lateral ptery-goid plate and the greater wing of sphenoid. Fibers course back to insert into the pterygoid fovea of the mandible (see Figure 4-39). Contraction of the lateral pterygoid muscle protrudes the mandible. The lateral and medial pterygoid muscles are innervated by the mandibular branch of the V trigeminal nerve.

The dual-bellied *digastricus* is described in Chapter 3, so it is dis-cussed only briefly here. Digastricus anterior originates on the inner surface of the mandible at the digastricus fossa, near the symphysis, and the digastricus posterior originates on the mastoid process of the temporal bone. The anterior fibers and posterior fibers join by means of an intermediate tendon that inserts into the hyoid at the juncture of the hyoid corpus and greater cornu. If the hyoid bone is held in position by other muscles, contraction of the digastricus depresses the mandible. The anterior belly is innervated by the mandibular branch of the V trigeminal nerve. The posterior belly is innervated by the VII facial nerve.

The *mylohyoid* (described in Chapter 3) originates on the mylohyoid line of the mandible and inserts into the median fibrous raphe and hyoid bone, forming the floor of the mouth. With the hyoid fixed in

FIGURE 4–38. Graphic representation of the temporalis muscle.

position, the mylohyoid depresses the mandible. The mylohyoid is innervated by the alveolar nerve, arising from the V trigeminal nerve, mandibular branch.

Also described in Chapter 3, the *geniohyoid muscle* originates at the mental spines of the mandible and inserts into the corpus hyoid. Contraction of the geniohyoid depresses the mandible if the hyoid is fixed. The geniohyoid is innervated by means of the XII hypoglossal nerve. The *platysma* is discussed in the section Muscles of the Face.

Summary

- Mandibular elevators include the masseter, temporalis, and medial pterygoid muscles, and the lateral pterygoid protrudes the mandible.
- Depression of the mandible is performed by the mylohyoid, geniohyoid, and platysma muscles. The grinding action of the molars requires coordinated and synchronized contraction of the muscles of mastication.

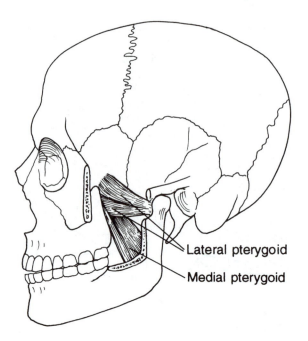

FIGURE 4-39. Lateral and medial pterygoid muscles.

Muscles of the Soft Palate

Only three speech sounds in English require that the soft palate be depressed (/m/, /ŋ/, and /n/). During most speaking time, the soft palate is actively elevated. We will discuss the general configuration of the soft palate and then discuss how we elevate and depress this important structure.

The *soft palate*, or *velum*, is actually a combination of muscle, aponeurosis, nerves, and blood supply covered by mucous membrane lining. The *palatal aponeurosis* makes up the mid-front of the soft palate, being an extension of an aponeurosis arising from the tensor veli palatini (described later). The palatal aponeurosis divides around the musculus uvulae, but serves as the point of insertion for other muscles of the soft palate. The *mucous membrane lining* is invested with lymph and mucous glands, and the oral side of the lining also has taste buds.

Muscles of the soft palate include elevators (levator veli palatini, musculus uvulae), a tensor (tensor veli palatini), and depressors (palatoglossus and palatopharyngeus). Although the superior constrictor muscle is a pharyngeal muscle, it is an important muscle for function of the soft palate. We will discuss the muscles of the pharynx following discussion of the muscles of the soft palate (see Figures 4-40 and 4-41).

The *levator veli palatini*, or *levator palati*, is the palatal elevator, making up the bulk of the soft palate (see Figure 4-40). This muscle arises from the petrous portion of the temporal bone and from the medial wall of the eustachian tube cartilage. The levator veli palatini courses down and forward to insert into the palatal aponeurosis of the soft palate. Contraction elevates and retracts the posterior velum. The levator veli palatini is innervated by the pharyngeal plexus, arising from the XI accessory and X vagus nerves.

The uvula makes up the medial and posterior portions of the soft palate, and the *musculus uvulae* is the muscle it embodies. This muscle arises from the posterior nasal spines of the palatine bones and from the palatal aponeurosis, and it inserts into the mucous membrane cover of the velum. Contraction of the uvula shortens the soft palate, effectively bunching it up. The musculus uvulae is innervated by the pharyngeal plexus, arising from the XI accessory and X vagus nerves.

The *tensor veli palatini* (tensor veli palati) may add some stability to the velum, but it is a major dilator of the eustachian tube. This muscle arises from the scaphoid fossa of the sphenoid bone and from the lateral eustachian tube wall. The fibers converge to course down to terminate in a tendon. The tendon passes around the pterygoid hamulus and then is directed medially. This tendon expands to become the palatal aponeurosis. Contraction of the tensor veli palatini stabilizes the soft palate and flattens it. It assists in dilating or opening the eustachian tube, thereby permitting aeration (exchange of air) of the middle ear cavity. This muscle is innervated by the V trigeminal nerve.

The *palatoglossus muscle* was discussed briefly as a muscle of the tongue. This muscle originates at the anterolateral palatal aponeurosis, coursing down to insert into the sides of the posterior tongue. This muscle helps to either elevate the tongue or depress the soft palate. The palatoglossus is innervated by the pharyngeal plexus, arising from the XI accessory and X vagus nerves.

Although classically considered a pharyngeal muscle, the *palatopharyngeus* is included in this discussion because of its role in velar

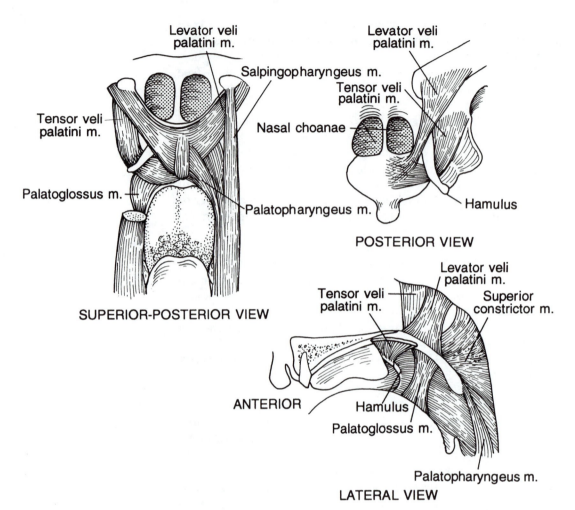

FIGURE 4-40. Muscles of the soft palate from superior-posterior (*left*), posterior (*top right*), and the side (*lower right*) views. (From data of Shprintzen & Bardach, 1995; Langley, Telford, & Christensen, 1969.)

function. Anterior fibers of the palatopharyngeus originate from the anterior hard palate, and posterior fibers arise from the midline of the soft palate posterior to the fibers of the levator veli palatini, attached to the palatal aponeurosis. Fibers of each muscle course laterally and down, forming the posterior faucial pillar and inserting into the posterior thyroid cartilage. It assists in narrowing the pharyngeal cavity and lowering the soft palate. The palatopharyngeus

FIGURE 4–41. **A.** Lateral view of pharyngeal constrictor muscles. **B.** Posterior view of pharyngeal constrictor musculature.

is innervated by the pharyngeal plexus, arising from the XI accessory and pharyngeal branch of the X vagus nerve.

Pharyngeal Musculature

Muscles of the pharynx are closely allied with those of the tongue, face, and larynx. It will help if you imagine the pharynx as a vertical tube. This tube is made of muscles wrapping more or less horizontally from the front to a midline point in the back, as well as by muscles and connective tissue running from skull structures. Thus, the pharynx is composed of a complex of muscles that when contracted constrict the pharynx to assist in deglutition.

Pharyngeal Constrictor Muscles

The superior, middle, and inferior constrictor muscles are the means by which the pharyngeal space is reduced in diameter. Of these, the superior constrictor is an important muscle of velopharyngeal function (see Figure 4-41).

The *superior pharyngeal constrictor* forms a tube originating at the *pterygomandibular raphe* (the point of attachment of the buccinator), the mylohyoid line of the mandible, and the sides of the tongue. It projects back from this structure on both sides to the median *pharyngeal raphe*, the midline tendonous component of the pharyngeal aponeurosis. This aponeurosis arises from the pharyngeal tubercle of the occipital bone and forms the upper sleeve of the pharyngeal wall by attaching to the temporal bone (petrous portion), medial pterygoid plate, and eustachian tube.

The median pterygoid plate gives rise to the uppermost fibers of the muscle, and these fibers are the "landing pad" for the soft palate, known as *Passavant's pad*. This pad of muscle at the posterior pharyngeal wall appears as a ridge at the point of articulation of the soft palate with the wall.

Contraction of the superior pharyngeal constrictor muscle pulls the pharyngeal wall forward and constricts the pharyngeal diameter, an especially prominent movement during swallowing. It assists in effecting the velopharyngeal seal. The superior pharyngeal constrictor is innervated by the XI accessory nerve in conjunction with the X vagus, via the pharyngeal plexus.

The *middle pharyngeal constrictor* arises from the horns of the hyoid bone and inserts into the median pharyngeal raphe. It narrows the diameter of the pharynx. The middle pharyngeal constrictor is innervated by the XI accessory nerve in conjunction with the X vagus, via the pharyngeal plexus.

The *inferior pharyngeal constrictor* arises from the cricoid and thyroid cartilages. The inferior portion, sometimes referred to as a separate muscle, the cricopharyngeal muscle, is an important muscle for swallowing. Contraction of the inferior constrictor reduces the diameter of the lower pharynx. The inferior pharyngeal constrictor is innervated by the XI accessory nerve in conjunction with the X vagus, via the pharyngeal plexus.

As the name implies, the *stylopharyngeus* arises from the styloid process of the temporal bone, coursing down between the superior and middle pharyngeal constrictors (see Figure 4-41). Some fibers insert into the constrictors, others insert into the posterior thyroid cartilage in concert with the palatopharyngeus muscle. The stylopharyngeus elevates and opens the pharynx, particularly during deglutition. The stylopharyngeus muscle is innervated by the muscular branch of the IX glossopharyngeal nerve.

Summary

- The levator veli palatini muscle elevates the soft palate, the musculus uvulae bunches the soft palate, and the tensor veli palatini tenses and shortens the palate.
- The soft palate is depressed by the palatoglossus and palatopharyngeus muscles.
- The superior pharyngeal constrictor assists in gaining velopharyngeal closure, and peristaltic movement of food is facilitated by the middle and inferior pharyngeal constrictors.
- The cricopharyngeal muscle, a component of the inferior constrictor, forms the muscular orifice of the esophagus.
- The stylopharyngeus assists in elevation of the pharynx.

Clearly, the structures of the articulatory system are extremely complex and mobile. We are capable of myriad movements that are incorporated into nonspeech and speech functions. Let us move on to articulatory physiology.

PHYSIOLOGY OF ARTICULATION AND RESONATION

In preparation for our discussion of the physiology of speech production, we will first discuss the biological functions from which the speech functions arise: mastication and deglutition. *Mastication* refers to the processes involved in food preparation, including moving unchewed food onto the grinding surface of the teeth, chewing it, and mixing it with saliva in preparation for swallowing. *Deglutition* refers to swallowing.

Mastication and Deglutition

Mastication and deglutition consist of a sequence of four events or stages: oral preparatory stage, oral stage of swallow, pharyngeal stage, and esophageal stage.

Oral Preparatory Stage

In the *oral preparatory stage*, food is prepared for swallowing (see Tables 4-4 and 4-5). First, we introduce food into the mouth and keep it there by tightly occluding the lips as we breathe through the nose. The tongue bunches up in back and the soft palate is pulled down to keep the food in the oral cavity with the aid of the palatoglossus muscle.

The food must be ground up so that it can pass through the esophagus for digestion. This is performed by the coordinated activity of the muscles of mastication and the lingual muscles. The tongue keeps food in the oral cavity by making a seal along the alveolar ridge. As it holds the food in place, it compresses it against the hard palate, partially crushing it in preparation for the teeth. The tongue then begins moving the food onto the grinding surfaces of the teeth, pulling the food back into the oral cavity to be mixed with saliva, and then moving it back to the teeth for more mastication. The salivary glands secrete saliva into the oral cavity to help form the mass of food into a bolus for swallowing. The risorius and buccinator muscles contract to keep the food from entering the lateral buccal cavity.

Oral Stage

When the bolus of food is finally ready to swallow, the *oral stage of swallowing* begins (Table 4-6). Several processes must occur sequentially.

Table 4–4. Muscles of the oral preparation stage required to effect oral seal, maintain buccal compression, tongue movements to move food onto grinding surface, and grinding action

Muscle	Function	Innervention (Cranial Nerve)
Facial Muscles		
Orbicularis oris	Maintain oral seal	VII
Mentalis	Elevate lower lip	VII
Buccinator	Flatten cheeks	VII
Risorius	Flatten cheeks	VII
Mandibular Muscles		
Masseter	Elevate mandible	V
Temporalis	Elevate mandible, retract, protrude	V
Medial pterygold	Elevate mandible, lateral movement, grind	V
Lateral pterygold	Protrude, grind	V
Tongue Muscles		
Mylohyoid	Elevate floor of mouth	V
Geniohyoid	Elevate hyoid, depress mandible	XII
Digastric	Elevate hyoid, depress mandible	V, XII
Superior longitudinal	Elevate tip, deviate tip	XII
Inferior longitudinal	Depress tip, deviate tip	XII
Vertical	Cupping and grooving of tongue	XII
Genioglossus	Tongue body movement, cupping of tongue	XII
Styloglossus	Elevate posterior tongue	XII
Palatoglossus	Elevate posterior tongue	IX, X, XI
Soft Palate Muscles		
Palatoglossus	Depress velum	IX, X, XI
Palatopharyngeus	Depress velum	X, XI

Table 4–5. Muscles of the oral stage required to propel the bolus into the oropharynx

Muscle	Function	Innervation (Cranial Nerve)
Mandibular Muscles		
Masseter	Elevate mandible	V
Temporalis	Elevate mandible	V
Internal Pterygoid	Elevate mandible	V
Tongue Muscles		
Mylohyoid	Elevate tongue and floor of mouth	V
Superior longitudinal	Elevate tip	XII
Vertical	Cupping and grooving of tongue	XII
Genioglossus	Tongue body movement, cupping of tongue	XII
Styloglossus	Elevate posterior tongue	XII
Palatoglossus	Elevate posterior tongue	IX, X, XI

Mastication stops and the anterior tongue elevates to the hard palate and squeezes the bolus back toward the faucial pillars.

Pharyngeal Stage

Propelling the bolus posteriorly during the oral stage causes the bolus to contact the fauces and the depressed velum. In younger individuals, the contact with the fauces and velum appears to trigger the reflexes of the pharyngeal stage; for the elderly these reflexes appear to be triggered as the bolus passes the region of the mandibular angle (viewed through fluoroscopy, in Logemann, 1998). The soft palate, which was depressed, elevates to close off the oropharynx from the nasopharynx. Respiration stops reflexively at this point. Both oral and nasal outlets are closed so air cannot escape or enter for respiration and food is ready to enter the pharynx. The airway must be protected. The vocal folds tightly adduct, and elevation of the larynx relative to the tongue base causes the epiglottis to drop over the laryngeal aditus. Simultaneously, the cricopharyngeus muscle relaxes, allowing the upper esophagus to open. When you are not swallowing it remains closed to keep food and gastric juices from escaping into the laryngopharynx (esophageal reflux). Elevation of the

Deficits of the Oral Preparatory Stage

Numerous problems arise when neuromuscular control and muscle strength associated with mastication are compromised. In addition, physical changes in the structure of the oral cavity can lead to problems of the oral preparation stage.

Loss of oral sensation and awareness, coupled with weak buccal musculature, can lead to pocketing of food in the buccal cavity (lateral sulcus) or between the teeth and the lip (anterior sulcus). Weak muscles of mastication can cause inadequately chewed food, and weak lingual muscles will result in poor mixture of saliva with the food, inadequate bolus generation, and difficulty compressing the bolus onto the hard palate. If the muscles of the soft palate are compromised, the velum may not be fully depressed and the tongue may not be elevated in the back, permitting food to escape into the pharynx prior to initiation of the pharyngeal reflexes. This is life-threatening because food entering the pharynx in absence of reflexive response may reach the open airway. Aspiration pneumonia (pneumonia secondary to aspirated matter) is a constant concern for individuals with **dysphagia** (a disorder of swallowing).

Dysphagia: Disorder of swallowing.

Deficits of the Oral Stage

Deficits of the oral stage can arise from sensory and motor dysfunction, as well as from structural problems. Weakened movements cause increased posterior transit time of the bolus toward the pharynx. Indeed, some people are so weak that they have difficulty propelling a thick bolus (for instance, mashed potatoes) to the pharynx. Structural problems, such as partial glossectomy (removal of a portion of the tongue) or palatal fistula (opening in the hard palate that is either developmentally present or secondary to a surgical procedure) can result in oral stage deficit as well.

Table 4–6. Muscles of the pharyngeal stage required to propel the bolus toward the esophagus, elevate larynx, and to close the airway

Muscle	Function	Innervation (Nerve)
Tongue Muscles		
Mylohyoid	Elevate hyoid and tongue	V
Geniohyoid	Elevate hyoid and larynx, depress mandible	C-1
Digastricus	Elevate hyoid and larynx	V, XII
Genioglossus	Retract tongue	XII
Styloglossus	Elevate posterior tongue	XII
Palatoglossus	Narrow fauces, elevate posterior tongue	IX, X, XI
Stylohyoid	Elevate hyoid and larynx	VII
Hyoglossus	Elevate hyoid	XII
Thyrohyoid	Elevate hyoid	XII
Superior longitudinal	Elevate tongue	XII
Inferior longitudinal	Depress tongue	XII
Transverse	Flatten tongue	XII
Vertical	Narrow tongue	XII
Soft Palate Muscles		
Levator veli palatini	Elevate soft palate	X, XI
Tensor veli palatini	Tense soft palate	V
Musculus uvulae	Shorten soft palate	X, XI
Pharyngeal Muscles		
Palatopharyngeus	Constrict oropharynx to channel bolus	X, XI
Salpingopharyngeus	Elevate pharynx	XI
Stylopharyngeus	Raise larynx	IX
Cricopharyngeus	Relax esophageal orifice	X, XI
Middle constrictor	Narrow pharynx	X, XI
Inferior constrictor	Narrow pharynx	X, XI
Laryngeal Muscles		
Lateral cricoarytenoid	Adduct vocal folds	X
Transverse arytenoid	Adduct vocal folds	X
Oblique arytenoid	Adduct vocal folds	X
Aryepiglottic	Retract epiglottis, constrict aditus	X
Thyroepiglottic	Retract epiglottis	X

Deficits of the Pharyngeal Stage

Sensory, motor, and structural deficits contribute to pharyngeal stage dysphagia. Slowed velar elevation during the pharyngeal swallow may result in **nasal regurgitation** (loss of food or liquid through the nose); reduced sensation at the fauces, posterior tongue, pharyngeal wall, and soft palate may result in an elevated threshold for triggering the swallowing reflex. Reduced function of the pharyngeal constrictors may result in slowed pharyngeal transit time of the bolus, in which case the individual may prematurely re-initiate respiration. Laryngeal elevation relative to the tongue normally causes the epiglottis to invert, covering the laryngeal aditus. Reduced laryngeal elevation during swallow may prevent the epiglottis from covering the larynx, resulting in residue left in the valleculae. Further, laryngeal elevation helps to open the relaxed esophageal sphincter, so that failure of elevation may result in food remaining in the airway at the level of the upper esophageal sphincter after respiration has resumed. This food can easily find its way into the airway, resulting in aspiration and life-threatening pneumonia.

Nasal regurgitation: Loss of masticated food through the nasal cavity.

---

larynx during the pharyngeal stage facilitates opening of the upper esophageal sphincter.

Food is propelled down the pharynx toward the esophagus by means of contraction of the pharyngeal constrictors. As food is forced into the oropharynx, the posterior faucial pillars move medially, effectively channeling the bolus downward.

After about 1 second of pharyngeal transit, the bolus reaches the laryngopharynx where it passes over the epiglottis. The bolus is divided into two roughly equal masses, passing on the sides of the larynx, through the pyriform sinuses, to recombine at the esophageal entrance.

Esophageal Stage

The *esophageal stage* is out of voluntary control. It begins when the bolus reaches the orifice of the esophagus. The bolus is transported through the esophagus to the inferior esophageal sphincter by peristaltic contraction and gravity, arriving at the stomach for the process of digestion after 10 to 20 seconds of transit time. When the bolus enters the esophagus, the cricopharyngeus again contracts, the larynx and soft palate drop down, and respiration begins again. In the normal swallow, respiration is suspended for only about a second. Because most individuals begin the pharyngeal swallow following a respiratory inspiration, they exhale when the swallow is completed. This expiration expels any residual food at the laryngeal entryway, which is blown clear and propelled to the esophagus.

Summary

- In the oral preparation stage, food is introduced into the oral cavity, moved onto the molars for chewing, and mixed with saliva to form a concise bolus between the tongue and hard palate.
- In the oral stage, the bolus is moved back by pressure of movement of the tongue on the hard palate.
- The pharyngeal stage begins when the bolus reaches the faucial pillars. The soft palate and larynx elevate, the vocal folds tightly adduct, the epiglottis depresses, the cricopharyngeal muscle relaxes, and the lower esophageal sphincter opens. Food passes through the valleculae at the base of the tongue, over the epiglottis, and through the pyriform sinuses to the esophagus.
- The esophageal stage involves peristaltic movement of the bolus through the esophagus to the lower esophageal sphincter.

Speech Function

Speech production requires execution of an extremely well-organized and well-integrated sequence of neuromotor events. The orbicularis oris is primarily responsible for ensuring a labial seal, but numerous facial muscles insert into it. The lower lip achieves a greater velocity and force than the upper lip, and it does most of the work in lip closure. Extra force is exerted by the mentalis muscle.

The mandible assists the lips, and changes its position for tongue movement. The mandible is an extremely important articulator in its supportive role of carrying the lips, tongue, and teeth to their targets in the maxilla (lips, teeth, alveolar ridge, hard palate), but its adjustments are rather minute in normal speech. In speech, the mandibular elevators and depressors stay in dynamic balance, so that slight

Mouth Breathing

Chronic mouth breathing is more than an unpleasant habit because it is at the root of facial malformation and hearing loss. Mouth breathing is attributed to hypertrophy of the tonsilar ring, prohibiting adequate nasal respiration. In children with this condition, the adenoids are frequently enlarged, blocking the nasal choanae and also the orifice of the eustachian tube. Inadequate ventilation of the middle ear cavity may result in otitis media (inflammation of the middle ear cavity). Chronic otitis media is often associated with fluid in the middle ear (serous otitis media), a condition resulting in conductive hearing impairment.

The hypertrophy also makes mouth breathing mandatory. During normal nasal respiration, the tongue maintains fairly constant contact with the upper alveolar ridge and hard palate; but with the mouth open constantly for respiration, the tongue exerts little pressure there. Without that pressure, the dental arch narrows and the palate bulges upward to an extreme vault as the facial bones develop. With narrow dental arches, the permanent teeth do not have adequate space, and so they become crowded and prone to caries (decay of bone or tooth). The narrowed maxillae cause the upper lip to pull up, exposing the upper front teeth. The nasal cavity becomes narrow, increasing the probability of later nasal obstruction. The look of "adenoid facies" includes an open mouth, narrow mandible, and dental crowding. Coupled with a persistent conductive hearing loss, mouth breathing presents a sizable (yet generally preventable) deficit to the developing child.

modification in muscle activation (and inhibition of antagonists) permits a quick adjustment of the mandible.

The tongue is the most important articulator. It is involved in production of the majority of English phonemes. A summary of tongue movements is presented in Table 4-7.

You can think of the tongue as a group of highly organized (intrinsic) muscles being carried on the "shoulders" of the extrinsic muscles. Much as the muscles of the legs and trunk move your upper body to a position where your arms and head can interact with the environment, the extrinsic muscles set the basic posture of the

Table 4-7. Muscles of Tongue Movement

Movement	Muscle
Elevate tongue tip	Superior longitudinal muscles
Depress tongue tip	Inferior longitudinal muscles
Deviate tongue tip	Simultaneous contraction of either left or right superior and inferior longitudinal muscles for left or right deviation
Relax lateral margin	Posterior genioglossus for protrusion; superior longitudinal for tip elevation; transverse intrinsic pulls sides medially
Narrow tongue	Transverse Intrinsic
Deep central groove	Genioglossus depresses tongue body; vertical intrinsic depresses central dorsum
Broad central groove	Moderate genioglossus to depress tongue body; vertical intrinsic depresses dorsum; superior longitudinal elevates margins
Protrude tongue	Posterior genioglossus advances body; vertical muscles narrow tongue; superior and inferior longitudinal balance and point tongue
Retract tongue	Anterior genioglossus retracts into oral cavity; superior and inferior longitudinal shorten tongue; styloglossus retracts into pharyngeal cavity
Elevate posterior tongue	Palatoglossus elevates sides; transverse intrinsic bunches tongue
Depress tongue body	Genioglossus contraction depresses medial tongue; hyoglossus and chondroglossus depress sides if hyoid is fixed by Infrahyoid muscles

Unilateral Tongue Weakness

One element of the oral-peripheral examination is evaluation of relative tongue strength. When you ask a client to push forcefully with his or her tongue sideways against a resistance, you are interested in identifying whether the client has adequate strength and symmetrical strength. If there appears to be greater strength in one direction than the other, the speech-language pathologist will consider activities to strengthen the musculature. Improving muscle strength will improve tone and muscle control.

tongue, whereas the intrinsic muscles have a great deal of responsibility for the microstructure of articulation. The two groups of muscles work together closely to achieve the target articulatory gesture.

Velum (Soft Palate)

Early in the history of our field we found it tempting to treat the velum as a binary element: It was either opened or closed. We have since realized that its function is more complex. The velum is capable of a range of motion and rate of movement that matches the needs of rapid speech and nonspeech functions.

The velum generally is closed for non-nasal speech, and this is the result of contraction of the levator veli palatini, a direct antagonist to the palatoglossus muscle. In speech, opening and closing of the velar port must occur precisely and rapidly, or the result will be hyper- or hyponasality. Failure to open the port turns a 70-ms nasal phoneme into a voiced stop consonant, an unacceptable result. The soft palate opens and closes in coordination with the other articulators, thus preventing nasal resonance on other phonemes (assimilation). In reality, some nasal assimilation is inevitable and acceptable, and in some geographic regions, dialectically appropriate.

Production of high-pressure consonants (such as fricatives and stops) requires greater velopharyngeal effort to seal air in the oral cavity. To accomplish this seal, additional help is needed from the tensor veli palatini, superior pharyngeal constrictor, and uvular muscles. Even then, the pressures for speech are far less than those

> ## Effects of Neuromuscular Disease on Velopharyngeal Function
>
> A deficit associated with the velum can have significant effects on speech. In neuromuscular disorders, such as amyotrophic lateral sclerosis and multiple sclerosis, muscular weakness arises from damage to the myelin sheath of the axons of motor neurons. When the weakness involves the muscles of the velum, the nasal cavity resonance is added to that of the oral cavity for non-nasal sounds. This "anti-resonance," as it is called, pulls energy out of the speech signal in the 1,500 Hz to 2,500 Hz range, causing a marked loss of clarity in the speech signal. Speech of the affected individual sounds muffled, monotone, and low in vocal intensity.
>
> It is not uncommon for the speech-language pathologist to be the first person approached by an individual with early signs of neuromuscular disease. The velum requires constant elevation for non-nasal sounds and is an early indicator of progressive muscular weakness. An individual may come to the clinician with the complaint that people say his or her speech sounds muffled. Your supervisor's oral-peripheral examination will reveal slow velar activity, and the person may be referred to a physician.

for, say, actions required in playing a wind instrument. Some individuals have difficulty avoiding nasal air escape when playing in the brass section but have perfectly normal speech.

Summary

- Movement of the mandible for speech is slight compared with movement for chewing. In addition, the mandibular posture for speech is one of sustained dynamic tension between antagonists.
- The tongue is an extremely versatile organ, with the extrinsic muscles providing the major movement of the body and the intrinsic muscles providing the shaping of the tongue. Muscle spindle and tactile sensors make the tongue quite sensitive to position and the forces placed on it by contact with other articulators.
- The soft palate must be maintained in a reasonably elevated position for most speech sounds, although it is capable of a range of movements.

Phonological Development and Motor Control

Certainly the development of a child's phonology is a marvel. It should now be fairly clear that the maturation of the motor speech system governs, in large part, the speech sounds a child is capable of making. The stops (/p,t,k,b,d,g/) are present in the child's repertoire fairly early in development, although their mastery occurs later than their emergence. The reason for this is apparently motoric. A child of 2 or 3 years is quite capable of the basic "valving" gesture of opening and closing the mouth (/ba/), raising and lowering the tongue on the alveolar ridge (/da/), or near the soft palate (/ga/). However, the controlled production of the stops requires the ability to differentiate labial, mandibular, and lingual movements, and thus mastery of the stops can occur as late as 6 years.

As the child develops greater motor control, he gains the ability to make graded movements with the tongue so that he can sustain one articulator against the other with a constant pressure. The "raspberry" you hear in the preverbal child is very likely the precursor to the fricatives. With graded control of lingual pressure comes the ability to make minute adjustments of an articulatory posture, such as those made with the dorsum of the tongue to differentiate /s/ and /ʃ/ through width of the tongue groove and tongue tip elevation.

Development of Articulatory Ability

The infant is faced with an enormous task during development. She begins life with no knowledge of the universe and with a motor system in which movement is governed by reflexes out of her control. She will spend the next several years (perhaps the rest of her life!) making sense of the world around her and learning to manipulate her environment. Fortunately, she is born with an innate "desire" to acquire information and learn about her environment, and it appears that this drives the often-painful process of development.

The primitive human motor system is actually an extremely complex network of protective reflexes. Reflexes provide the means for an immature infant to respond to the environment in a stereotyped manner, without volition. This is not to argue that infants have no will, but rather to point out that they cannot express it voluntarily. If a breast touches the lips of an infant, the infant will orient to the breast and start sucking reflexively (you can stimulate this reflex with a stroke of your fingers). The infant does not need to think, "Gee, I'm hungry. I wonder if there is anything to eat around here?" Rather, nature has "hard-wired" the infant to meet its needs.

This reflexive condition results in what Langley and Lombardino (1991) refer to as "primitive mass patterns of movement." Movements are gross responses to environmental stimuli that help the infant meet his or her basic needs. Development is a process of gaining cortical control of the motor patterns for volitional purposes, and the development of the articulatory system has its roots in learning to walk.

Cephalo-caudal: Development occurs from head to tail.

Proximo-distal: Development occurs from medial to distal structures.

The most pervasive postnatal experience an infant has is gravity. Always present, gravity provides the ultimate challenge to an infant who wants to experience a universe that is out of reach. Reflexive movement against gravity provides the child with information about the effects of movement. He can see his hands as he moves them and learns that there is a relationship between the sensation and the hands he sees. These are the essential elements of motor development: reflexive response to environmental stimuli, providing feedback to an intact neuromotor system. Motor development is a process of refining gross movements, and this refinement occurs **cephalo-caudally** (from head to tail) and **proximo-distally** (from medial structures to distal structures). The infant will develop gross mandibular movements before fine mandibular movements and will have head control before she develops trunk control. She will develop posterior tongue control before anterior tongue control. Four vital elements of basic motor control support later speech development: experience with gravity, flexor-extensor balance, trunk control, and differentiation.

During the *reflexive period* (roughly birth to 6 months), the infant's vestibular system is being stimulated by handling by the caregiver. *Vestibular stimulation* causes changes in muscle tone relative to gravity, setting the stage for the tonic activity of the postural muscles.

The baby begins life in a general state of flexion, and the advent of extension heralds an infant's ability to attend actively to her environment. When the newborn is placed on her stomach, her weight shifts to her face. When she is pulled up from a supine position by her hands, her head flops back with no control. The 3-month-old has

Apraxia

Apraxia is a deficit in the neural "programming" of musculature for voluntary movement in the absence of muscular weakness or paralysis. There appear to be many types and subtypes of apraxia. Limb apraxia is identified as the inability to perform volitional gestures using the limbs. A person with limb apraxia might reveal deficits in voluntarily using multiple objects to perform a sequence of acts upon request, such as making a sandwich. The act may be fluent, but the object is used inappropriately. The person's ability to perform the act by imitation would be much less impaired.

A person with oral apraxia might have difficulty programming the facial and lingual muscles for nonspeech acts. When this individual is asked to blow out a candle, she may go through many effortful attempts (groping) to find the right gesture with the lips in coordination with the outward flow of air. Often the individual with oral apraxia also has a verbal apraxia.

Verbal apraxia is a deficit in programming the articulators for speech sound production. The individual with verbal apraxia makes errors in correct articulation of the sounds of speech, although the errors vary widely from one attempt to another. The individual is aware of the error and makes frequent attempts at production, so that the flow of speech is greatly impeded. This person has more difficulty with multisyllabic than monosyllabic words, and semiautomatic speech (such as greetings) may be quite fluent.

By definition, apraxias do not involve muscular weakness, although muscular weakness or paralysis may occur with the apraxia. Apraxias may arise from lesions to a variety of brain structures. Damage to the premotor region of the cerebral cortex appears to have the greatest probability of producing apraxia, and the specific premotor region involved with speech is known as Broca's area. Damage to the supramarginal gyrus of the parietal lobe also results in verbal apraxia, with the errors being more pure phonemic errors than those seen with damage in Broca's area, which contains more distortions.

a great deal of extensor balance and can now control her head when pulled from supine. Soon her trunk muscles will be under sufficient control that she can rotate her trunk and reach for objects in her environment while sitting.

The combination of trunk stability and extensor–flexor balance gives her the tools for standing and walking—and talking. It is no surprise that the infant's speech begins to develop in concert with her loco-motor skills. If you remember that the tongue is intimately related to the hyoid and larynx, you will realize that it is unreasonable to expect a child to control the complex, refined movements of the tongue until the trunk and neck muscles are stabilized.

Following stabilization, the infant must develop differential motor control. In the articulatory system, the manifestations of this control are evident in the rapidly increasing complexity of his speech pro-duction. The simple consonant-vowel syllable represents the most basic valving of the articulatory system. All the child must do to pro-duce this syllable is begin phonation and open and close the mouth repeatedly. Tongue contact will approximate a velar or alveolar stop, or lip contact will produce a bilabial plosive. In any case, this infant has babbled, much to the delight of her parents!

The simple valving gives way to refined control of the tongue. With mandible stability accomplished, the child can begin the process of differentiating the tongue movements from those of the mandible. Following this, the infant differentiates tongue body and tip move-ments, as well as lateralization.

This development is hierarchical. The infant must balance muscle tone before being able to sit, and must sit before he can establish independent head and neck control. With control of neck muscles comes the freedom to move the mandible and tongue independently, and with that freedom comes the ability to differentially move the articulators.

Does this mean that a child with deficits of motor development will never develop speech? The answer, fortunately, is "no." The task is doubly difficult for this child, however, and still depends on gaining the voluntary control and differentiation of those muscles.

Summary

- Primitive patterns of muscle movement gradually develop with voluntary control patterns to facilitate control of trunk, neck, and limbs.

- With this control comes the ability to make graded movements of the mandible and, subsequently, differentiated lingual movements.

CHAPTER SUMMARY

Articulators have both speech and nonspeech functions. Biological (nonspeech) functions fulfilled by the articulators include mastication and deglutition. There are four stages of mastication and deglutition. Food is introduced into the oral cavity, masticated, and formed into a bolus during the oral preparation stage. During the oral stage, the bolus is moved back on the hard palate, and the pharyngeal stage begins when the bolus reaches the fauces. The reflexive swallow includes elevation of the soft palate and larynx, propulsion of the bolus through the pharynx, closure of the laryngeal sphincter, and opening of the esophageal sphincter. The esophageal stage involves peristaltic movement of the bolus through the esophagus.

Movement of the mandible for speech is slight compared with movement for chewing. The mandibular posture for speech is one of sustained dynamic tension between antagonists. The tongue is versatile, with the extrinsic muscles providing the major movement of the body and the intrinsic muscles providing the shaping of the tongue. The soft palate must be maintained in a reasonably elevated position for most speech sounds, although it is capable of a range of movements.

Development of articulatory function involves gaining control of postural muscles that provide trunk stability and differentiation of muscle group function. Reflexive responses are protective and nurturant, and these primitive patterns gradually develop with voluntary control patterns to facilitate control of trunk, neck, and limbs, and finally differentiation for graded oral movement.

The source-filter theory states that speech is the product of sending an acoustic source, such as the sound produced by the vibrating vocal folds, through the filter of the vocal tract that shapes the output. Sources may be voicing, as in the case of vowels, or the product of turbulence, as in fricatives. Articulators may be movable (such as the tongue, lips, pharynx, mandible, and velum) or immobile (such as the teeth, hard palate, and alveolar ridge).

Facial bones and those of the skull work together to produce the structures of articulation. The mandible provides the lower dental arch, alveolar regions, and the resting location for the tongue. The maxillae provide the bulk of the hard palate, alveolar ridge, upper dental arch, and dominant structures of the nasal cavities, and the palatine bones provide the rest of the hard palate and the point of attachment for the soft palate. The midline vomer articulates with the perpendicular plate of ethmoid and the cartilaginous septum to form the nasal septum. The zygomatic bone articulates with the frontal bone and maxillae to form the cheekbone. The small nasal bones form the upper margin of the nasal cavity. The ethmoid bone serves as the core of the skull and face, with the prominent crista galli protruding into the cranium and the perpendicular plate dividing the nasal cavities. The frontal, parietal, temporal, and occipital bones of the skull overlie the lobes of the brain of the same name. The sphenoid bone has a marked presence in the braincase, with the prominent greater and lesser wings of sphenoid lateral to the corpus. The hypophyseal fossa houses the pituitary gland.

Incisors, cuspids, bicuspids, and molars are housed in the alveoli of the maxillae and mandible. Teeth have roots and crowns, and the exposed tooth surface is covered with enamel. Each tooth has medial, lateral, lingual, buccal (or labial), and occlusal surfaces. Clinical eruption of the deciduous arch begins between 6 and 9 months, and eruption of the permanent arch begins at 6 years. Class I occlusion refers to normal orientation of mandible and maxillae. Class II malocclusion refers to a relatively retracted mandible, and Class III malocclusion refers to a relatively protruded mandible. Individual teeth may have aberrant orientations within the alveolus, including torsiversion, labioversion, linguaversion, distoversion, and mesioversion. Inadequately erupted or hypererupted teeth are referred to as infraverted and supraverted, respectively.

The cavities of the articulatory and resonatory system can be envisioned as a series of linked tubes. The vertically directed pharynx comprises the laryngopharynx, oropharynx, and nasopharynx. The nasal cavities arise from the nasopharynx, with the nasal and nasopharyngeal regions entirely separated from the oral cavity by the soft palate. The oral cavity is flanked by the small buccal cavities. The shape and size of the oral cavity is altered through movement of the tongue and mandible, and the nasal cavity may be coupled with the oral and pharyngeal cavities by means of the soft palate. The shape of the pharyngeal cavity is altered by the pharyngeal constrictor muscles, but it is secondarily changed by elevation or depression of the larynx.

Facial muscles are important for articulation that involves the lips. Numerous muscles insert into the orbicularis oris inferior and superior muscles, permitting lip protrusion, closure, retraction, elevation, and depression. The risorius and buccinator muscles retract the lips and support entrapment of air in the oral cavity. The levator labii superioris, zygomatic minor, levator labii superioris alaeque nasi, and levator anguli oris elevate the upper lip, and the depressor labii inferioris depresses the lower lip. The zygomatic major muscle elevates and retracts the corner of the mouth. The depressor labii inferioris pulls the lips down and out. The depressor anguli oris muscle depresses the corner of the mouth, and the mentalis muscle pulls the lower lip out. The platysma depresses the mandible.

The tongue occupies the floor of the mouth, being divided into dorsum, apex (tip), and base. Fine movements are the product of the intrinsic musculature (transverse, vertical, inferior longitudinal and superior longitudinal muscles of the tongue). Larger adjustments of lingual movement requires extrinsic muscles. The genioglossus retracts, protrudes, or depresses the tongue, and the hyoglossus and chondroglossus depress the tongue. The styloglossus and palatoglossus elevate the posterior tongue.

Muscles of mastication include mandibular elevators and depressors, as well as muscles to protrude the mandible. The masseter, temporalis, and medial pterygoid muscles elevate the mandible, and the lateral pterygoids protrude it. Mandibular depression is achieved by the mylohyoid, geniohyoid, and platysma muscles.

The soft palate, or velum, is attached to the posterior hard palate. The levator veli palatini muscle elevates the soft palate and the musculus uvulae bunches it. The tensor veli palatini tenses and shortens the palate. The soft palate is depressed by the palatoglossus and palatopharyngeus. The superior pharyngeal constrictor assists in gaining velopharyngeal closure, while peristaltic movement of food is facilitated by the middle and inferior pharyngeal constrictors. The cricopharyngeus forms the muscular orifice of the esophagus. The salpingopharyngeus elevates the pharyngeal wall, and the stylopharyngeus assists in elevation of the pharynx.

Study Questions

1. The _____ theory of vowel production states that the voicing source is routed through the vocal tract where it is shaped into the sounds of speech by the articulators.

2. On the following figure, identify the indicated bones and landmarks.

A. _____ (bone)

B. _____ (bone)

C. _____ bone

D. _____ bone

E. _____ bone

F. _____ process

G. _____ process

H. _____

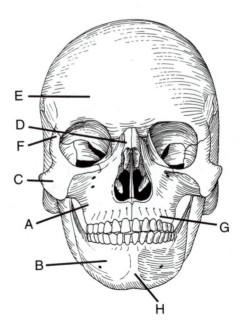

3. On the following figure, identify the indicated bones and land-marks.

A. _____ (bone)

B. _____ bone

C. _____ bone

D. _____

E. _____

F. _____

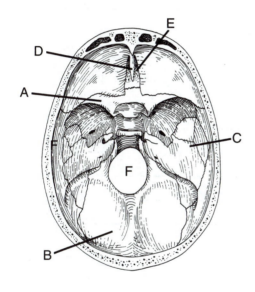

4. On the following figure, identify the indicated bones and land-marks.

A. _____ bone

B. _____ bone

C. _____ (bone)

D. _____ (bone)

E. _____ bone

F. _____ bone

G. _____ bone

H. _____ bone

I. _____

J. _____

K. _____ process

L. _____ process

M. _____ process

N. _____

O. _____ process

P. _____ process

Q. _____

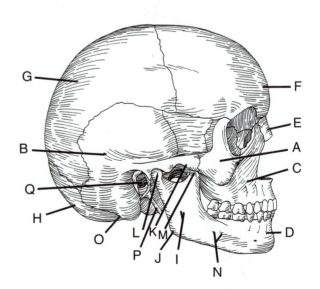

5. On the following figure, identify the indicated structures.

A. _____ process

B. _____ (bone)

C. _____ bone

D. _____

E. _____ foramen

F. _____ suture

G. _____ process

H. _____ plate

I. _____ plate

J. _____ process

K. _____

L. _____

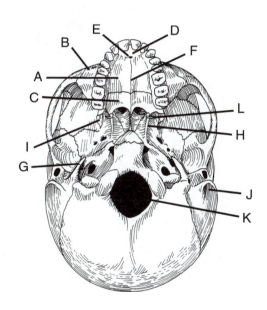

6. On the following figure, identify the indicated muscles.

A. _____

B. _____

C. _____

D. _____

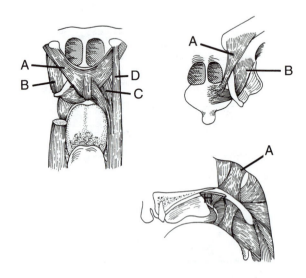

7. On the following figure, identify the indicated muscles.

A. _____

B. _____

C. _____

D. _____

E. _____

F. _____

G. _____

H. _____

I. _____

J. _____

K. _____

L. _____

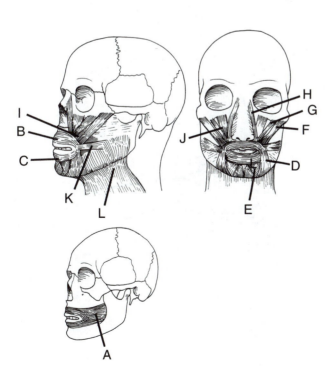

8. On the following figure, identify the indicated muscles.

A. _____

B. _____

C. _____

D. _____

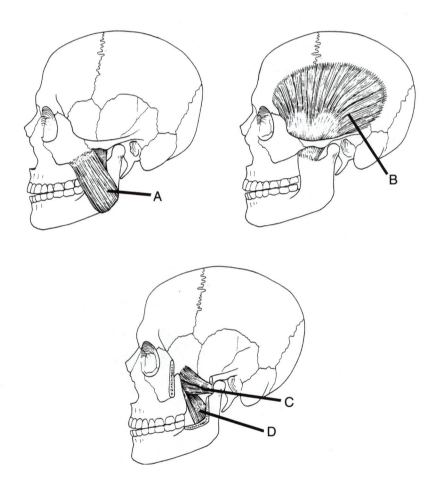

9. On the following figure, identify the indicated muscles.

A. _____

B. _____

C. _____

D. _____

E. _____

F. _____

G. _____

H. _____

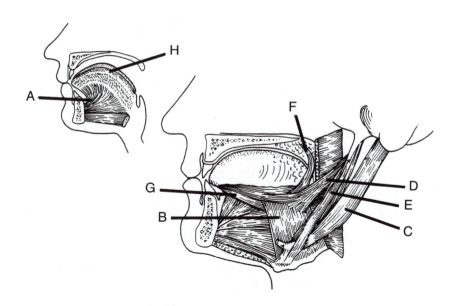

10. On the following figure, identify indicated structures.

A. _____ (bone)

B. _____ process

C. _____ plate

D. _____ plate

E. _____

F. _____ bone

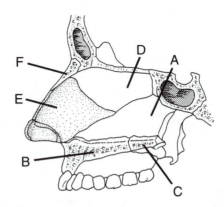

11. _____ refers to the processes involved in food preparation, such as chewing food, moving the food onto the molars, and so forth.

12. _____ refers to swallowing.

13. In the _____ stage of swallowing, food is prepared for swallowing.

14. In the _____ stage of swallowing, mastication ceases, the tongue drops down and pulls posteriorly, and the anterior tongue elevates to the hard palate and squeezes the bolus back toward the faucial pillars.

15. In the _____ stage of swallowing, the bolus contacts the anterior faucial pillars, the soft palate elevates, respiration stops, the vocal folds tightly adduct, the larynx elevates and moves forward, and the cricopharyngeus relaxes as food enters the pharynx.

16. During the _____ stage of swallowing, the bolus is transported through the esophagus.

17. Identify the muscle that best fits the statement. (In some cases more than one muscle fills the bill.)

 A. _____ Elevates tongue tip

 B. _____ Depresses tongue tip

 C. _____ Protrudes tongue

 D. _____ Retracts tongue

 E. _____ Elevates posterior tongue

 F. _____ Narrows tongue

 G. _____ Flattens tongue

 H. _____ Depresses soft palate

 I. _____ Tenses soft palate

 J. _____ Constricts esophageal opening

 K. _____ Constricts upper pharynx

 L. _____ Elevates soft palate

18. Motor control in the body develops from _____ (head/tail) to _____ (head/tail) and from _____ (proximal/distal) to _____ (proximal/distal).

19. Tongue movement depends on the graceful balance of many muscles. Which muscles are involved in elevation of the back of the tongue? As you think of this, ponder the muscles that must work as antagonists to help structures as well.

REFERENCES

Abbs, J. H., & Cole, K. J. (1991). Consideration of bulbar and suprabulbar afferent influences upon speech motor coordination and programming. In S. Grillner, B. Lindblom, J. Lubker, & A. Persson (Eds.), *Speech motor control* (pp. 159–186). Oxford: Pergamon.

Abrahams, P. H., McMinn, R. M. H., Hutchings, R. T., Sandy, C., Mark, S. (2003). *McMinn's color atlas of human anatomy* (5th ed.). Philadelphia: Mosby.

Baken, R. J., & Orlikoff, R. F. (1999). *Clinical measurement of speech and voice* (2nd ed.). San Diego: Singular Publishing Group.

Barlow, S. M., & Netsell, R. (1986). Differential fine force control of the upper and lower lips. *Journal of Speech and Hearing Research, 29,* 163–169.

Barlow, S. M., & Rath, E. M. (1985). Maximum voluntary closing forces in the upper and lower lips of humans. *Journal of Speech and Hearing Research, 28,* 373–376.

Basmajian, J. V. (1975). *Grant's method of anatomy.* Baltimore: Williams & Wilkins.

Bateman, H. E. (1977). *A clinical approach to speech anatomy and physiology.* Springfield, IL: Charles C. Thomas.

Bateman, H. E., & Mason, R. M. (1984). *Applied anatomy and physiology of the speech and hearing mechanism.* Springfield, IL: Charles C. Thomas.

Beck, E. W., Monson, H., & Groer, M. (1982). *Mosby's atlas of functional human anatomy.* St. Louis: Mosby.

Bly, L. (1983). *The components of normal movement during the first year of life and abnormal motor movement.* Chicago: Neuro-Developmental Treatment Association.

Bly, L. (1994). *Motor skills acquisition in the first year.* Tucson, AZ: Therapy Skill Builders.

Bunton, K., & Weismer, G. (1994). Evaluation of a reiterant force-impulse task in the tongue. *Journal of Speech and Hearing Research, 37,* 1020–1031.

Chusid, J. G. (1985). *Correlative neuroanatomy and functional neurology* (17th ed.). Los Altos, CA: Lange Medical Publications.

DeNil, L. F., & Abbs, J. H (1991). Influence of speaking rate on the upper lip, lower lip, and jaw peak velocity sequencing during bilabial closing movements. *Journal of the Acoustical Society of America, 89* (2), 845–849.

Duffy, J. R. (1995). *Motor speech disorders.* St. Louis: Mosby.

Ettema, S. L., & Kuehn, D. P. (1994). A quantitative histologic study of the normal human adult soft palate. *Journal of Speech and Hearing Research, 37,* 303–313.

Fairbanks, G. (1954). A theory of the speech mechanism as a servosystem. *Journal of Speech and Hearing Disorders, 19,* 133–139.

Flege, J. E. (1988). Anticipatory and carry-over nasal coarticulation in the speech of children and adults. *Journal of Speech and Hearing Research, 31,* 525–536.

Folkins, J. W., Linville, R. N., Garrett, J. D., & Brown, C. K. (1988). Interactions in the labial musculature during speech. *Journal of Speech and Hearing Research, 31,* 253–264.

Ganong, W. F. (2003). *Review of medical physiology* (21st ed.). New York: McGraw-Hill/Appleton & Lange.

Garcia-Colera, A., & Semjen, A. (1988). Distributed planning of movement sequences. *Journal of Motor Behavior, 20* (3), 341–367.

Gelb, H. (1985). *Clinical management of head, neck and TMJ pain and dysfunction.* Philadelphia: Saunders.

Goffman, L., & Smith, A. (1994). Motor unit territories in the human perioral musculature. *Journal of Speech and Hearing Research, 37,* 975–984.

Gosling, J. A., Harris, P. F., Humpherson, J. R., Whitmore, I., & Willan, P. L. T. (1985). *Atlas of human anatomy.* Philadelphia: Lippincott.

Gracco, V. L. (1988). Timing factors in the coordination of speech movements. *Journal of Neuroscience, 8* (12), 4628–4639.

Gracco, V. L. (1994). Some organizational characteristics of speech movement control. *Journal of Speech and Hearing Research, 37,* 4–27.

Gracco, V. L., & Abbs, J. H. (1989). Sensorimotor characteristics of speech motor sequences. *Experimental Brain Research, 75,* 586–598.

Gray, H., Bannister, L. H., Berry, M. M., & Williams, P. L. (Eds.). (1995). *Gray's anatomy.* London: Churchill Livingstone.

Grobler, N. J. (1977). *Textbook of clinical anatomy (Vol. 1).* Amsterdam: Elsevier Scientific.

Groher, M. E. (1997). *Dysphagia* (3rd ed.). St. Louis, MO: Butterworth-Heinemann Hall, P. K., Hardy, J. C., & LaVelle, W. E. (1990). A child with signs of developmental apraxia of speech with whom a palatal lift prosthesis was used to manage palatal dysfunction. *Journal of Speech and Hearing Disorders, 55,* 454–460.

Hauser, G., Daponte, A., & Roberts, M. J. (1989). Palatal rugae. *Journal of Anatomy, 124,* 237–249.

Hellstrand, E. (1981). The neuromuscular system of the tongue. In S. Grillner, B. Lindblom, J. Lubker, & A. Persson (Eds.), *Speech motor control* (pp. 141–157). Oxford: Pergamon.

Horak, M. (1992). The utility of connectionism for motor learning: A reinterpretation of contextual interference in movement schemas. *Journal of Motor Behavior, 24* (1), 58–66.

Jordan, M. I. (1990). Motor learning and the degrees of freedom problem. In M. Jeannerod (Ed.), *Attention and performance XIII: Motor representation and control.* Hillsdale, NJ: Lawrence Erlbaum.

Kahane, J. C., & Folkins, J. F. (1984). *Atlas of speech and hearing anatomy.* Columbus, OH: Charles E. Merrill.

Kapetansky, D. I. (1987). *Cleft lip, nose, and palate reconstruction.* Philadelphia: Lippincott.

Kaplan, H. (1960). *Anatomy and physiology of speech.* New York: McGraw-Hill.

Katz, W. F., Kripke, C., & Tallal, P. (1991). Anticipatory coarticulation in the speech of adults and young children: Acoustic, perceptual, and video data. *Journal of Speech and Hearing Research, 34,* 1222–1249.

Kelso, J. A. S., Tuller, B., Vatikiotis-Bateson, E., & Fowler, C. A. (1984). Functionally specific articulatory cooperation following jaw perturbations during speech: Evidence for coordinative structures. *Journal of Experimental Psychology: Perception and Performance, 19,* 812–832.

Kelso, J. A., & Ding, M. (1993). Fluctuations, intermittency, and controllable chaos in biological coordination. In K. M. Newell & D. M. Corcos (Eds.), *Variability and motor control* (pp. 291–316). Champaign, IL: Human Kinetics.

Kent, R. D. (1997). *The speech sciences.* San Diego: Singular Publishing Group.

Kent, R. D., Kent, J. F., & Rosenbek, J. C. (1987). Maximum performance tests of speech production. *Journal of Speech and Hearing Disorders, 52,* 367–387.

Kuehn, D. P., Lemme, M. L., & Baumgartner, J. M. (1989). *Neural bases of speech, hearing, and language.* Boston: Little, Brown.

Kuehn, D. P., Templeton, P. J., & Maynard, J. A. (1990). Muscle spindles in the velopharyngeal musculature of humans. *Journal of Speech and Hearing Research, 33,* 488–493.

Landgren, S., & Olsson, K. A. (1981). Oral mechanoreceptors. In S. Grillner, B. Lindblom, J. Lubker, & A. Persson (Eds.), *Speech motor control* (pp. 129–139). Oxford: Pergamon.

Langley, M. B., & Lombardino, L. J. (1991). *Neurodevelopmental strategies for managing communication disorders in children with severe motor dysfunction.* Austin, TX: Pro-Ed.

Lashley, K. S. (1951). The problem of serial order in behavior. In L. A. Jerrers (Ed.), *Cerebral mechanisms in behavior* (pp. 506–528). New York: Wiley.

Lieberman, P. (1977). *Speech physiology and acoustic phonetics: An introduction.* New York: Macmillan.

Liss, J. M. (1990). Muscle spindles in the human levator veli palatini and palatoglossus muscles. *Journal of Speech and Hearing Research, 33,* 736–746.

Logemann, J. (1998). *Evaluation and treatment of swallowing disorder* (2nd ed.). Austin, TX: Pro-Ed.

Love, R. J., Hagerman, E. L., & Taimi, E. G. (1980). Speech performance, dysphagia, and oral reflexes in cerebral palsy. *Journal of Speech and Hearing Disorders, 45,* 59–75.

McClean, M. (1973). Forward coarticulation of velar movement at marked junctural boundaries. *Journal of Speech and Hearing Research, 16,* 286–296.

McMinn, R. M. H., Hutchings, R. T., & Logan, B. M. (1994). *Color atlas of head and neck anatomy.* London: Mosby-Wolfe.

McNeil, M. R., Weismer, G., Adams, S., & Mulligan, M. (1990). Oral structure nonspeech motor control in normal, dysarthric, aphasic, and apraxic speakers: Isometric force and static position control. *Journal of Speech and Hearing Research, 33,* 255–268.

Minifie, F. (1973). Speech acoustics. In F. D. Minifie, T. J. Hixon, & F. Williams (Eds.), *Normal aspects of speech, hearing, and language* (pp. 11–72). Englewood Cliffs, NJ: Prentice-Hall.

Moore, C. A. (1993). Symmetry of mandibular muscle activity as an index of coordinative strategy. *Journal of Speech and Hearing Research, 36,* 1145–1157.

Moore, C. A., Smith, A., & Ringel, R. L. (1988). Task-specific organization of activity in human jaw muscles. *Journal of Speech and Hearing Research, 31,* 670–680.

Moore, K. L. (1988). *The developing human.* Philadelphia: Saunders.

Netsell, R. (1973). Speech physiology. In F. D. Minifie, T. J. Hixon & F. Williams (Eds.), *Normal aspects of speech, hearing, and language* (pp. 134–211). Englewood Cliffs, NJ: Prentice-Hall.

Netsell, R. (1986). A neurobiologic view of speech production and the dysarthrias. San Diego: College-Hill.

Netter, F. H. (1983). *The CIBA collection of medical illustrations.* Vol. 1. Nervous System. Part I. Anatomy and physiology. West Caldwell, NJ: CIBA Pharmaceutical Company.

Netter, F. H. (1989). *Atlas of human anatomy*. Summit, NJ: CIBA Pharmaceuticals Division.

Netter, F. H. (1997). *Atlas of human anatomy*. Los Angeles: Icon Learning Systems.

Perlman, A. L., Grayhack, J. P., & Booth, B. M. (1992). The relationship of vallecular residue to oral involvement, reduced hyoid elevation, and epiglottic function. *Journal of Speech and Hearing Research, 35,* 734–741.

Perlman, A. L., Luschei, E. S., & DuMond, C. E. (1989). Electrical activity from the superior pharyngeal constrictor during reflexive and nonreflexive tasks. *Journal of Speech and Hearing Research, 32,* 749–754.

Pickett, J. M. (1980). *The sounds of speech communication*. Baltimore: University Park Press.

Rademaker, A. W., Pauloski, B. R., Logemann, J. A., & Shanahan, T. K. (1994). Oropharyngeal swallow efficiency as a representative measure of swallowing function. *Journal of Speech and Hearing Research, 37,* 314–325.

Rohen, J. W., & Yokochi, C. (1993). *Color atlas of anatomy*. New York: Igaku-Shoin.

Rohen, J. W., Yokochi, C., Lutjen-Drecoll, E. L., & Romrell, L. J. (2002). *Color atlas of anatomy: A photographic study of the human body* (5th ed.). Philadelphia: Lippincott, Williams & Wilkins.

Rosenbaum, D. A., Kenny, S. B., & Derr, M. A. (1983). Hierarchical control of rapid movement sequences. *Journal of Experimental Psychology: Human Perception and Performance, 9* (1), 86–102.

Rosenbek, J. C., Robbins, J., Fishback, B., & Levine, R. L. (1991). Effects of thermal application on dysphagia after stroke. *Journal of Speech and Hearing Research, 34,* 1257–1268.

Rosse, C., Gaddum-Rosse, P., & Rosse, G. (1997). *Hollinshead's textbook of anatomy*. Philadelphia: Lippincott-Raven.

Saltzman, E. (1986). Task dynamic coordination of the speech articulators: A preliminary model. *Experimental brain research* (pp. 129–144). Berlin-Heidelberg: Springer-Verlag.

Sawashima, M., & Cooper, F. S. (1977). *Dynamic aspects of speech production*. Tokyo: University of Tokyo Press.

Schmidt, R. A. (1975). A schema theory of discrete motor skill learning. *Psychological Review, 82,* 225–260.

Shaffer, L. H. (1976). Intention and performance. *Psychological Review, 33* (5), 375–393.

Shprintzen, R. J., & Bardach, J. (1995). *Cleft palate speech management*. St. Louis: Mosby.

Shriberg, L. D., & Kent, R. D. (2002). *Clinical phonetics* (3rd ed.). Boston: Allyn & Bacon.

Small, A. M. (1973). Acoustics. In F. D. Minifie, T. J. Hixon, & F. Williams (Eds.), *Normal aspects of speech, hearing, and language*. Englewood Cliffs, NJ: Prentice-Hall.

Smith, A., McFarland, D. H., & Weber, C. M. (1986). Interactions between speech and finger movements: An exploration of the dynamic pattern perspective. *Journal of Speech and Hearing Research, 29,* 471–480.

Snell, R. S. (1978). *Gross anatomy dissector*. Boston: Little, Brown.

Square-Storer, P., & Roy, E. A. (1989). The apraxias: Commonalities and distinctions. In P. Square-Storer (Ed.), *Acquired apraxia of speech in aphasic adults: Theoretical and clinical issues*. London: Taylor & Francis.

Weber, C. M., & Smith, A. (1987). Reflex responses in human jaw, lip, and tongue muscles elicited by mechanical stimulation. *Journal of Speech and Hearing Research, 30*, 70–79.

Westbury, J. R. (1988). Mandible and hyoid bone movements during speech. *Journal of Speech and Hearing Research, 31*, 405–416.

Wickens, J., Hyland, B., & Anson, G. (1994). Cortical cell assemblies: A possible mechanism for motor programs. *Journal of Motor Behavior, 26* (2), 66–82.

Wohlert, A. B., & Goffman, L. (1994). Human perioral muscle activation patterns. *Journal of Speech and Hearing Research, 37*, 1032–1040.

Zemlin, W. R. (1998). *Speech and hearing science. Anatomy and physiology* (4th ed.). Needham Heights, MA: Allyn & Bacon.

Zickefoose, W. (1989). *Techniques of oral myofunctional therapy*. Sacramento, CA: O.M.T. Materials.

CHAPTER

5

Anatomy and Physiology of Hearing

OUTLINE

I. Anatomy of Hearing

  A. Outer ear

      1. Landmarks of the pinna

         a. Helix

         b. Antihelix

         c. Concha

         d. Lobe

         e. Tragus

2. External auditory meatus
    a. One third cartilage
    b. Two thirds bone
3. Tympanic membrane

B. Middle ear
  1. Middle ear
  2. Ossicles
    a. Malleus
    b. Incus
    c. Stapes
  3. Stapedius muscle
  4. Tensor tympani muscle
  5. Landmarks of the middle ear
    a. Oval window
    b. Round window
    c. Lateral semicircular canal
    d. Entrance to the eustachian tube
    e. Stapedial pyramid

C. Inner ear
  1. Osseous labyrinth
    a. Osseous semicircular canals
    b. Osseous cochlear canal
    c. Scala vestibuli
    d. Scala tympani
    e. Osseous spiral lamina
    f. Helicotrema
    g. Round window
    h. Oval window
    i. Cochlear aqueduct
  2. Membranous labyrinth
    a. Vestibular organ
    b. Ampulla
    c. Crista ampularis
    d. Utricle and saccule
  3. Cochlear Duct
    a. Between the scala vestibuli and tympani
    b. Reissner's membrane
    c. Basilar membrane
    e. Organ of corti
    f. Hair cells, outer and inner
    g. Innervation

II. Auditory Physiology

    A. Outer and middle ear functions

        1. Localization

        2. Resonant frequencies

        3. Impedance matching

    B. Inner ear function

        1. Cochlear function

            a. Spectral (frequency) and temporal analyses

            b. Movement of fluid in the scala vestibuli

            c. Disturbance at basilar membrane causes the traveling wave

            d. Frequency selectivity

            e. Stiffness, thickness, and width of basilar membrane

            f. Shearing effect on the cilia of outer hair cells

            g. Fluid flow and turbulence of endolymph activates inner hair cells

        2. Neural Responses

            a. Low-threshold and high-threshold neurons

            b. Frequency specificity

            c. Characteristic frequency

            d. Tuning curve

THE STRUCTURES OF HEARING

The physical structures of the ear are deceptively simple, especially in light of their exquisite function. The ear is an energy transducer, which means that it converts acoustic energy into electrochemical energy.

We will talk about the ear in terms of its basic elements: outer ear, middle ear, inner ear, and auditory pathways (see Figure 5-1).

Outer Ear

The outer ear is composed of two basic components with which you are quite familiar (Table 5-1). The *pinna* (or auricle) is the prominence we colloquially refer to as the ear, although it serves primarily as a collector of sound to be processed at deeper levels (e.g., the eardrum and cochlea). The structure of the pinna is provided by cartilage (see Figure 5-2 and Table 5-1).

Table 5–1. Landmarks of the Outer Ear

Auricle
Helix
Auricular tubercle (Darwin's tubercle)
Antihelix
Crura
Crura anithelicis
Triangular fossa
Scaphoid fossa
Concha
    Cymba conchae
    Cavum conchae
Tragus
Intertragic incisure
Antitragus
Lobule

External Auditory Meatus
Cartilagenous meatus
Osseous meatus
Isthmus
Tympanic membrane

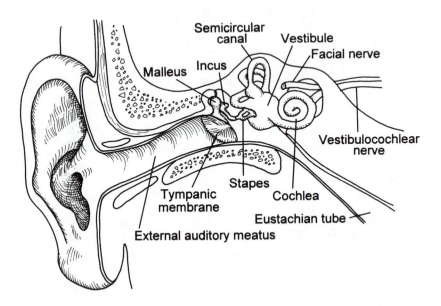

FIGURE 5–1. Schematic of frontal section revealing outer, middle, and inner ear structures.

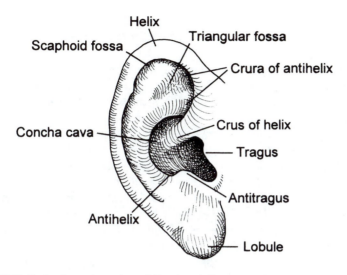

FIGURE 5–2. Landmarks of the auricle.

The pinna has several important functions, including aiding local-ization of sound in space and "capturing" sound energy. The *helix* forms the curled margin of the pinna, and immediately ahead of the helix is the *antihelix*, a similar fold of tissue that marks the entrance to the *concha*. The concha is the entrance to the ear canal, known as the *external auditory meatus* (abbreviated EAM). A flap of epithelium-covered cartilage known as the *tragus* may have at one time served as a partial cover the entrance to the *meatus*, or opening. The *lobule* has no cartilage; it is the prominence at the inferior pinna made up of epithelial tissue and fat.

The external auditory meatus is approximately 7 mm in diameter and 2.5 cm long when measured from the depth of the concha, or 4 cm. The lateral one third of the canal is cartilage and is about 8 mm long; the medial two thirds is the bony meatus of the temporal bone. At the end of the EAM is the *tympanic membrane,* or eardrum, a thin tri-laminar sheet of tissue that sits at an oblique angle in the EAM. The epithelial cover of the pinna continues into the EAM and serves as the outer layer of the tympanic membrane, to be discussed later.

Because the adult ear canal takes a turn downward, you cannot see the medial end of the canal without some effort. If you were to look into the ear canal, you would see that the outer third of the EAM is lined with hairs, and has cerumen, or ear wax. These are both quite functional additions to the canal because they trap insects and dirt, protecting the medial-most point of the outer ear, the tympanic membrane.

Otitis Externa and Cerumen

The epithelial lining of the pinna and EAM is tightly bound to the cartilage and bone of these structures, which accounts for the pain when the tissue swells. Otitis externa is inflammation of the skin of the external ear. When tissue is inflamed, it responds by edema, or swelling. If the epithelium is tightly bound to its underlying structure, as it is in the EAM and pinna, the swelling increases the tension on the epithelium, making it quite painful.

Otitis externa may result from bacterial infection following trauma or abrasion. Failure to clean probe tips and specula could result in transmission of the infection between clients. Otitis externa can also result from viral infection, including infection with herpes zoster virus. This painful infection may lead to facial paralysis or hearing loss if the facial or vestibulocochlear nerves are involved.

The EAM is invested with cilia and ceruminous glands, largely restricted to the cartilaginous portion of the canal. Cerumen (ear wax) is secreted by the glands into the ear canal, trapping insects and dirt that would otherwise threaten the tympanic membrane. Individuals with overly active ceruminous glands may find that the EAM becomes occluded, and removal of the cerumen may be required. A person's attempts to remove the cerumen with cotton swabs often results in cerumen and dirt being packed against the inferior boundary of the tympanic membrane; the oblique angle forms a perfect "pocket" to catch the matter.

The interested student and budding audiologist or audiology assistant would be well advised to read the descriptions of these and other conditions provided by Martin (1981).

The *tympanic membrane* marks the boundary between the outer and middle ears. It completely separates the two spaces, being an extremely thin three-layered tissue. The epithelial lining of the EAM continues as the external layer of the tympanic membrane, while the lining of the middle ear provides the inner layer. Sandwiched between these two delicate epithelial linings is a layer of fibrous tissue that provides structure for the tympanic membrane.

The tympanic membrane is approximately 55 mm^2 in area and has a number of important landmarks (see Figure 5-3). If you view the

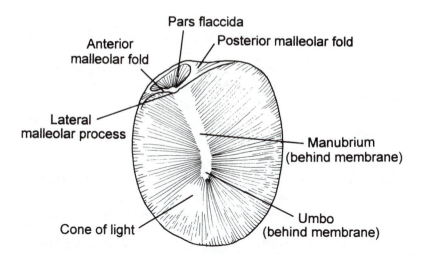

FIGURE 5-3. Tympanic membrane of the left ear, as viewed from the external auditory meatus.

tympanic membranes, you will see the *umbo,* which is the most distal point of attachment of the inner tympanic membrane to one of the bones of the middle ear, the *malleus.* The tympanic membrane is particularly taut at this point, and the location inferior and anterior to this is referred to as the *cone of light.* You may be able to see the handle, or *manubrium,* of malleus behind the tympanic membrane, appearing as a streak on the membrane.

The tympanic membrane is slightly concave when viewed from the EAM, and the umbo is the most depressed portion of this concavity. Although most of the tympanic membrane is invested with fibrous tissue, the *pars flaccida* is not, and this "flaccid part" can be seen in the superior quadrant of the tympanic membrane. On each side of the pars flaccida is a recess, consisting of the anterior and posterior malleolar folds. These folds and the region at the cone of light are the result of the malleus pushing distally on the membrane, much as if you were to stretch an unfilled balloon and push it from behind. This tight binding between membrane and malleus permits ready transmission of acoustic energy from the tympanic membrane to the ossicular chain. If the tympanic membrane is particularly transparent, you may also be able to see the long process of the incus parallel to the lateral process of malleus. In addition, the *chorda tympani* can sometimes be seen through the superior tympanic membrane.

Atresia: Absence.

Stenosis: Narrowing.

Aplasia: Lack of development.

Microtia: Small ear.

Malformations of the Pinna and EAM

If the pinna is subjected to trauma, as in that inflicted during the "sport" of boxing, the result can be permanent deformation of its structure. Trauma can cause hemorrhaging between the epithelium and cartilage, and if left untreated, the resulting swelling might cause a permanent distortion.

Several congenital conditions can be manifested in the EAM and pinna. **Atresia**, or congenital absence, of the EAM may signal absence of middle ear structures as well. **Stenosis**, or narrowing, of the ear canal reduces its ability to transmit sound to the middle ear structures. **Aplasia** of the pinna occurs when it fails to develop or does not develop completely. If the pinna is abnormally small, it is termed **microtia**. If something interferes with development, the pinnae may remain set low on the sides of the head.

A number of genetic syndromes cause auricular anomalies. Children affected by branchio-oto-renal syndrome often have cupped ears or microtia in conjunction with disarticulation of the bones of the middle ear and conductive or sensorineural hearing loss. A high proportion of individuals with Down syndrome (trisomy 21) show microtia, have small earlobes and helix malformation, and occasionally have stenosis of the ear canal.

Summary

- The outer ear is composed of the pinna, the structure that serves primarily as a sound collector, and the external auditory meatus, or ear canal.
- Landmarks of the pinna include the margin of the auricle, the helix, the lobule, and the tragus.
- The external auditory meatus has both osseous and cartilaginous parts.
- At the terminus of the external auditory meatus is the tympanic membrane, the structure that separates the outer and middle ears.

Middle Ear

Structure of the Tympanic Membrane

The tympanic membrane is a slightly oval structure, being approximately 10 mm in diameter in the superior-inferior dimension. The anterior-posterior dimension is slightly smaller (about 9 mm in diameter), and the entire membrane is placed in the canal at a 55° angle with the floor. The circumference of the membrane is a fibro-cartilaginous ring that fits into the tympanic sulcus, a groove in the temporal bone. The sulcus is incomplete in the superior aspect, accommodating the anterior and posterior malleolar folds.

The tympanic membrane is made up of three layers of tissue: outer, intermediate, and inner. The outer (cuticular) layer is a continuation of the epithelial lining of the EAM and pinna. The intermediate (fibrous) layer is made up of two parts: (1) The superficial layer is composed of fibers that radiate out from the handle of the malleus to the periphery. (2) The deep layer is made up of circular fibers that are found mostly in the periphery of the membrane. The inner (mucous) layer is continuous with the mucosa of the middle ear.

The middle ear is a small but extremely important space occupied by three of the smallest bones of the body. First, let us examine these bones and their attachments, then we will explore their attachments, and then we will explore the landmarks of the cavity itself (Table 5-2).

Table 5-2. Landmarks of the Middle Ear

Ossicles

Malleus
　Manubrium (handle)
　Head (caput)
　Lateral process
　Anterior process
　Facet for incus
　Ligaments
　　Superior ligament
　　Lateral ligament
　　Anterior ligament
Incus
　Short process (crus breve)
　Long process (crus longum)
　Lenticular process
　Facet for malleus
　Superior ligament of incus
　Posterior ligament of incus
Stapes
　Head (caput)
　Neck
　Posterior crus (crus posterius)

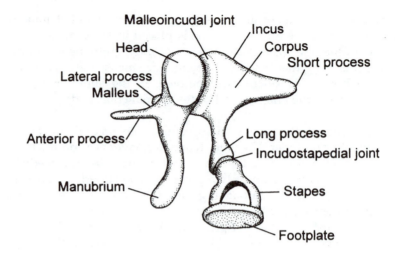

MEDIAL VIEW

FIGURE 5-4. Articulated ossicular chain of the right ear in medial view.

Ossicles

The bones of the ear, known as the *ossicles*, include the *malleus, incus,* and *stapes* (see Figures 5-4 and 5-5). This ossicular chain of three articulated bones provides the means for transmission of acoustic energy by impinging on the tympanic membrane to the inner ear. The malleus, the largest ossicle, provides the point of attachment with the tympanic membrane.

As you can see in Figure 5-4, the handle, or manubrium, of malleus is a long process, separated from the head by a thin neck. The anterior and lateral processes provide points of attachment for ligaments. The manubrium attaches to the tympanic membrane along its length, terminating with the lateral process.

The incus (fancied to be shaped like an anvil) provides the intermediate link of the ossicular chain. The body of the incus articulates with the head of the malleus by means of the malleolar facet in such a way that the long process of the incus is nearly parallel to the long process of the malleus. The long process bends medially, forming the lenticular process with which the stapes articulate.

The stapes, or "stirrup," is the third bone of this chain. The head (caput) of the stapes articulates with the lenticular process of incus,

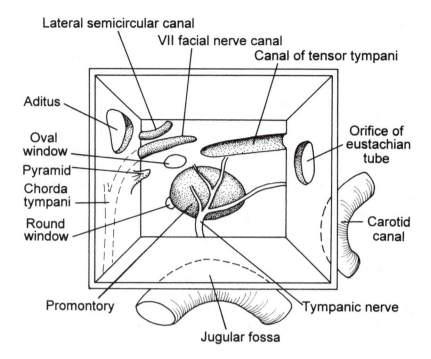

FIGURE 5–5. Schematic representation of the middle ear cavity of the right ear, as viewed from the external auditory meatus. (Redrawn by permission. From *Anatomy: A Regional Study of Human Structure*, 5th ed., by E. Gardner, D. J. Gray, & R. O'Rahilly, 1986, p. 623. Copyright © 1986 by R. O'Rahilly. Philadelphia: W. B. Saunders.)

and the neck of the stapes bifurcates to become the crura. The arch formed by the anterior and posterior crura converges on the footplate, or base, of the stapes. The footplate of the stapes rests in the oval window of the temporal bone, held in place by the annular ligament.

Tympanic Muscles

Two important muscles of the middle ear are attached to the ossicles. These are the smallest muscles of the human body.

Stapedius. The *stapedius muscle*, approximately 6 mm long, is embedded in the bone of the posterior wall of the middle ear, with only its tendon emerging from the pyramidal eminence in the middle ear space. The muscle inserts into the posterior neck of stapes, so that when it contracts, the stapes is rotated posteriorly. Innervation of the stapedius is by means of the stapedial branch of VII facial nerve.

Tensor Tympani. The *tensor tympani* is approximately 25 mm long, arising from the anterior wall of the middle ear space, superior to the orifice of the eustachian tube. As with the stapedius, only the tendon of the tensor tympani is found in the middle ear space, with the muscle housed in bone. The muscle originates from the cartilaginous part of the eustachian tube, as well as from the greater wing of sphenoid, coursing through the canal for the tensor tympani in the anterior wall of the middle ear. Contraction of this muscle reduces the range of movement of the tympanic membrane by placing indirect tension on it. Indeed, both tensor tympani and stapedius muscles stiffen the middle ear transmission system, thereby reducing transmission of acoustical information in the lower frequencies. Innervation of the tensor tympani is by the V trigeminal nerve.

Landmarks of Middle Ear

The middle ear space is invested with numerous landmarks of importance in the study of auditory function. Figure 5-5 is a schematic of the right middle ear represented as a box, to help our discussion.

Medial Wall. On the medial wall of Figure 5-5 you can see the *oval window* in which the *footplate of the stapes* is embedded, and the *round window*. Between these two is the *promontory*, a bulge created

Otitis Media with Effusion

Serous (secretory) otitis media is any condition in which fluid accumulates in the middle ear cavity. The typical sequence is as follows. The eustachian tube stops functioning properly, allowing the middle ear space to become anaerobic as tissue within the space absorbs the available oxygen. Parallel to this, the poorly functioning eustachian tube does not allow equalization of pressure between the middle ear space and the environment. In either condition, a relatively negative pressure can ensue in the middle ear space, pulling serous fluid from the blood of the middle ear tissues (termed transudation). The negative air pressure can also stimulate secretion of mucus from the middle ear tissue. This state, termed middle ear effusion, places a barrier to sound transmission in that the movement of the tympanic membrane is greatly inhibited.

by the basal turn of the cochlea. Immediately above the oval window is the prominence of the *lateral semicircular canal* of the vestibular mechanism.

Examination of the anterior wall reveals the entrance to the eustachian tube, and within that wall the internal carotid artery courses. The canal for the tensor tympani arises from the medial-most aspect of this wall, marked by the trochleariform process.

The eustachian tube is the sole means of bringing oxygen to the middle ear space (aeration), an important process for maintaining equilibrium between middle ear and atmospheric pressure. The eustachian tube is about 36 mm long, coursing anteriorly and medially on its way to the nasopharynx. The eustachian tube is capable of expanding by pulling the inferior margins away from each other, a function performed by the tensor veli palatine.

On the posterior wall is the prominence of the stapedial pyramid, from which the tendon of stapedius arises en route to the neck of

Acoustic Reflex

The acoustic reflex (also known as the stapedial reflex) is a staple of the audiologist's diagnostic toolkit. The stapedius muscle applies a force on the footplate of the stapes that reduces the amplitude of the footplate's movement, thereby reducing the sound pressure level reaching the cochlea. It is thought that this is a basic protective mechanism for the cochlea because it is triggered by loud sounds, typically greater than 85 dB SPL. The acoustic reflex can also include response by the tensor tympani muscle.

The neural circuit for the acoustic reflex is such that stimulation of either ear results in response by both ears, although attenuation of the signal by the ipsilateral ear (the ear closest to the sound) is stronger than the attenuation in the contralateral ear. As outlined by Møller (1983), a stimulus entering the right ear is transduced by the right cochlea, right ventral cochlear nucleus, and right medial superior olive, consecutively. The right medial superior olive communicates with both the right- and left-side nuclei of the VII facial and V trigeminal nerves, so that the appropriate stimulus triggers a response in stapedius muscles on both left and right sides.

stapes. Within the posterior wall courses the chorda tympani, and the VII facial nerve prominence continues on the medial wall.

Summary

- The malleus is the largest of the ossicles and provides the point of attachment with the tympanic membrane.
- The incus provides the intermediate communicating link of the ossicular chain, and the stapes is the third bone of this chain.
- The ossicular chain is held in place by the superior, anterior, and lateral ligaments of malleus and the posterior and superior ligaments of incus.
- The stapedius muscle inserts into the posterior neck of stapes and pulls the stapes posteriorly.
- The tensor tympani muscle inserts into the upper manubrium malli and pulls the malleus anteromedially.
- Landmarks of the medial wall of the middle ear cavity include the oval window, the round window, the promontory of the cochlea, and the prominence of facial nerve.
- The anterior wall houses the entrance to the eustachian tube, and the posterior wall houses the prominence of the stapedial pyramid.

Inner Ear

The inner ear houses the sensors for balance (the vestibular system) and hearing (the cochlea) (see Table 5-3). The entryway to the cochlea is the *vestibule*. Depicted in Figure 5-6 is the osseous, or bony labyrinth, representing the cavities (tunnels) in which the inner ear structures (the membranous labyrinth) are housed. The *osseous labyrinth* is made up of the entryway to the labyrinth, the vestibule, *semicircular canals*, and the *osseous cochlear canal*.

Osseous Semicircular Canals

The osseous semicircular canals house the sense organs for movement of the body in space. These consist of the anterior, posterior, and horizontal semicircular canals, each canal's name describing its orientation. You can envision the canals as a series of three rings attached to a ball (the vestibule), and lying behind and above that ball. Each ring is in a plane at right angles to one other ring, so that the interaction of the three permits the brain to code movement in three-dimensional space. The semicircular canals all open onto the vestibule.

Table 5–3. Landmarks of the Inner Ear

Vestibule
Saccule
Utricle
Macula
Otolithic membrane
Stereocilia
Kinocilium
Ductus reunien
Endolymphatic duct

Semicircular Canals
Lateral semicircular canal
Anterior vertical semicircular canal
Posterior vertical semicircular canal
Ampulla
Crista ampularis
Stereocilia
Kinocilium

Cochlea
Scala vestibuli
Scala tympani
Scala media (cochlear duct)
    Reissner's membrane
    Basilar membrane
    Spiral ligament
    Stria vascularis
    Organ of Corti
        Inner and outer hair cells
        Deiter's cells
        Tunnel of Corti
        Spiral limbus
        Inner spiral sulcus
        Tectorial membrane
        Reticular lamina
        Hensen's cells
        Cells of Claudius
        Rods of Corti

Osseous Spiral Lamina
Habenula perforata

Helicotrema

The anterior vertical canal is oriented so that it senses movement in the plane roughly perpendicular to the length of the temporal bone. This configuration transduces lateral movement of the head such as rocking your head from one shoulder to the other. The posterior vertical semicircular canal is oriented roughly parallel to the length of the temporal bone; it senses movement in the anterior-posterior

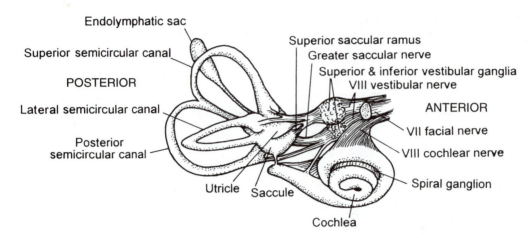

FIGURE 5-6. The osseous labyrinth, revealing components of the inner ear.

dimension, as in nodding your head "yes." The lateral horizontal semicircular canal senses movement roughly in the transverse plane of the body, as in shaking your head "no."

Binaural orientation of the two semicircular canals is such that the anterior semicircular canal of one ear is parallel to the posterior canal of the other. The horizontal canals lie in the same plane, but the ampullae are in mirror-image locations. As we will see, this horizontal orientation of the canal helps your brain differentiate rotary movement toward the left and right.

Osseous Cochlear Labyrinth

The osseous labyrinth has the appearance of a coiled snail shell. It coils out from a base near the vestibule, wrapping around itself $2\frac{3}{4}$ times before reaching its apex. The core of the osseous labyrinth, the *modiolus*, is finely perforated bone. Fibers of the VIII vestibulo-cochlear nerve pass through these perforations en route to ganglion cells within the modiolus. The core of the modiolus is continuous with the *internal auditory meatus* of temporal bone, through which the vestibulocochlear nerve passes.

The labyrinth is partially divided into two chambers, the *scala vestibuli* and the *scala tympani*, by an incomplete bony shelf protruding from the modiolus. This shelf is called the *osseous spiral lamina*. This structure forms the point of attachment for the scala media, which houses the sensory organ for hearing. The osseous spiral lamina becomes progressively smaller as it approaches the apex, such that the space between it and the opposite wall of the labyrinth increases. At the apex, the two chambers formed by the incomplete lamina become hooklike, forming the *helicotrema*, the region through which the scala tympani and scala vestibuli communicate.

The osseous labyrinth has three prominent openings. The *round window* (*foramen rotunde*) provides communication between the scala tympani and the middle ear. The oval window, within which the stapes is placed, permits communication between the scala vestibuli and the middle ear space. The *cochlear canaliculus*, or *cochlear aqueduct*, is a minute opening between the scala tympani in the region of the round window and the subarachnoid space of the cranial cavity. The fluid that fills the scala vestibuli and scala tympani passes through this duct.

Summary

- The inner ear houses the sensors for balance (the vestibular system) and hearing (the cochlea).
- The entryway to these structures is the vestibule.
- The osseous labyrinth is made up of the entryway to the labyrinth, the vestibule, semicircular canals, and the osseous cochlear canal.
- The semicircular canals in the inner ear are organs of balance.
- The osseous labyrinth has the appearance of a coiled snail shell.
- The labyrinth is divided into two incomplete chambers, the scala vestibuli and the scala tympani, by an incomplete bony shelf protruding from the modiolus, the osseous spiral lamina.
- The round window provides communication between the scala tympani and the middle ear.
- The oval window permits communication between the scala vestibuli and the middle ear space.
- The cochlear aqueduct connects the upper duct and the subarachnoid space.

Membranous Labyrinth

The structure of the *membranous labyrinth* parallels that of the *bony labyrinth*. First, orient yourself to the oval window, recognizing its link to the stapes of the middle ear. Beneath it, but not quite visible, is the round window. The *vestibule*, or entryway, to the inner ear is a space shared by the sense organ of hearing (the *cochlea*) and the sense organs of balance (the semicircular canals). Let us examine the sensory components of the inner ear (see Figure 5-7).

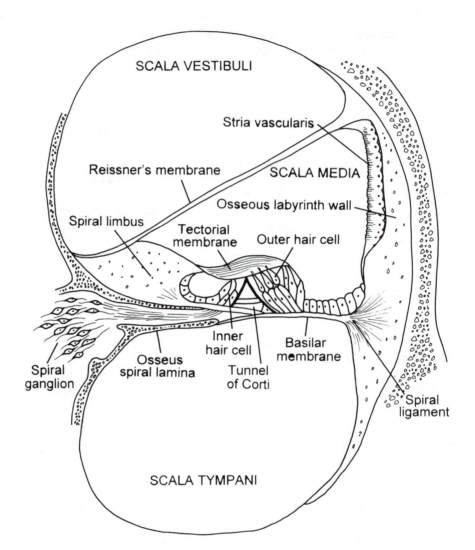

FIGURE 5-7. Cross section of the cochlea, revealing scala vestibuli, scala media, and scala tympani.

Vestibular System

The membranous labyrinth can be thought of as a fluid-filled sac that rests in the cavity of the osseous labyrinth. This sac does not completely fill the labyrinth, but rather forms an additional space in the already fluid-filled region. The duct forms only a small portion of the labyrinth and contains *endolymph*, fluid of a slightly different composition.

In the vestibular system, the membranous labyrinth houses the vestibular organ. Each *ampulla* houses a *crista ampularis*, which is the receptor organ for movement. From each of the 6,000 vestibular receptor cells protrude approximately 50 stereocilia, minute hairs that sense movement in fluid, and one kinocilium. A *cupula* overlays the crista ampularis such that the cilia are embedded in the cupula.

The *utricle* and *saccule* lie within the vestibule, the housing for the otolithic membrane of the vestibular system. The *otolithic membrane* is a layer of gelatinous material in which the cilia of the hair cells are embedded, and which has the effect of distending the cilia when the fluid is moved (Bhatnagar & Andy, 2002). The *utricular macula* is the sensory organ, which is endowed with hair cells and cilia. It is covered by the otolithic membrane, which is invested with crystals (*otoliths*). The saccule lies near the scala vestibuli in the vestibule, and it is similarly endowed with macula and otolithic membrane. The saccule and utricle communicate by means of the *endolymphatic duct*, which is embedded in the *dura mater*. The saccule communicates with the cochlea by means of the minute *ductus reuniens*.

Cochlear Duct

The membranous labyrinth of the cochlea, the cochlear duct, resides between the scala vestibuli and tympani, making up the intermediate scala media. This structure houses the sensory apparatus for hearing.

A cross section through the region of the scala media reveals its extraordinary structure, as shown in Figure 5-8. The osseous spiral lamina courses across the extent of the osseous labyrinth, forming the major point of attachment for the cochlear duct. Again, looking at Figure 5-7, you can see Reissner's membrane, an extremely thin separation between the perilymph of the scala vestibuli and the endolymph of the scala media. One end is continuous with the stria vascularis, which is highly vascularized tissue that is firmly attached to the spiral ligament.

As you can see in Figure 5-8, the *basilar membrane* forms the "floor" of the scala media, separating the scala media and scala tympani. It is on this membrane that the organ of hearing is found (the organ of Corti). The *organ of Corti* is similar to the vestibular organs. There are four rows of hair cells. The three rows of *outer hair cells* (OHC) are separated from the single row of *inner hair cells* (IHC) by *the tunnel of Corti*, the product of pillar cells of Corti. The *spiral limbus* arises from

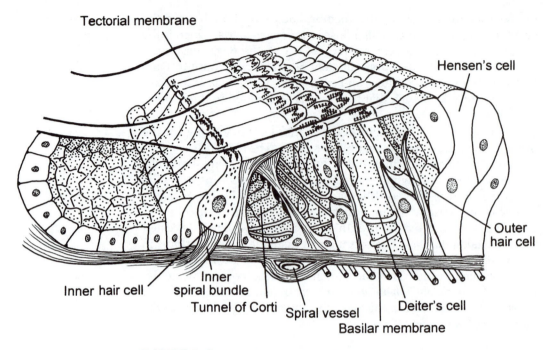

FIGURE 5–8. Landmarks and structures of the organ of Corti.

the *tectorial membrane*, which overlays the hair cells. The outer hair cells are embedded in the tectorial membrane but the inner hair cells do not make physical contact with it.

The 3,500 inner hair cells form a single row stretching from the base to apex of the cochlear duct. The three rows of outer hair cells (approximately 12,000) broaden to four rows in the apical end.

The hair cells of the cochlea receive both sensory and motor innervation. Clearly afferent information relates to the business of the cochlea (receiving and processing sound), but the motor innervation has a surprising function, discussed in the next section.

Innervation

There is sensory information transmitted through the auditory pathway that relates to vestibular sense and stimulation by sound. There is also motor innervation of the outer hair cells that is inhibitory, reducing the sensory activity caused by hair cell stimulation. The *olivocochlear bundle* comprises about 1,600 fibers, consisting of the crossed olivocochlear bundle (COCB) and uncrossed olivocochlear bundle (UCOB). When activated, these fibers reduce the response of the hair cells to sound. That is, they serve to reduce the effects that sound has on the cells they inhibit. It appears that this system helps us to "tune out" irrelevant information in noisy environments.

Summary

- The membranous labyrinth can be thought of as a fluid-filled sac that rests in the cavity of the osseous labyrinth and is filled with endolymph.
- In the vestibular system, the membranous labyrinth houses the vestibular organ.
- The ampulla is the expanded region of the semicircular canals that contains the crista ampularis. Within the vestibule lie the utricle and saccule.
- The membranous labyrinth of the cochlea resides between the scala vestibuli and tympani, making up the intermediate scala media.
- Reissner's membrane forms the upper boundary of the scala media, and the basilar membrane forms the floor.
- The organ of Corti has four rows of hair cells.
- The outer hair cells are separated from the inner row of hair cells by the tunnel of Corti.
- The upper surface of each hair cell is graced with a series of stereocilia.

AUDITORY PHYSIOLOGY

The auditory mechanism processes the acoustic signal of speech. Auditory stimuli can arrive at the tympanic membrane with an amazingly wide range of sound pressures, from the whisper of a leaf blowing in the breeze to the pressures associated with a jet engine. Likewise, the human auditory mechanism has a frequency range of approximately 10 octaves, spanning 20 Hz to 20,000 Hz. Within these broad requirements are much finer tasks, including differentiating small increments in frequency and intensity.

The field of audiology owes a great deal to the extraordinary scientist, Georg von Békésy, whose work resulted in a Nobel prize. Von Békésy (1960) performed exceedingly intricate measurements on the auditory mechanism, being forced to create tools where none existed. We refer frequently to his work, which defined the function of the middle and inner ears, as we discuss the basic physiological principles involved in transmission of an acoustic stimulus to a form that is interpretable by the brain. The simplified version of the process of hearing includes the following steps: (1) The outer ear collects sound and "shapes" its frequency components some-what; (2) the middle ear matches the airborne acoustic signal with the fluid medium of the cochlea; (3) the inner ear performs tempo-ral and spectral analysis on the ongoing acoustical signal; (4) the auditory pathway conveys and further processes that signal; and (5) the cerebral cortex interprets the signal.

Outer Ear Function

The outer ear can be seen primarily as a collector of sound. The pinna, with its ridges, grooves, and dished-out regions, is an excel-lent funnel for information directed toward the head from the front or side, although less effective for sound arising from behind the head.

Indeed, the crevices and crannies of the pinna are functional. Because the human outer ear cannot move as a cat's ear can; it can have only a passive effect on the input stimulus. The pinna acts as a "sound funnel," focusing acoustic energy into the external auditory meatus, and the external auditory meatus funnels sound to the tym-panic membrane. Both of these structures, however, have shapes that boost the relative strength of the signal through resonance, with the result being relatively enhanced signal intensity between 1,500 Hz and 8,000 Hz. The components of the pinna contribute a net gain reaching 20 dB at approximately 2,000 Hz.

Middle Ear Function

The cochlea is a fluid-filled cavity, and were it not for the presence of the middle ear mechanism, talking to each other would be like trying to talk to someone under water: The sound energy would reflect off the oval window because of the vast differences in the liq-uid and gaseous media of perilymph and air. Somewhere in our evo-lution, a mechanism arose to improve our plight.

The middle ear mechanism has evolved to increase the pressure arriving at the cochlea, thereby overcoming the resistance to flow of energy. Resistance to flow of energy is *impedance*, and the middle ear system overcomes a great deal of this resistance through three sig-nificant mechanisms. You will recall that sound intensity is a direct function of increase in sound pressure. Since pressure is equal to force divided by area $(P = F/A)$, to increase the sound pressure you would have to either increase the force applied or decrease the area over which the force is applied. In reality our middle ear does both of these things, using area benefits and lever benefits.

The tympanic membrane has an area of about 55 mm^2, and the area of the oval window is about 3.2 mm^2, making the tympanic membrane 17 times larger, depending on species size. Sound energy reaching the tympanic membrane is funneled to the much smaller area of the oval window, so there is a gain of 17:1, which translates to an increase of about 25 dB.

The second impedance-matching function is achieved by a lever effect. The length of the manubrium is approximately 9 mm and that of the long process of stapes is about 7 mm, giving an overall gain of about 1:2. The lever effect arising from this gain is nearly 2 dB.

Combined, the area and lever effects result in a signal gain of about 27 dB, from tympanic membrane to cochlea, depending on the stimulus frequency. Again, were the middle ear removed, a signal entering the external auditory meatus would have to be 27 dB more intense to be heard.

A third effect arises from the buckling of the tympanic membrane. As it moves in response to sound, the tympanic membrane buckles somewhat so that the arm of the malleus moves a shorter distance than the surface of the tympanic membrane. This results in a reduction in velocity of the malleus, with an increased force that provides a 4 dB to 6 dB increase in effective signal increase.

Summary

- The outer and middle ears serve as funneling and impedance-matching devices.
- The pinna funnels acoustical information to the external auditory meatus and aids in localization of sound in space.
- The resonant frequencies of the pinna and external auditory meatus are important components of the speech signal, between 1,500 Hz and 8,000 Hz.
- Resistance to flow of energy is impedance.
- The middle ear mechanism is an impedance-matching device, increasing the pressure of a signal arriving at the cochlea.
- The area ratio between the tympanic membrane and the oval window provides a 25-dB gain.
- The lever advantage of the ossicles provides a 2-dB gain.

- The buckling effect of the tympanic membrane relative to the malleus provides a 4-dB to 6-dB gain.

Inner Ear Function

Vestibular Mechanism

The semicircular canals are uniquely designed to respond to rotatory movement of the body. By virtue of their orientation, each canal is at right angles to one other canal, so that all movements of the head can be mapped by combinations of outputs of the sensory components, the cristae ampulares. As your head rotates, the fluid in the semicircular canals tends to remain in the same location, and the cilia are stimulated by relative movement of the fluid during rotation. The utricle and saccule sense acceleration, rather than rotation, of the head during body or head tilting. Taken together, the vestibular mechanisms provide the major input to the proprioceptive system that provides the sense of one's body in space. This information is integrated with joint sense, muscle spindle afferents, and visual input to form the perception of body position.

Auditory Mechanism: Mechanical Events

Spectral analysis: Analysis of a signal that identifies frequency components of that signal.

The inner ear is responsible for spectral and temporal acoustic analyses of incoming acoustical signals. By **spectral analysis** we refer to the process of extracting or defining the various frequency components of a given signal.

Sound causes the tympanic membrane to move, and that movement is translated to the oval window. When the tympanic membrane moves inward or outward, the stapes footplate in the oval window follows. When the stapes compresses the perilymph of the scala vestibuli, Reissner's membrane is distended toward the scala media, and the basilar membrane is distended toward the scala tympani. Since the frequency of a sound is determined by the number of oscillations or vibrations per second, a 100-Hz signal results in the footplate moving inward and outward 100 times per second, and that periodic vibration is translated to the basilar membrane, where it initiates a wave action known as the *traveling wave*.

Georg von Békésy discovered that when high-frequency sounds impinge on the inner ear, they cause vibration of the basilar membrane closer to the vestibule, the basal end of the cochlea. Low-frequency sounds result in a long traveling wave that reaches toward the apex, covering a greater distance along the basilar membrane. In this way, the traveling wave separates out the frequency components

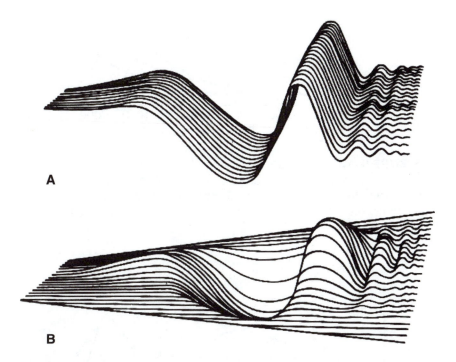

FIGURE 5–9. Traveling wave patterns. **A.** Pattern of oscillation in absence of lateral restraints. **B.** Pattern of vibration arising from stimulation, but accounting for lateral attachment of basilar membrane. (Reprinted with permission from "Shearing Motion in Scala Media of Cochlear Models" by J. Tonndorf, 1960, p. 241. *Journal of the Acoustical Society of America, 32*(5). Copyright © 1960 Acoustical Society of America.)

of complex sounds because high-frequency sounds are processed in basal regions, whereas low-frequency sounds are processed nearer the apex (see Figure 5-9). When a sound has both high- and low-frequency components, those components are separated out and processed at their respective portions of the basilar membrane (see Figures 5-10 and 5-11). The traveling wave moves along the basilar membrane, growing and swelling as it travels, until it reaches a point of maximum growth.

Excitation of the hair cells occurs as the result of the traveling wave's effect on the basilar membrane. The cilia of the outer hair cells are embedded in the tectorial membrane, and as the traveling wave moves along the basilar membrane, the hair cells are displaced relative to the tectorial membrane. This produces a shearing action that is greatest at the point of maximum perturbation of the basilar membrane.

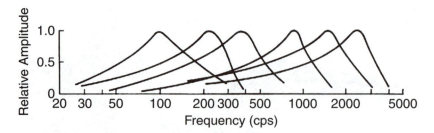

FIGURE 5–10. Resonance curves of six regions along the basilar membrane. CPS, cycles per second. (Reprinted by permission from *Experiments in Hearing* by G. von Békésy, 1960, p. 454. Copyright © 1960 by McGraw-Hill. New York: McGraw-Hill Book Company.)

FIGURE 5–11. Vibratory pattern of the basilar membrane at two instants within a cycle of vibration. Input stimulus is 200 Hz signal. (Reprinted by permission from *Experiments in Hearing* by G. von Békésy, 1960, p. 462. Copyright © 1960 by McGraw-Hill. New York: McGraw-Hill Book Company.)

Summary

- The inner ear is responsible for spectral (frequency) and temporal acoustic analyses of incoming acoustical signals.
- Movement of the tympanic membrane is translated into analogous movement of the stapes footplate and the fluid in the scala vestibuli.

- Compression in the fluid of the scala vestibuli is translated directly to the basilar membrane, and the disturbance at the basilar membrane initiates the traveling wave.
- The cochlea is arranged so that high-frequency sounds are resolved at the base and low-frequency sounds are processed at the apex.

Neural Responses

There are two basic types of VIII nerve neuron: low spontaneous rate (high-threshold) and high spontaneous rate (low-threshold) fibers. High-threshold neurons require a higher level of stimulation to fire, respond to the higher end of our auditory range of signal intensity, and have little or no random background firing noise. (Background "neural noise" is caused by random firing of neurons in absence of stimulation and is a widespread phenomenon in the nervous system.) Low-threshold fibers, on the other hand, respond at very low signal intensities and display random firing even when no stimulus is present. Thus, it appears that the low-threshold neurons may be a mechanism for hearing sound at near-threshold levels, whereas high-threshold fibers may pick up where the low-threshold fibers stop, as the signal increases.

Because neurons are all-or-none devices, every unit response is equal to the next in intensity and duration. Thus, the only way neurons can provide differential response is in rate of firing. When an VIII nerve fiber responds to tonal stimulation, there is an initial burst of strong activity followed by a decline to a plateau of discharge over the duration of the tone. When the tone is terminated, the response of the fiber drops below baseline levels, rising up the baseline "noise" level after recovery. This fairly straightforward poststimulus time histogram has provided us with very important verification of the *frequency specificity*, the ability of the cochlea to differentiate spectral components of a signal.

Researchers who study auditory perceptual abilities as they relate to the physical mechanism (*psychoacousticians*) have found that, in general, humans can discriminate change in frequency of signals of about 2%. Figure 5-12 shows a tuning curve for a single unit recording. A tuning curve is basically a composite of the responses of a single fiber at each frequency of presentation. For instance, researchers placed an electrode on a neuron and presented different frequencies of stimulation. They then recorded the stimulus intensity at which the neuron began to fire in response to the stimulus (its threshold) and plotted that intensity. In Figure 5-12, you can see that the fiber

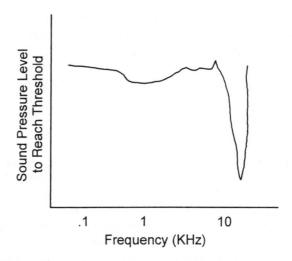

FIGURE 5-12. Schematic representation of tuning curve for VIII nerve fiber with characteristic frequency of 10,000 Hz.

was most sensitive to the 10,000-Hz signal. This is its *characteristic frequency*, or *CF*. As the signal frequency decreased to 8,000 Hz, the signal had to be of greater intensity to cause the neuron to fire. The signal at 5,000 Hz had to be 60 dB stronger than that at the CF for that neuron.

This tuning curve is a measure of neural specificity in one sense, but probably as much a measure of basilar membrane response. The electrode is, in effect, measuring the activity at one point on the basilar membrane (10,000 Hz, near the base), and activity farther up the cochlea toward the apex has less and less effect on the neuron we are recording. The sharper the tuning curve is, the greater is the frequency specificity of the basilar membrane. Indeed, when Khanna and Leonard (1982) compared the tuning curves of the basilar membrane and the auditory nerve, they found that the two curves were quite similar. That is, the basilar membrane is a very finely tuned filter capable of fine differentiation.

What happens when the stimulation to the cochlea is more complex than a simple sinusoidal tone? For instance, if a tone complex including 500 Hz, 1,000 Hz, 1,500 Hz, and 2,000 Hz were presented to the ear, how would the cochlea and VIII nerve respond? Essentially, the nerve fibers with characteristic frequencies of the stimulus components (i.e., 500 Hz, 1,000 Hz, etc.) will respond, whereas fibers with CF at other frequencies (i.e., 510 Hz, 511 Hz, 512 Hz, etc.) will take much more stimulation to fire. We judiciously avoided 505 Hz in our list of off-stimulus CF because that difference is probably not discriminable. That is, the cochlea generally cannot differentiate a difference smaller than 1% of its CF (i.e., 5 Hz in this situation), so the fibers at 502 Hz would respond the same as those at 500 Hz. To the brain, these two frequencies are indiscriminable.

As the intensity of stimulation increases, rate of firing increases, up to a point. Because neurons are limited by the refractory period, they typically cannot fire more than once per millisecond. The dynamic range for intensity that can be encoded in rate of firing is in the order of 30 to 40 dB, far too low for encoding of intensity. We are capable of differentiating a much greater range of intensities than this. Recall that different neurons have different thresholds of response (low- and high-threshold neurons). Apparently, intensity is coded by using both types of neuron: Low-threshold neurons can process low-intensity signals and high-threshold neurons carry the load of higher intensity sound.

Recall that we mentioned the motor system of the auditory mechanism earlier, stating that it helps to reduce the response of some hair cells. When this system of nerve fibers, called the *crossed-olivocochlear bundle (COCB)* and *uncrossed-olivocochlear bundle (UOCB)*, is stimulated, the firing rate of neurons innervated by them is reduced dramatically. This has the effect of reducing response to unwanted information, perhaps permitting the nervous system to "focus" on a desired signal while damping the response to noise. The motor system also appears to have a role in frequency discrimination.

Summary

- There are two basic types of VIII nerve neuron, and specific techniques have been developed to assess their functions.
- High-threshold neurons require a higher intensity and encompass the higher end of our auditory range of signal intensity.
- Low-threshold fibers respond at very low signal levels and display random firing even when no stimulus is present.
- Low-threshold neurons may process near-threshold sounds, whereas high-threshold fibers process higher level sounds.
- Frequency specificity is the ability of the cochlea to differentiate the spectral components of a signal.

- The characteristic, or best, frequency of a neuron is the frequency to which it responds best.
- A tuning curve is a composite of the responses of a single fiber at each frequency of presentation.
- The sharper the tuning curve is, the greater is the frequency specificity of the basilar membrane.
- As the intensity of stimulation increases, rate of firing increases.
- When the crossed-olivocochlear and uncrossed-olivocochlear bundles are stimulated, the firing rate of neurons innervated by them is reduced dramatically.

Auditory Pathway Responses

The cochlea and VIII nerve represent only the first stage of information extraction of the auditory signal. Temporal and tonotopically arrayed information is passed to progressively higher centers for further extraction of information (see Figure 5-13). Researchers have identified a wide variety of responses at every level of the auditory pathway, indicating very detailed information processing by the auditory nervous system, but let us focus on only one aspect of that processing.

The *superior olivary complex (SOC)* has the primary responsibility for localization of sound in space. It receives information from both ears and compares that information to determine the origination of the sound in space. One portion of the SOC (the lateral superior olive, or 'S segment') compares the intensity between the two ears to identify the location of high-frequency sounds. The *medial superior olive (MSO)* compares the time patterns of low-frequency sounds to identify the locations based on phase differences between the two signals.

The cerebral cortex receives input primarily from the contralateral ear via the thalamus (specifically, the medial geniculate body, or MGB). The cerebral cortex then proceeds to make sense of this acoustical information.

Summary

- Temporal and tonotopically arrayed information is passed to progressively higher centers for further extraction of information.
- The superior olivary complex (SOC) is the primary site of localization of sound in space.
- The medial geniculate body (MGB) is a relay of the thalamus.

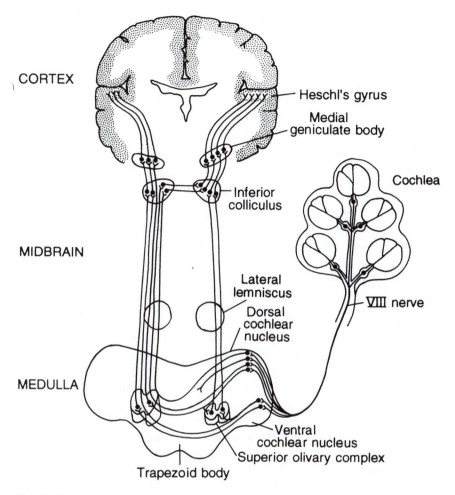

FIGURE 5–13. Course of the VIII vestibulocochlear nerve and auditory pathway.

▪ The cortex completes the analysis of the auditory signal that is accomplished by the auditory pathway.

CHAPTER SUMMARY

The outer ear is composed of the pinna and the external auditory meatus. Landmarks of the pinna include the margin of the auricle, the helix, and the auricular tubercle on the helix. The external auditory meatus has both osseous and cartilaginous parts: The cartilaginous portion makes up one third of the ear canal, while the other two thirds is housed in bone. At the terminus of the external auditory meatus is the tympanic membrane, the structure that separates the outer and middle ears.

The middle ear cavity houses the middle ear ossicles. The malleus is the largest ossicle, providing the point of attachment with the tympanic membrane. The incus provides the intermediate communicating link of the ossicular chain, and the stapes is the third bone of this chain. The ossicular chain is held in place by a series of important ligaments. The stapedius muscle inserts into the posterior neck of stapes and pulls the stapes posteriorly, and the tensor tympani muscle inserts into the upper manubrium malli, pulling the malleus anteromedially. Landmarks of the medial wall of the middle ear cavity include the oval window, the round window, the promontory of the cochlea, and the prominence of facial nerve. The anterior wall houses the entrance to the eustachian tube, and the posterior wall houses the prominence of the stapedial pyramid.

The inner ear contains the sense mechanism for balance (the vestibular system) and hearing (the cochlea). The entryway to these structures is the vestibule. The osseous labyrinth is made up of the entryway to the labyrinth, the vestibule, semicircular canals, and the osseous cochlear canal. It has the appearance of a coiled snail shell, and it is divided into two incomplete chambers, the scala vestibuli and the scala tympani, by an incomplete bony shelf protruding from the modiolus, the osseous spiral lamina. The round window provides communication between the scala tympani and the middle ear. The oval window permits communication between the scala vestibuli and the middle ear space. The cochlear aqueduct connects the upper duct and the subarachnoid space.

The membranous labyrinth is an endolymph-filled sac that rests within the cavity of the osseous labyrinth. In the vestibular system, the membranous labyrinth contains the vestibular organ. The ampulla is the expanded region of the semicircular canals and contains the crista ampularis. Within the vestibule lie the utricle and saccule. The membranous labyrinth of the cochlea resides between the scala vestibuli and scala tympani, making up the intermediate scala media. Reissner's membrane forms the distal boundary of the scala media, and the basilar membrane forms the proximal boundary. The organ of Corti has four rows of hair cells resting on a bed of Deiters' cells for support. The outer hair cells are separated from the row of inner hair cells by the tunnel of Corti. The upper surface of each hair cell is graced with a series of stereocilia. Each inner hair cell innervates as many as ten VIII nerve fibers, while each outer hair cell shares its innervation with ten other outer hair cells, all being innervated by the same VIII nerve fiber.

The outer and middle ears serve as funneling and impedance-matching devices. The pinna funnels acoustical information to the external auditory meatus and aids in localization of sound in space. Resistance to flow of energy is termed impedance. The middle ear mechanism is an impedance-matching device, increasing the pressure of a signal arriving at the cochlea. The area ratio between the tympanic membrane and the oval window provides a significant gain in output over input, and the lever advantage of the ossicles provides a smaller gain.

The inner ear is responsible for performing spectral (frequency) and temporal acoustic analyses of incoming acoustical signals. Movement of the tympanic membrane is translated into parallel movement of the stapes footplate and the fluid in the scala vestibuli. Movement of the fluid of the scala vestibuli is translated directly to the basilar membrane, and the disturbance at the basilar membrane causes the initiation of the traveling wave. The cochlea has a tonotopic arrangement, with high-frequency sounds resolved at the base and low-frequency sounds processed toward the apex. The point of maximum displacement of the basilar membrane determines the frequency information transmitted to the brain. The traveling wave quickly damps after reaching its point of maximum displacement. The frequency analysis ability of the basilar membrane is determined by graded stiffness, thickness, and width. The basilar membrane is stiffer, thinner, and more narrow at the base than apex. Excitation of the outer hair cells occurs primarily as the result of a shearing effect on the cilia. Excitation of the inner hair cells is produced by the effect of fluid flow and turbulence of endolymph.

There are two basic types of VIII nerve neuron. High-threshold neurons require a higher intensity and encompass the higher end of our auditory range of signal intensity. Low-threshold fibers respond at very low signals and display random firing even when there is no stimulus. Low-threshold neurons may process near-threshold sounds, whereas high-threshold fibers process higher level sounds. Frequency specificity is the ability of the cochlea to differentiate spectral components of a signal. A tuning curve is a composite of the responses of a single fiber at each frequency of presentation. The sharper the tuning curve is, the greater is the frequency specificity of the basilar membrane.

Study Questions

1. The _____ of the outer ear is important for localization of sound in space.

2. Resistance to flow of energy is called _____.

3. The area ratio between the tympanic membrane and the oval window provides a _____ dB gain, and the lever advantage gives a _____ dB gain.

4. The cochlea performs both _____ analysis and _____ analysis.

5. Compression in the fluid of the scala vestibuli is translated directly to the basilar membrane, and the disturbance at the basilar membrane causes the initiation of _____ wave.

6. High-frequency sounds are resolved at the base of the cochlea, with progressively lower sounds processed at progressively higher positions on the cochlea. This array is called _____.

7. The frequency analysis ability of the basilar membrane is determined by graded _____, _____, and _____.

8. At the apex, the basilar membrane is thinner/thicker (circle one) than at the base.

9. At the apex, the basilar membrane is wider/narrower (circle one) than at the base.

10. T/F The cilia of the outer hair cells are embedded in the tectorial membrane.

11. T/F The cilia of the inner hair cells are embedded in the tectorial membrane.

12. _____ neurons require a higher intensity and encompass the higher end of our auditory range of signal intensity, whereas _____ neurons respond at very low signal levels and display random firing even when there is no stimulus.

13. _____ refers to the ability of the cochlea to differentiate spectral components of a signal.

14. The _____ frequency of a neuron is the frequency to which it responds best.

15. Tuning curves are composites of the responses of a single fiber at each frequency of presentation. The sharper the tuning curve is, the greater is the _____ of the basilar membrane.

16. Rate of firing of neurons increases as the _____ increases.

17. Stimulation of the _____ bundle and the _____ bundle reduces the firing rate of neurons innervated by them.

18. The _____ meatus is a conduit for sound reaching the tympanic membrane.

19. The _____ meatus is a conduit for the VIII nerve fibers coursing to the brainstem.

20. The tympanic membrane (or eardrum) is made up of _____ layers of tissue.

21. The outer layer of the tympanic membrane is continuous with the _____.

22. The _____ layer of the tympanic membrane is made up primarily of radiating fibers.

23. The _____ is a landmark produced by the most distal part of the manubrium malli.

24. The _____ is the bone of the middle ear directly attached to the tympanic membrane.

25. The _____ is the bone of the middle ear directly communicating with the oval window.

26. The _____ of the malleus attaches to the tympanic membrane.

27. The _____ of the stapes articulates with the oval window.

28. The _____ muscle pulls the stapes posteriorly.

29. The _____ muscle pulls the malleus anteromedially.

30. The entryway to the cochlea and vestibular system is via the space known as the _____.

31. The _____ is the system of cavities within bone that houses the membranous labyrinth.

32. The scala _____ and scala _____ are incomplete spaces in the osseous labyrinth.

33. The _____ window provides communication between the scala tympani and the middle ear.

34. The _____ window permits communication between the scala vestibuli and the middle ear space.

35. The _____ is a fluid-filled sac attached to the walls of the osseous labyrinth and is filled with endolymph.

36. The _____ membrane separates the scala vestibuli and the scala media; the _____ membrane separates the scala media from the scala tympani.

37. There is/are _____ row(s) of outer hair cells and _____ row(s) of inner hair cells.

38. The hair cells are innervated by the _____ nerve.

39. Microsurgery procedures have advanced rapidly in recent years, permitting re-articulation of ossicles that have become disarticulated. Considering how well protected the ossicles are, what could cause them to become disarticulated?

40. Comparative anatomy provides insight into function. What differences in the cochlea would you predict when comparing the cochlea of a human with that of a mammal that used ultra-high-frequency sound to echo-locate, such as a fruit bat? What differences would you predict that you would find when comparing an elephant's cochlea with that of a human?

REFERENCES

Altschuler, R. A., Bobbin, R. P., & Hoffman, D. W. (1986). *Neurology of hearing: The cochlea.* New York: Raven.

Anson, B. J., & Donaldson, J. R. (1973). *Surgical anatomy of the temporal bone and ear.* Philadelphia: Saunders.

Bhatnagar, S. C., & Andy, O. J. (2002). *Neuroscience for the study of communicative disorders* (2nd ed.). Baltimore: Williams & Wilkins.

Carpenter, M. B. (1991). *Core text of neuroanatomy* (4th ed.). Baltimore: Williams & Wilkins.

Cazals, Y., Demany, L., & Horner, K. (1991). *Auditory physiology and perception.* Oxford: Pergamon.

Chusid, J. G. (1985). *Correlative neuroanatomy and functional neurology* (17th ed.). Los Altos, CA: Lange Medical Publications.

Cianfrone, G., & Grandori, F. (1985). Cochlear mechanics and otoacoustic emissions. *Scandinavian Audiology (Suppl. 25).*

Dallos, P. (1973). *The auditory periphery.* New York: Academic.

Dallos, P., Billone, M. C., Durrant, J. D., Wang, C-Y., & Raynor, S. (1972). Cochlear inner and outer hair cells: Functional differences. *Science, 177,* 356–358.

Davis, H. (1958). Transmission and transduction in the cochlea. *Laryngoscope, 68,* 359–382.

Duifhuis, H., Horst, J. W., van Dijk, P., & van Netten, S. M. (1993). *Biophysics of hair cell sensory systems.* Singapore: World Scientific.

Durrant, J. D., & Lovrinic, J. H. (1995). *Bases of hearing science.* Baltimore: Williams & Wilkins.

Engstrom, H., Ades, H. W., & Andersson, A. (1966). *Structural pattern of the organ of corti.* Baltimore: Williams & Wilkins.

Gardner, E., Gray, D. J., & O'Rahilly, R. (1986). *Anatomy: A regional study of human structure* (5th ed.). Philadelphia: Saunders.

Gelfand, S. A. (2001). *Essentials of audiology* (2nd ed.). New York: Thieme Medical.

Gray, H., Bannister, L. H., Berry, M. M., & Williams, P. L. (Eds.). (1995). *Gray's anatomy.* London: Churchill Livingstone.

Green, D. (1976). *An introduction to hearing.* Hillsdale, NJ: Lawrence Erlbaum.

Gulick, W. L. (1971). *Hearing physiology and psychophysics.* New York: Oxford University Press.

Henson, O. W. (1974). Comparative anatomy of the middle ear. In H. Autrum, R. Jung, W. R. Loewenstein, D. M. MacKay, & H. L. Teuber (Eds.), *Handbook of sensory physiology* (pp. 40–110). New York: Springer-Verlag.

Javel, E. (1986). Basic response properties of auditory nerve fibers. In R. A. Altschuler, R. P. Bobbin, & D. W. Hoffman (Eds.), *Neurobiology of hearing: The cochlea* (pp. 213–245). New York: Raven.

Kandel, E. R., Schwartz, J. H., & Jessell, T. M. (2000). *Principles of neural science* (4th ed.). New York: McGraw Hill.

Khanna, S. M., & Leonard, D. G. B. (1982). Basilar membrane tuning in the cochlea. *Science, 215,* 305–306.

Kiang, N. Y-S. (1965). *Discharge patterns of single fibers in the cat's auditory nerve.* Cambridge, MA: M.I.T. Press.

Kiang, N. Y-S., Liberman, M. C., Sewell, W. F., & Guinan, J. J. (1986). Single unit clues to cochlear mechanisms. *Hearing Research, 22,* 171–182.

Kuehn, D. P., Lemme, M. L., & Baumgartner, J. M. (1991). *Neural bases of speech, hearing, and language.* Boston: Little, Brown.

Lewis, E. R., Leverenz, E. L., & Bialek, W. S. (1985). *The vertebrate inner ear.* Boca Raton, FL: CRC Press.

Lim, D. J. (1980). Cochlear anatomy related to cochlear micromechanics: A review. *Journal of the Acoustical Society of America, 67* (5), 1686–1695.

Martin, F. N. (1981). *Medical audiology.* Englewood Cliffs, NJ: Prentice-Hall.

Minifie, F. (1973). Speech acoustics. In F. D. Minifie, T. J. Hixon, & F. Williams (Eds.), *Normal aspects of speech, hearing, and language* (pp. 11–72). Englewood Cliffs, NJ: Prentice-Hall.

Minifie, F. D., Hixon, T. J., & Williams, F. (Eds.). (1992). *Normal aspects of speech, hearing, and language.* Englewood Cliffs, NJ: Prentice-Hall.

Møller, A. R. (1973). *Basic mechanisms of hearing.* New York: Academic.

Møller, A. R. (1983). *Auditory physiology.* New York: Academic.

Netter, F. H. (1989). *Atlas of human anatomy.* Summit, NJ: CIBA Pharmaceuticals Division.

Parkins, C. W., & Anderson, S. W. (1983). Cochlear prostheses. *Annals of the New York Academy of Sciences, 405.*

Pickles, J. O. (1988). *An introduction to the physiology of hearing* (2nd ed.). London: Academic.

Rhode, W. W. (1985). The use of intracellular techniques in the study of the cochlear nucleus. *Journal of the Acoustical Society of America, 78,* 320–327.

Rosse, C., Gaddum-Rosse, P., & Rosse, G. (1997). *Hollinshead's textbook of anatomy.* Philadelphia: Lippincott-Raven.

Ryan, A., & Dallos, P. (1976). Physiology of the inner ear. In J. L. Northern (Ed.), *Hearing disorders* (pp. 89–101). Boston: Little, Brown.

Shaw, E. A. G. (1974). The external ear. In W. D. Keidel & W. D. Neff (Eds.), *Handbook of sensory physiology* (pp. 455–490). New York: Springer-Verlag.

Spoendlin, H. (1978). The afferent innervation of the cochlea. In R. F. Naunton & C. Fernandez (Eds.), *Evoked electrical activity in the auditory nervous system.* New York: Academic.

Syka, J., & Masterton, R. B. (1988). *Auditory pathway structure and function.* New York: Plenum.

Tobias, J. V., & Schubert, E. D. (1983). *Hearing research and theory (Vol. 2).* New York: Academic.

Tonndorf, J. (1958). The hydrodynamic origin of aural harmonics in the cochlea. *Annals of Otology, 67,* 754–774.

Tonndorf, J. (1960). Shearing motion in scala media of cochlear models. *Journal of the Acoustical Society of America, 32* (5), 238–244. Von Békésy, G. (1960). *Experiments in hearing.* New York: McGraw-Hill.

Wever, E. G., & Bray, C. W. (1930). Action currents in the auditory nerve in response to acoustical stimulation. *Proceedings of the National Academy of Science, 16,* 344–350.

Wilson, J. P., & Kemp, D. T. (1989). *Cochlear mechanisms: Structure, function, and models.* New York: Plenum.

Winans, S. S., Gilman, S., Manter, J. T., & Gatz, A. J. (2002). *Manter and Gatz's essentials of clinical neuroanatomy and neurophysiology* (10th ed.). Philadelphia: Davis.

Yost, W. A. (2000). *Fundamentals of hearing: An introduction* (4th ed). New York: Academic.

Zemlin, W. R. (1998). *Speech and hearing science. Anatomy and physiology* (4th ed.). Needham Heights, MA: Allyn & Bacon.

CHAPTER

6

Neuroanatomy and Neurophysiology

OUTLINE

I. Anatomy of the Central and Peripheral Nervous Systems

    A. Functional divisions of the nervous system

        1. The autonomic nervous system (ANS)

            a. Sympathetic system

            b. Parasympathetic system

2. The somatic system controls the conscious and voluntary bodily functions
    a. Pyramidal system
    b. Extrapyramidal system

B. Anatomic divisions of the nervous system
  1. The central nervous system (CNS) includes the brain (cerebrum, cerebellum, subcortical structures, and brainstem) and spinal cord
  2. The peripheral nervous system (PNS) includes 12 pairs of cranial nerves and 31 pairs of spinal nerves, as well as the sensory receptors

C. Meningeal linings

D. Cerebral cortex
  1. Two hemispheres connected by corpus callosum
  2. Gyri and sulci
  3. Frontal lobe
  4. Parietal lobe
  5. Temporal lobe
  6. Occipital lobe
  7. Insular cortex
  8. Limbic lobe

E. Medial surface of cerebral cortex
  1. Myelinated fibers
    a. Projection fibers
    b. Association fibers
    c. Commissural fibers
  2. Basal ganglia
  3. Diencephalic structures

F. Cerebrovascular system
  1. Life-blood of the brain
  2. Anterior cerebral arteries
  3. Middle cerebral artery
  4. Superior and anterior inferior cerebellar arteries
  5. Posterior inferior cerebellar artery
  6. Basilar artery
  7. Circle of Willis

G. Cerebellum
  1. Coordinates motor commands
  2. Divided into superior, middle, and inferior peduncles

H. Brainstem
  1. Medulla, pons, and midbrain
  2. Pyramidal decussation
  3. Reticular formation

I. Cranial nerves
    1. Sensory, motor, or mixed sensorimotor
    2. I olfactory
    3. II optic nerve
    4. III oculomotor
    5. IV trochlear
    6. V trigeminal
    7. VI abducens
    8. VII facial
    9. VIII vestibulocochlear
    10. IX glossopharyngeal
    11. X vagus
    12. XI spinal accessory
    13. XII hypoglossal

II. Neurophysiology

A. Neuron function
    1. Synaptic communication
    2. Excitatory and inhibitory functions
    3. Action potential and polarization
    4. Absolute refractory period
    5. Resting membrane potential
B. Propagation
    1. Saltatory conduction
    2. Temporal summation
    3. Convergence and divergence
C. Muscle function
D. Higher neural functioning
    1. Cerebrum
        a. Primary reception for somatic sense, primary motor area, primary auditory cortex, and primary region of visual reception
        b. Higher-order areas
        c. Association areas
    2. Prefrontal area
    3. Temporal-occipital-parietal association area
    4. Limbic association area
D. Hemispheric specialization
    1. Left hemisphere processes language and speech
    2. Right hemisphere processes holistic information
E. Motor control of speech
    1. Precentral gyrus
    2. Motor strip
    3. Premotor regions

There is nothing in nature as awe inspiring as the nervous system. Although humans have been studying the brain for thousands of years (there is evidence that the Pueblo Indians of prehistoric New Mexico performed surgical procedures on the skull), we have only begun to understand this very complex system. There are at least 100 billion nerve cells in the nervous system, and each of these may communicate directly with as many as 2,000 other neurons, providing at least one trillion points of communication. The brain is the control center and processor for all of the functions of communication and life. It is at the very heart of communication.

ANATOMY OF THE CENTRAL AND PERIPHERAL NERVOUS SYSTEMS

While it is an understatement to say that the central nervous system (CNS) is extremely complex, it may be a comfort to realize that there is a common denominator to all of the structures of the nervous system: All structures are made of neurons.

Neurons

Neurons (nerve cells): Tissue specialized for communication.

Glia (glial cells): Nervous system tissue that provides support and nutrients within the nervous system.

Soma: The cell body of a neuron.

Dendrite: The component of a neuron that generally receives input from another neuron or sensor.

Axon: The terminal point of a neuron, through which information passes.

Neurons, also known as nerve cells, are the communicating elements of the nervous system. **Glia**, also known as glial cells, are structural and nutrient-bearing cells that support the neurons. Neurons are the functional building blocks of the nervous system and are unique among tissue types.

While different types of neurons have different structures, there are some commonalities. Most neurons have a **soma** (cell body), a **dendrite** (receiver of information), which transmits information toward the soma, and an **axon**, which transmits information away from the soma (see Figure 6-1). We will discuss the function of the neurons later in this chapter.

Neuron Landmarks

If a neuron has many dendrites, it is often referred to as a dendritic tree because it looks "bushy." Most neurons have only one axon. The *axon hillock* is the junction of the axon and soma. Many axons are covered with a white fatty wrapping called the *myelin sheath*. Myelin speeds up neural conduction. Myelin is segmented, and the areas between the myelinated segments are known as *nodes of Ranvier* (see Table 6-1). At the end of the axon are the *telodendria*, which are long, thin projections. At the tips of the telodendria are

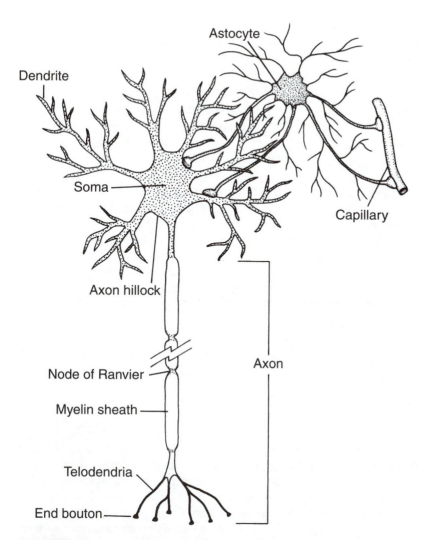

FIGURE 6-1. Schematic of basic elements of a neuron. Note that the astrocyte is a glial cell that supports transport of nutrients to the neuron while shielding it from toxins via the blood-brain barrier.

terminal end boutons (buttons), and inside the boutons are *synaptic vesicles*. Synaptic vesicles contain special chemicals called *neurotransmitters*. There are many types of neurotransmitters, and they are responsible for activating the next neuron in a chain of neurons. Neurotransmitters are released into the gap between two neurons (known as the *synaptic cleft*), which causes the next neuron in the

Table 6–1. Basic Components of the Neuron

Component	Function
Dendrite	Receptor region
Soma	Contains metabolic organelles
Axon	Transmits Information from neuron
Hillock	Generator site for action potential
Myelin sheath	Insulates axons
Schwann cells	Forms myelin in PNS
Oligodendrocytes	Forms myelin in CNS
Nodes of Ranvier	Permit saltatory conduction
Telodendria	Processes from axon
Terminal end boutons	Contain synaptic vesicles
Neurotransmitter	Facilitates synapse
Synaptic cleft	Region between pre- and postsynaptic neurons

chain to be activated. Groups of gray cell bodies are referred to as *gray matter; white matter* refers to myelin.

Glial Cells

There are many more glial cells than neurons. They provide support and nutrients to neurons and make up the myelin sheath. Different types of glia have different functions. *Astrocytes* provide the primary support for neurons, help suspend neurons, and transport nutrients from a capillary supply to the neuron. They also provide the important blood-brain barrier, a filter system that prohibits some toxins from passing from the brain's blood supply (*cerebrovascular system*) to neurons.

Oligodendrocytes are glia that make up the myelin in the central nervous system, and *Schwann cells* are glia that make up the myelin in the peripheral nervous system. Microglia perform the housekeeping process that scavenges dead (**necrotic**) tissue that is found after damage (**lesion**) in the nervous system. Astrocytes then form scars around this dead tissue, isolating it from the rest of the brain.

Necrotic tissue: Dead tissue.
Lesion: Damage to tissue.

Summary

▪ The nervous system is a complex, hierarchical structure made of neurons.

Hematoma

A hematoma is a pooling of blood, typically caused by breakage of a blood vessel. Subdural hematoma involves intracranial bleeding beneath the dura mater of the brain, caused by rupture of cortical arteries or veins, usually the result of trauma to the head. Pressure from the pooling blood displaces the brain, shifting and compressing the brainstem, forcing the temporal lobe under the tentorium cerebelli, and compressing cerebral arteries. This critically dangerous condition may not be immediately recognized because it may take several hours before pooling blood compresses the brain sufficiently to produce symptoms such as reduced consciousness, hemiparesis, or pupillary dilation. Epidural hematoma, a hematoma above the dura mater, may result in a person's being initially lucid but displaying progressively decreasing levels of consciousness, reflecting compression of the brain.

Hematomas are characterized by location of insult. Frontal epidural hematomas are caused by blows to the frontal bone and may result in personality changes. Posterior fossa epidural hematomas are caused by blows to the back of the head, resulting in visual and coordination deficits.

- Neurons communicate through synapse by means of neurotransmitter substance, and the postsynaptic neuron may be excited or inhibited by the transmitting neuron.
- Glial cells make up the myelin sheath and provide support for neurons.

FUNCTIONAL VIEW: AUTONOMIC AND SOMATIC NERVOUS SYSTEMS

A functional view of the nervous system categorizes the brain into autonomic and somatic nervous systems. The **autonomic nervous system (ANS)** governs involuntary activities of the visceral muscles (or viscera), including glandular secretions, heart function, digestive function, and so forth. You have little control over what happens to that triple chili cheeseburger as you digest it, although you may occasionally be aware of the digestive process.

The ANS can be divided into two subsystems, the sympathetic and the parasympathetic nervous systems. The **sympathetic nervous system**

Autonomic nervous system: The division of the central nervous system that is responsible for involuntary functions.

Sympathetic nervous system: The component of the autonomic nervous system responsible for body system responses that prepare the body to cope with stressful situations by increasing states of physiological vigilance and preparedness for muscular action.

Parasympathetic nervous system: The component of the autonomic nervous system responsible for body system responses that reverse autonomic responses, thereby preserving energy.

responds to stimulation by expending energy, and the **parasympathetic nervous system**, or craniosacral system, reduces the sympathetic response. When you have had a significant scare, such as a near collision in an automobile, your body's sympathetic responses include vasoconstriction (constriction of blood vessels), increase in blood pressure, dilation of pupils, cardiac acceleration, sweating, and "goose bumps." You may be less aware of the parasympathetic system response that is responsible for counteracting the effects of sympathetic response, such as slowing of the heart rate, reduction of blood pressure, and pupillary constriction.

Somatic nervous system: The subdivision of the nervous system responsible for voluntary motor function and nonvisceral sensation.

The **somatic nervous system** (voluntary component) is very important to the discipline of speech pathology. The somatic system controls the conscious and voluntary bodily functions, including control of all skeletal (somatic) muscles. The CNS's control of muscles arises mostly from the precentral region of the cerebral cortex. Neural impulses are conveyed through descending motor tracts of the brainstem and spinal cord. Cranial nerves of the brainstem and spinal nerves of the spinal cord are activated and cause muscles to contract. Likewise, the sensory component of the somatic nervous system monitors information about the function of the skeletal muscles, their environment, and other "nonvisceral" activities.

Direct (pyramidal) motor system: The motor system under voluntary control.

Indirect (extrapyramidal) motor system: The motor system that provides background support for the direct motor system.

The motor component of the somatic system can be divided into pyramidal and extrapyramidal systems. The **direct**, or **pyramidal, motor system** is responsible for initiating voluntary motor acts. The **indirect**, or **extrapyramidal, motor system** also is responsible for the background tone and movement that supports the primary acts.

Sensation is an essential part of communication. Without sensation, a perfectly functioning brain would be worthless as a communicating system. Likewise, since communication requires some sort of muscular activity or glandular secretion, the absence of motor activity would signal the end of communication. Fortunately, the large number of sensors in the human body permits us to use various pathways for receiving communication and for passing information to another person. We are rarely completely cut off from communication with others. Let us now examine the components of this system.

ANATOMICAL VIEW: CENTRAL AND PERIPHERAL NERVOUS SYSTEMS

Anatomically, the nervous system can be divided into the central nervous system and peripheral nervous system (see Table 6-2). The

Table 6–2. Divisions of the Nervous System from Anatomical and Physiological Perspectives

Anatomical Divisions of Nervous System

    Central Nervous System*:* Cerebrum, cerebellum, brainstem, spinal cord, thalamus, subthalamus, basal ganglia, etc.

    Peripheral Nervous System*:* Spinal nerves, cranial nerves, sensors

Functional Divisions of Nervous System

    Autonomic Nervous System*:* Involuntary bodily function

        Sympathetic nervous system: Expends energy (e.g., vaso-constriction when frightened)

        Parasympathetic nervous system: Conserves energy (e.g., vaso-dilation upon removal of fearful stimulation)

    Somatic Nervous System*:* Voluntary bodily function

---

central nervous system (CNS) includes the brain (cerebrum, cerebellum, subcortical structures, brainstem) and spinal cord. The **peripheral nervous system (PNS)** includes 12 pairs of *cranial nerves* and 31 pairs of *spinal nerves*, as well as the sensory receptors. All of the CNS components are housed in bone (skull or vertebral column), but most of the PNS components are outside of bone. We will spend a great deal of time with this organizational structure as we discuss the anatomy of the nervous system.

Central nervous system (CNS): The division of the nervous system that contains the brain and spinal cord.

Peripheral nervous system (PNS): The division of the nervous system that contains cranial and spinal nerves.

ANATOMY OF THE CEREBRAL CORTEX

The *cerebral cortex*, or *cerebrum* is the largest structure of the nervous system, weighs approximately 3 pounds, and contains billions of neurons. The cerebrum is divided into left and right hemispheres. In exploring the cerebral cortex we will start at the outside and work toward the center.

Meningeal Linings

Brain structures of the CNS are surrounded by a three-layer *meningeal lining* that protects neurons. Three meningeal linings cover the brain. The *dura mater* is the tough outer meningeal lining. The *arachnoid mater* is the middle meningeal lining through which many blood vessels for the brain pass. The inner lining is the *pia mater*, which is a thin, filmy covering that follows the contour of the brain. The major arteries and veins serving the surface of the brain course within this layer. Together the meningeal linings provide an

An Ounce of Prevention

If you choose to work in a trauma center, a significant portion of your caseload will arise from traumatic brain injury (TBI). Traumatic brain injury is a leading cause of death of individuals younger than 24 years old, with motor vehicle accidents far exceeding all other causes (falls, assaults, sport, firearms). The addition of safety belts to automobiles has reduced death in automobile accidents caused by brain injury by nearly 50%. Unfortunately, use of alcohol is related to reduced seatbelt use and increased death due to head injury during accidents. Mandatory use of helmets has reduced the frequency of brain injury in motorcycle accidents by 20% to 50% and up to 85% in bicycle accidents.

Gunshot wounds to the head result in most deaths attributable to firearms, and handguns are involved in more than 60% of homicides. More than 40,000 people in the United States are killed by firearms annually. While laws that restrict access to firearms are being hotly debated as a constitutional issue, trigger lock systems could greatly reduce the carnage that occurs in the United States, where nearly 50% of households have firearms. You can refer to Mackay and colleagues (1997) for an extremely thorough review of causes and treatment of TBI.

excellent means of nurturing and protecting the central nervous system structures.

Landmarks of the Cerebral Cortex

The cerebral cortex is divided into two hemispheres or roughly equal halves of the brain (see Figure 6-2). The term *cortex* actually means "bark," referring to the bark or outer surface of a tree, and the cerebral cortex is the outer surface of the brain.

The surface of the brain is quite convoluted (see Figure 6-3). Early in development, the cerebral cortex has few of these furrows and bulges, but as brain growth outstrips skull growth, the cerebral cortex doubles in on itself. The result is greatly increased surface area, translating into more "neural horsepower." You can think of the surface as a topographical map with mountains and valleys. The mountains (convolutions) in this case are called **gyri** (singular, gyrus) and

Gyri: Outfolding of tissue on the cerebral or cerebellar cortex.

FIGURE 6–2. Major landmarks of the cerebrum as seen from above and from the side. Note that the insular cortex (insula, *bottom left*) is typically hidden from view.

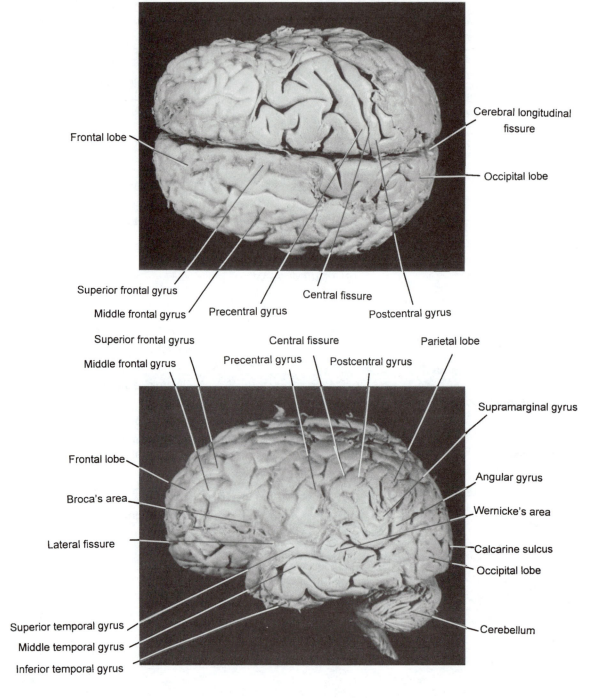

FIGURE 6-3. Lateral (*lower*) and superior (*upper*) views of cerebral cortex. Note that the pia mater can be seen in portions of both photographs.

the infolding valleys that separate the gyri are called **sulci** (singular, sulcus). If the groove is deeper and more pronounced it is a **fissure**. These gyri, sulci, and fissures, are the major landmarks of the cerebral cortex.

We divide the cerebral cortex into six lobes. Four of them are reasonably easy to recognize, but the other two are less obvious.

Before we differentiate the lobes of the brain, it will help to identify some major landmarks. The *lateral fissure*, also known as the *Sylvian fissure*, divides the temporal lobe from the frontal and anterior parietal lobes. The *central sulcus* separates the frontal and parietal lobes.

Sulci: Minor infolding of tissue on the cerebral or cerebellar cortex.

Fissure: Significant infolding or complete separation of two structures of the cerebral or cerebellar cortex.

Amyotrophic Lateral Sclerosis

There are a number of demyelinating diseases, conditions that cause degeneration of the brain myelin. Amyotrophic lateral sclerosis (ALS, Lou Gehrig's disease), a form of motor neuron disease, is a progressive, demyelinating condition of unknown etiology with a typical course of 2 to 5 years from date of diagnosis to death. People typically develop ALS in their fourth or fifth decade of life, and they experience initial weakness in a limb, with fatigue and cramping. As the disease progresses, limb function is lost, although sensory function typically is retained. Motor symptoms indicate both upper and lower motor neuron degeneration, which sometimes produces alternating spasticity and flaccidity. As the myelin deteriorates, it is replaced with a sclerosis or a covering of hardened tissue that markedly increases neural conduction time. In the later stages of the disease, the person experiences difficulty with respiration, requiring alteration of posture to accommodate reduced ability to work against gravity. The individual eventually experiences dysphagia and paralysis of muscles of speech while retaining full cognitive function. For a very moving account of the effects of the disease, read *Tuesdays with Morrie*, by Mitch Albom.

Frontal Lobe

The *frontal lobe* is the largest lobe, making up one third of the cortex (see Figure 6-2). This lobe controls the planning, initiation, and inhibition of voluntary motions, as well as thought processes.

The *pars opercularis*, or simply the *frontal operculum*, (see Figure 6-2) is beneath the inferior frontal lobe; it conceals one of the "hidden lobes," the *insular cortex*. The frontal operculum is commonly referred to as **Broca's area**, an extremely important region for speech motor planning within the dominant hemisphere. The anterior portion of the frontal lobe, particularly the area just above the eyes, is associated with memory, emotion, motor inhibition, and thought processes.

Another important landmark of the frontal lobe is the *precentral gyrus*, or *motor strip*, which is the site of initiation of voluntary motor movement. Anterior to the motor strip is the *premotor region*, generally involved in motor planning (see Figure 6-2). Axons from the motor strip make up the corticospinal and corticobulbar tracts, the major motor tracts of voluntary movement.

Different regions of the motor strip serve different regions of the body (see Figure 6-4). The face, head, and laryngeal regions are on the far lateral edge, while leg, thigh, and thorax are represented on the more medial surface of the superior cortex. If you compare this with the location of Broca's area on the side view of the hemisphere in Figure 6-5, you will see that these two regions are in close proximity. The area for motor function for the speech mechanisms (larynx, lips, facial muscles, muscles of mastication) is immediately adjacent

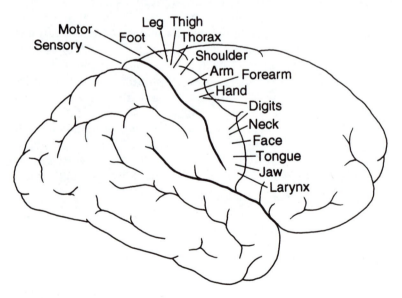

FIGURE 6-4. Right hemisphere, displaying regions of motor strip governing activation of specific muscle groups.

FIGURE 6–5. A. Landmarks of the left cerebral hemisphere. **B**. Effects upon function of lesion at different cerebral locations.

to Broca's area, the region responsible for planning the motor act for speech.

Parietal Lobe

The *parietal lobe* is the primary reception site for somatic (body) sense. All senses that reach consciousness terminate in the parietal lobe.

The *postcentral* gyrus receives somatic sensation from various body regions. The distribution of sensory function by body region is quite close to that of the motor strip. The *inferior parietal lobule* is a cortical association area that integrates visual information, auditory information, and somatic sense. The *angular gyrus* is important for comprehension of written material, and the *supramarginal gyrus* is involved in motor planning for speech.

Temporal Lobe

The *temporal lobe* is the site of auditory reception and is important for auditory and receptive language processing. The *superior temporal gyrus* is of great importance in both speech-language pathology and audiology. The upper surface of the superior temporal lobe is *Heschl's gyrus*, the location of the brain to which all auditory information is projected. The posterior portion of the superior temporal gyrus is *Wernicke's area*. This area is responsible for processing receptive language, within the dominant hemisphere. Damage to this site results in profound disturbances of language.

Occipital Lobe

The *occipital lobe* is the region responsible for receiving visual stimulation, as well as some of the higher level visual processing. The regions surrounding the *calcarine sulcus* are the primary reception areas for visual information.

Insular Cortex

The *insular cortex* (insula) is beneath the region of the cerebrum known as the operculum. To see the insular cortex, one would have to pull the temporal lobe laterally and lift the frontal and parietal opercula. Upon doing that, you would see the circular sulcus, which surrounds the insula. The insula is directly involved in **gustation** (sense of taste) and motor planning.

Gustation: Sense of taste.

Limbic Lobe

The *limbic lobe* (limbic system) is not an anatomically distinct region, but a system of structures with functional relationships associated with motivation, sex drive, emotional behavior, and affect. The limbic lobe includes the *uncus* (formed by the *amygdala*), *parahippocampal gyrus, cingulate gyrus, olfactory bulb* and *tract*, and the *hippocampal formation*.

Summary

- The gyri and sulci of the hemisphere provide important landmarks for lobes and other regions of the cerebral cortex.
- The anterior-most region is the frontal lobe, the site of most voluntary motor activation and the important speech region known as Broca's area.
- Adjacent to the frontal lobe is the parietal lobe, the region of somatic sensory reception.
- The temporal lobe is the prominent lateral lobe separated from the parietal and frontal lobes by the lateral (Sylvian) fissure.
- The temporal lobe is the site of auditory reception and Wernicke's area.
- The occipital lobe is the most posterior of the regions and is the site of visual input to the cerebrum.
- The insular lobe lies deep in the lateral sulcus and is revealed by deflecting the temporal lobe.
- The operculum overlies the insula, and the functionally defined limbic lobe includes the cingulate gyrus, uncus, parahippocampal gyrus, and other deep structures.

Medial Surface of Cerebral Cortex

Viewing a sagittal section of the brain reveals the *corpus callosum* (literally, "large body"). It is the large structure immediately inferior to the cerebral gray matter (see Figure 6-6). The corpus callosum is the "information superhighway" of the brain. It provides communication concerning sensation and memory among the diverse regions of the two hemispheres by means of myelinated fibers. Any information arising in the left postcentral gyrus can be potentially shared by the right postcentral gyrus, so that each hemisphere "knows" what the other one knows.

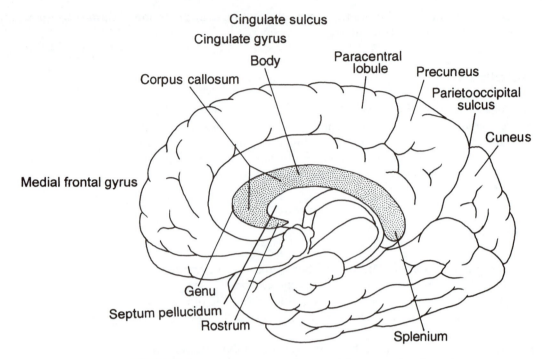

FIGURE 6-6. Medical surface of the cerebral cortex.

Myelinated Fibers

The gray matter of the cortex is made up mostly of neuron bodies, while the white matter of the brain represents myelinated axon fibers. These fibers make up the communication link among the neurons; without them there would be no neural function. In diseases that cause demyelination of the fibers, dysfunction of the areas served is virtually guaranteed. There are three basic types of fiber: projection, association, and commissural.

Projection Fibers

The tracts running to and from the cortex to the brainstem and the spinal cord are made up of projection fibers. Projection fibers connect the cortex with distant locations.

Association Fibers

Association fibers provide communication between regions of the same hemisphere. *Short association fibers* connect neurons of one gyrus to the next, traversing the sulcus. *Long association fibers* interconnect the lobes of the brain in the same hemisphere. The *arcuate fasciculus* is one group of association fibers that permits the superior and middle frontal gyri to communicate with the temporal, parietal, and occipital lobes. A lesion of the arcuate fasciculus can result in conduction aphasia, in which expressive and receptive language remain essentially intact, but the individual remains unable to repeat information presented auditorily.

Commissural Fibers

Commissural fibers run from one location on a hemisphere to the corresponding location on the other hemisphere, such as from the supramarginal gyrus of the left parietal lobe to the supramarginal gyrus of the right parietal lobe. We have already discussed one group of commissural fibers, the corpus callosum.

ANATOMY OF THE SUBCORTEX

Although the following structures are extremely important, an extensive discussion of them is beyond the scope of this introductory view of neuroanatomy.

Basal Ganglia

The *basal ganglia*, or *basal nuclei*, are a group of cell bodies related to control of background movement and initiation of movement patterns. The basal ganglia structures are the *caudate nucleus* (including head, body, and tail), the *putamen*, and the *globus pallidus*. Some consider the *amygdaloid body*, or *amygdala*, to be part of the basal ganglia, but it is generally included with the limbic system (see Figure 6-7).

Diencephalic Structures

The *diencephalon* includes the thalamus, hypothalamus, and subthalamus. The *thalamus* is the largest structure of the diencephalon and is the final, common relay for sensory information directed toward the cerebral cortex. The *hypothalamus* provides the organizational structure for the limbic system to regulate reproductive behavior and physiology, the perception of need for food and water, perception of satiation, control of digestive processes, and metabolic functions including maintenance of water balance and body temperature. The *subthalamus* modulates all output of the basal ganglia.

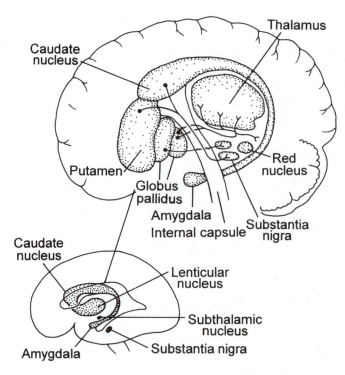

FIGURE 6-7. The basal ganglia consist of the caudate nucleus, amygdala, globus pallidus, and putamen. The basal ganglia are shown in relation to the other subcortical structures, including the diencephalic thalamus and hypothalamus, as well as the red nucleus and substantia nigra.

Summary

- The corpus callosum provides direct communication between components of the left and right cerebral hemispheres.
- The basal ganglia are subcortical structures involved in control of movement, and the hippocampal formation of the inferior temporal lobe is implicated in memory function.
- The thalamus of the diencephalon is the final relay for somatic sensation directed toward the cerebrum and other diencephalic structures.
- The subthalamus interacts with the globus pallidus to control movement, and the hypothalamus controls many bodily functions and desires.
- The regions of the cerebral cortex are connected by a complex network of projection fibers, which connect the cortex with other

structures; association fibers, which connect regions of the same hemisphere; and commissural fibers, which provide communication between corresponding regions of the two hemispheres.

CEREBROVASCULAR SYSTEM

Although the brain makes up only 2% of body weight, it consumes 20% of the oxygen transported by the vascular system to meet the high metabolic requirements of nervous tissue. The vascular system of the brain (the **cerebrovascular system**) maintains the constant circulation required by the nervous system. Disruption of this supply for a few seconds will begin cellular changes in neurons, and longer vascular deprivation has devastating effects.

Cerebrovascular system: The vascular supply of the central and peripheral nervous systems.

The vascular supply of the brain originates in the carotid and vertebral arteries, both of which branch from the aorta. There are some major divisions of the cerebrovascular supply that we should point out (see Figure 6-8). The *anterior cerebral artery* supplies the medial surfaces of the frontal and parietal lobes, the corpus callosum, the basal ganglia, and the anterior limb of the internal capsule. The *middle cerebral artery* provides blood to the lateral surface of the hemispheres, including the temporal lobe, motor strip, Wernicke's area, sensory reception regions, and association areas. The *superior cerebellar* and *anterior inferior cerebellar arteries* serve the cerebellum. The *basilar artery* serves the brainstem structures. The *posterior cerebral artery* serves the inferior temporal and occipital lobes, the medial occipital lobe and primary visual cortex, upper midbrain, diencephalon, and cerebellum.

Circle of Willis

The Circle of Willis is a series of **anastomoses**, or points of communication between arteries, that completely encircles the optic chiasm. It helps equalize locally high or low blood pressure and promotes equal distribution of blood.

Anastomoses: Points of communication among arteries.

Summary

■ The anterior cerebral arteries serve the medial surfaces of the brain, while the middle cerebral artery serves the lateral cortex, including the temporal lobe, motor strip, Wernicke's area, and much of the parietal lobe.

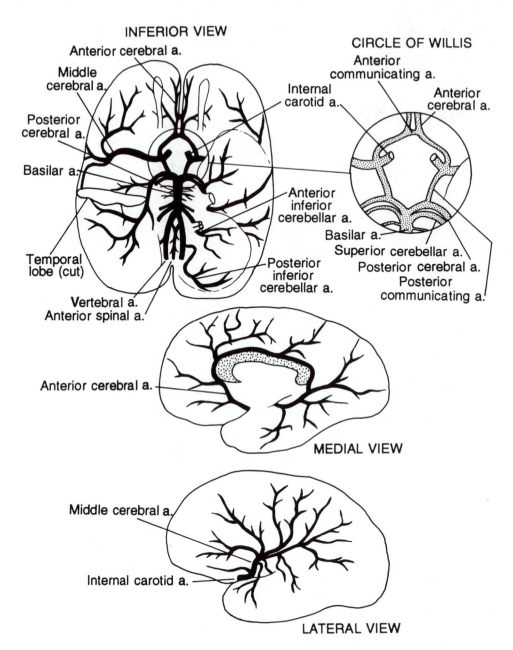

FIGURE 6-8. Major vascular supply of the cerebral cortex.

- The superior and anterior inferior cerebellar arteries serve the cerebellum, and the posterior inferior cerebellar artery arises from the vertebral artery.
- The basilar artery divides to become the posterior cerebral arteries, serving the inferior temporal and occipital lobes, upper midbrain, and diencephalon.
- The Circle of Willis is a series of communicating arteries that provides redundant pathways for blood flow to regions of the cerebral cortex, equalizing pressure and flow of blood.

CEREBELLUM

The cerebellum is the largest component of the hindbrain, immediately inferior to the posterior cerebral cortex. The cerebellum coordinates motor commands with sensory inputs to control movement, and it communicates with the brainstem, spinal cord, and cerebral cortex by means of superior, middle, and inferior cerebellar peduncles (see Figure 6-9).

Cerebellar Function

The cerebellum is a vital "silent partner" in integration of body movement with the internal and external environment of the body. Although it is incapable of initiating movement, it is intimately related to control of rate and range of movement, as well as the force with which that movement is executed.

Summary

- The cerebellum is an important structure for motor function.
- Information about the state of the muscles and structures of the body is integrated with the motor plan to provide smooth execution of movement.

ANATOMY OF THE BRAINSTEM

The brainstem consists of the *medulla oblongata, pons,* and *midbrain.* The brainstem reflects an intermediate stage of organization between the simple reflexive responses at the level of the spinal cord and the exquisitely complex responses generated by the cerebral cortex. Cranial nerves and their nuclei arise from the brainstem, and basic

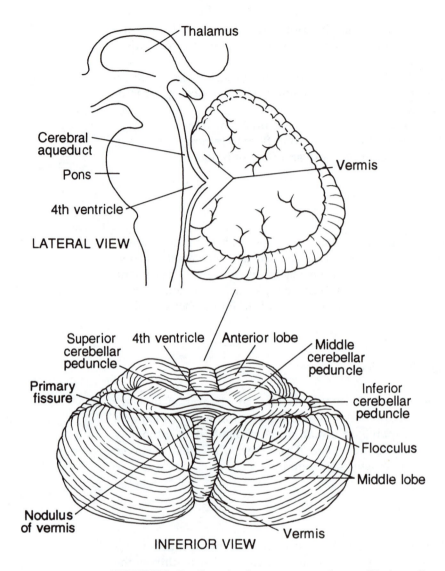

FIGURE 6-9. Cerebellum as seen in sagittal section and from beneath.

bodily functions for life are maintained here. It will help to refer to Figures 6-10 through 6-13 during the discussion of the brainstem.

Brainstem Landmarks

Medulla Oblongata

The *medulla oblongata*, or *medulla*, is the inferior-most segment of the brainstem. It looks like an enlargement of the upper spinal

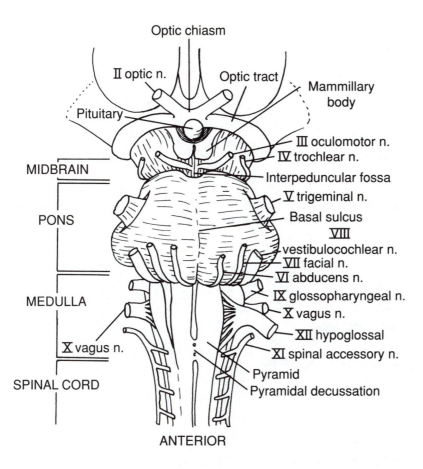

FIGURE 6-10. Anterior view of brainstem.

cord, and is about 2.5 cm long and 1 cm in diameter. This is a small but mighty structure; damage to the medulla is imminently life threatening.

If you look at the *pyramidal decussation* (see Figure 6-10), you will see the point in the medulla at which fibers of the corticospinal tract cross from one side to the other. That is, most of the axons carrying the motor command from the left hemisphere cross to the right side of the medulla to continue down through the spinal cord on the right side. The significance of this will not be lost on you if you remember meeting an individual with left-hemisphere stroke who had right-side hemiparesis. That is, unilateral paralysis signals a neuropathology on the side opposite the lesion. The point of decussation marks the lower border of the medulla, roughly at the level of the foramen magnum of the skull.

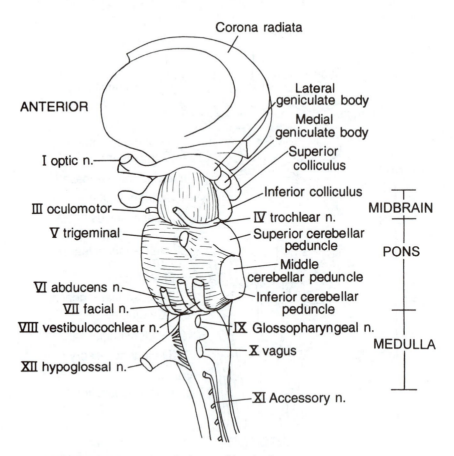

FIGURE 6-11. Lateral view of brainstem.

Pons and Midbrain

The pons is above the medulla, serving as the bridge between medulla and midbrain, as well as to the cerebellum. The pons is the site of four cranial nerve nuclei. The superior-most structure of the brainstem is the midbrain. The midbrain contains the important cerebral peduncles that provide communication between lower pathways and the cerebrum. The midbrain is also the point of origin for the III and IV cranial nerves.

The reticular formation is the mid-posterior "core" of the brainstem, housing some of the phylogenetically oldest structures of the brainstem. It contains nuclei responsible for inspiration, expiration, chewing, and swallowing. It also contains the reticular activating

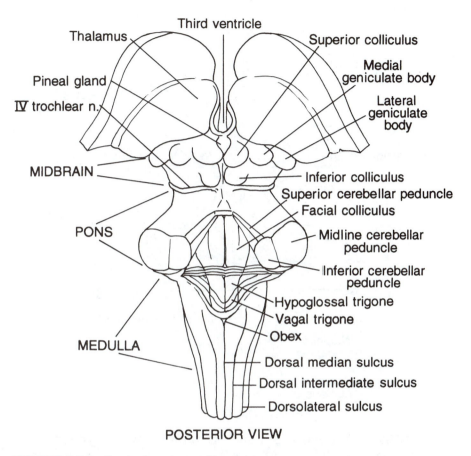

FIGURE 6-12. Posterior view of brainstem.

system (RAS), which works with the thalamus to keep the cerebrum conscious.

Summary

- The brainstem is divided into medulla, pons, and midbrain. It is more highly organized than the spinal cord, mediating higher level body functions such as vestibular responses.
- The medulla contains the important pyramidal decussation, the point at which the motor commands originating in one hemisphere of the cerebral cortex cross to serve the opposite side of the body. The IX, X, XI, and XII cranial nerves emerge at the level of the medulla, and the inferior cerebellar peduncle arises there. The fourth ventricle enlargement is a prominent brainstem landmark

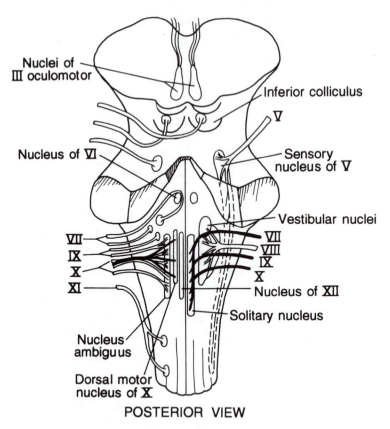

Nuclei of III oculomotor

Inferior colliculus

V

Nucleus of VI

Sensory nucleus of V

Vestibular nuclei

VII
IX
X
XI

VII
VIII
IX
X

Nucleus of XII

Solitary nucleus

Nucleus ambiguus

Dorsal motor nucleus of X

POSTERIOR VIEW

FIGURE 6-13. Posterior view of brainstem revealing orientation of major nuclei and cranial nerves supplied by those nuclei (from views of Carpenter, 1978).

in cross section. The pons contains the superior and middle cerebellar peduncles, as well as four cranial nerve nuclei, the V, VI, VII, and VIII nerves.

■ The midbrain contains the important cerebral peduncles and is the point of origin for the III and IV cranial nerves.

■ The reticular formation is a phylogenetically old set of nuclei essential for life function, including respiration, mastication, deglutition, and consciousness.

Cranial Nerves

A working knowledge of the cranial nerves is important for speech and hearing professionals because most of these nerves affect speech production and reception (see Table 6-3).

Table 6-3. Cranial Nerves

Classes of Cranial Nerves

GSA	**General Somatic Afferent**	Related to pain, temperature, mechanical stimulation of somatic structures (skin, muscle, joints)
GVA	**General Visceral Afferent**	From receptors in visceral structures (e.g., digestive tract)
GVE	**General Visceral Efferent**	Autonomic efferent fibers
GSE	**General Somatic Efferent**	Innervates skeletal (striated) muscle
SSA	**Special Somatic Afferent**	Special senses—sight, hearing, equilibrium
SVA	**Special Visceral Afferent**	Special senses of smell, taste
SVE	**Special Visceral Efferent**	Innervation of muscle of branchial arch origin: larynx, pharynx, face

Cranial Nerves, Sources, and Functions

I. Olfactory

SVA: Sense of smell

Source: Mitral cells of olfactory bulb

II. Optic

SSA: Vision

Source: Rod and cone receptor cells synapse with bipolar interneurons, which synapse with multipolar ganglionic neuron; optic nerve is axon of multipolar ganglionic neurons; nerve becomes myelinated after exit from eye socket and entrance into cranium; left and right nerves decussate at chiasm and project as optic tract to lateral geniculate body; projects to occipital cortex via optic radiations; left nasal nerve portion and right temporal nerve portion join after chiasm; left temporal nerve portion and right nasal aspect of nerve join after chiasm; visual field result is that left nasal and right temporal visual fields (right portion of image) project to left cerebral cortex; left temporal and right nasal visual fields (left portion of image) project to right cerebral cortex).

III. Oculomotor

GSE: All extrinsic ocular muscles except superior oblique and lateral rectus

Source: Oculomotor nucleus

GVE: Light and accommodation reflexes

Source: Edinger-Westphal nucleus

IV. Trochlear

GSE: Superior oblique muscle of eye (turns eye down when eye is adducted)

Source: Trochlear nuclei

V. Trigeminal

GSA: Exteroceptive afferent for pain, thermal, tactile from face, forehead, mucous membrane of mouth and nose, teeth, cranial dura; proprioceptive (deep pressure, kinesthesis) from teeth, gums, temporomandibular joint, stretch receptors of mastication

Source: Sensory nucleus of trigeminal nerve

(continues)

SVE: To muscles of mastication, tensor tympani, tensor veli palatini

Source: Motor nucleus of trigeminal nerve

Components of V Trigeminal

Ophthalmic branch: Sensory only

> **GSA:** From cornea, iris, upper eyelid, front of scalp

Maxillary branch: Sensory only

> **GSA:** From lower eyelid, nose, palate, upper jaw

Mandibular branch: Sensory and motor

> **GSA:** From lower jaw and teeth, mucosa, cheeks, temporomandibular joint, anterior two thirds of tongue

> **SVE:** To muscles of mastication (internal and external pterygoid, temporalis, masseter), tensor tympani

VI. Abducens

> **GSE:** Lateral rectus muscle for ocular abduction
>
> **Source:** Abducens nucleus

VII. Facial

> **SVE:** To facial muscles of expression, platysma, buccinator
>
> **Source:** Motor nucleus of VII
>
> **SVA:** Taste, anterior two thirds of tongue
>
> **Source:** Solitary nucleus
>
> **GSA:** Cutaneous sense of EAM and skin of ear
>
> **Source:** Trigeminal nuclei
>
> **GVE:** Lacrimal gland (tears); mucous membrane of mouth and nose
>
> **Source:** Superior salivatory and lacrimal nuclei

VIII. Vestibulocochlear

> **SSA:** Vestibular and cochlear sensation
>
> **Cochlear (auditory) portion:** Sensors are hair cells; cell bodies in spiral ganglion; axons are VIII nerve, auditory portion; low-frequency (apical) fibers terminate at ventral cochlear nucleus (VCN) and high-frequency fibers (basal) terminate at dorsal cochlear nucleus (DCN); transfer of auditory sensation to central nervous system
>
> **Source:** Spiral ganglion
>
> **Vestibular portion:** From semicircular canals, utricle, saccule; project to vestibular nuclei of medulla and subsequently to all levels of brainstem, spinal cord, cerebellum, thalamus, and cerebral cortex; maintenance of extensor tone, anti-gravity responses, balance, sense of position in space; coordinated eye/head movement through projection to III Oculomotor, IV Trochlear, VI Abducens cranial nerves;
>
> **Source:** Vestibular ganglion

(continues)

IX. Glossopharyngeal

GVA: Somatic (tactile, thermal, pain sense) from posterior one third of tongue, tonsils, upper pharynx, eustachian tube, mastoid cells

Source: Solitary nucleus

SVA: Taste, posterior one third of tongue

Source: Inferior salivatory nucleus

GSA: Somatic sense of EAM and skin of ear

Source: Trigeminal nuclei

SVE: Innervation of stylopharyngeus, superior pharyngeal constrictor

Source: Inferior salivatory nucleus

GVE: Parotid gland

Source: Inferior salivatory nucleus

X. Vagus

GSA: Cutaneous sense from external auditory meatus

Source: Trigeminal nuclei

GVA: Sensory from pharynx, larynx, trachea, esophagus, viscera of thorax, abdomen

Source: Solitary nucleus

SVA: Taste buds near epiglottis and valleculae

Source: Solitary nucleus

GVE: To parasympathetic ganglia, thorax, and abdomen

Source: Dorsal motor nucleus of X

SVE: Striated muscle of larynx and pharynx

Source: Nucleus ambiguus

XI. Accessory

SVE, Cranial portion: Joins with X vagus to form recurrent laryngeal nerve to innervate intrinsic muscles of larynx

Spinal portion: Innervates sternocleidomastoid and trapezius

Source: Cranial portion: Nucleus ambiguus of medulla

SVE: Spinal portion: Anterior horn of C1 through C5 spinal nerves; unite and ascend; enter skull via foramen magnum; exit with vagus at jugular foramen

XII. Hypoglossal

GSE: Muscles of tongue

Source: Nucleus of hypoglossal nerve

Clinical note: Lesion of LMN produces ipsilateral damage (tongue deviates to side of damage)

Cranial Nerve Classification

Cranial nerves are referred to by name, number, or both. By convention, roman numerals are used when discussing cranial nerves, and the number represents inverse height in the brainstem. Cranial nerves I through IV are at the level of the midbrain, V through VIII are pons level, and IX through XII are in the medulla. Nerves can be efferent (motor), afferent (sensory), or mixed efferent/afferent.

Although all of the cranial nerves are important, not all of them are relevant to speech-language pathology or audiology. Therefore we will only lightly cover nonessential cranial nerves, focusing instead on those that will be critical for your career.

Olfaction: Sense of smell.

Damage to the I Olfactory Nerve

The most common trauma resulting in *anosmia* (loss of sense of smell and taste) is an injury involving frontal impact. This often causes damage to the sensory apparatus itself, especially as a result of shearing forces applied to the I olfactory nerve at the cribriform plate.

The *I olfactory nerve* mediates the sense of smell and the *II optic nerve* mediates the sense of vision. The *III oculomotor nerve* innervates all but two of the muscles responsible for eye movement, and the *IV trochlear* and *VI abducens nerves* innervate the other eye muscles.

In more detail, following are the cranial nerves that affect speech and hearing. Motor cranial nerves are activated by means of the corticobulbar tract, a motor pathway from the cerebrum to the brainstem. Individual cranial nerve motor nuclei reside in the brainstem.

V Trigeminal Nerve. The V trigeminal nerve is an extremely important nerve for speech production because it provides motor supply to the muscles of mastication and transmits sensory information from the face. The V trigeminal divides into the ophthalmic, the maxillary, and the mandibular branches (see Figure 6-14).

The *ophthalmic branch* is the small, superior nerve of the trigeminal. It is entirely afferent (sensory) and transmits information from the skin of the upper face, forehead, and scalp, cornea, iris, upper eyelid, conjunctiva, nasal cavity mucous membrane, and lacrimal gland.

Lesions of V Trigeminal Nerve

The V trigeminal nerve has both motor and sensory components, and all trigeminal nerves can be affected by lesions. With a lesion of the cerebral cortex in the area innervating the muscles of mastication you may see increased jaw jerk reflex (elicited by pulling down on the passively opened mandible). Damage to the V trigeminal nerve itself results in atrophy (wasting) and weakness on the affected side. When your client closes his or her mouth, the jaw will deviate toward the side of the lesion as a result of the action of the intact internal pterygoid muscle. The jaw will hang open with bilateral LMN damage, which has an extreme effect on speech. The tensor veli palatine is also innervated by the trigeminal, and weakness or paralysis may result in hypernasality because of this muscle's role in maintaining the velopharyngeal sphincter.

Damage to the sensory component of the V cranial results in loss of tactile sensation for the anterior two thirds of the tongue, loss of the corneal blink reflex, and alteration of sensation at orifice eustachian tube, external auditory meatus, and tympanic membrane, teeth, and gums. Sensation of the forehead, upper face, and nose region are lost with ophthalmic branch lesion, and the sensation to the skin region roughly lateral to the zygomatic arch and over the maxilla is lost with maxillary branch lesion. Damage to the mandibular branch affects sensation from the side of the face down to the mandible. Trigeminal neuralgia (Tic doulereux) may also arise from damage to the V cranial nerve. The result is severe and sharp shooting pain along the course of the nerve, which may be restricted to areas served by only one of the branches.

The *maxillary nerve* is also only afferent. It transmits information from the lower eyelid, skin on the sides of the nose, upper jaw, teeth, and lip, mucosal lining of buccal and nasal cavities, maxillary sinuses, and nasopharynx.

The *mandibular branch* is both afferent and efferent (motor). This largest branch of the trigeminal exits the skull via the *foramen ovale of sphenoid* and divides into a number of branching nerves. The afferent component conducts sensory information from a region roughly encompassing the mandible, including the skin, lower teeth, gums and lower lip, a portion of the skin and mucosal lining of the cheek,

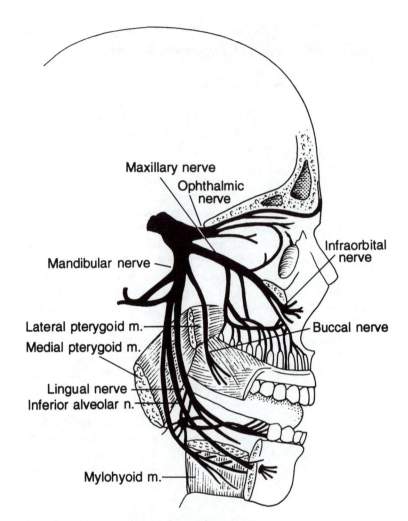

FIGURE 6-14. Ophthalmic, maxillary, and mandibular branches of the V trigeminal nerve.

external auditory meatus and auricle, temporomandibular joint, and the region of the temporal bone. It also transmits kinesthetic and proprioceptive sense of muscles of mastication. The lingual nerve conducts somatic sensation from the anterior two thirds of the mucous membrane of the tongue and floor of the mouth.

The efferent component of the mandibular branch serves the muscles of mastication (masseter, temporalis, lateral and medial pterygoids), as well as the tensor veli palatine and tensor tympani of the middle ear.

VII Facial Nerve. The VII facial nerve supplies motor innervation to the facial muscles of expression and tear glands, as well as sense of taste for a portion of the tongue (see Figure 6-15).

The facial nerve also transmits the sense of taste (gustation) from the anterior two thirds of the tongue.

Lesions of VII Facial Nerve

Lesions of the facial nerve can significantly affect articulatory function. Because the upper motor neuron supply to the upper face is bilateral, unilateral cortical damage does not result in upper face paralysis. It may, however, paralyze all facial muscles below the eyes. Even then, muscles of facial expression (*mimetic muscles*) may be contracted involuntarily in response to emotional stimuli because these motor gestures are initiated at regions of the brain that differ from those of speech.

Damage directly to the VII cranial nerve causes upper- and lower-face paralysis on the side of the lesion. This may involve the inability to close the eyelid and results in muscle sagging, loss of tone, and reduction in wrinkling around the lip, nose, and forehead. When the individual attempts to smile, the affected corners of the mouth will be drawn toward the unaffected side. The person may drool due to loss of the ability to hold back saliva with the lips, and the cheeks may puff out during expiration due to a flaccid buccinator.

Bell's palsy (*palsy* means "paralysis") may result from any compression of the VII nerve or even from cold weather. It results in paralysis of facial musculature, which remits in most cases within a few months.

Damage to the facial nerve following penetrating facial or cranial trauma is quite common. Both damage to the middle ear and skull fractures of the temporal bone result in facial nerve damage. Most fractures of the temporal bone occur along the long axis of the temporal bone, although facial paralysis is much more likely if the fracture is transverse (see Mackay et al., 1997).

VIII Vestibulocochlear Nerve. This nerve, also known as the auditory nerve, is extremely important in both speech-language pathology and audiology because it mediates both auditory information and sense of movement in space. The nerve consists of both

Lesions of VIII Vestibulocochlear Nerve

Damage to the VIII nerve results in ipsilateral hearing loss reflecting the degree of trauma. Damage to the VIII nerve can arise from a number of causes, including physical trauma (skull fracture), tumor growth compressing the nerve, and vascular incident.

Traumatic injury to the VIII vestibulocochlear nerve is usually caused by a fracture of the temporal bone or a penetrating injury, such as a gunshot wound. If the fracture is along the long axis of the temporal bone, it often results in sensorineural loss and vertigo without VIII nerve compression or apparent damage to the labyrinth. If the fracture is in the transverse dimension, the VII and VIII nerves may well be sheared or compressed. Vertigo and nystagmus in head injury often occur when the head position is changed. In absence of evidence of physical damage to the labyrinth, it is hypothesized that the vertigo and nystagmus arise from disturbance of calcium particles used in the sensory mechanisms of the vestibular system. Fortunately, most trauma-induced vertigo remits over time (see Mackay et al., 1997).

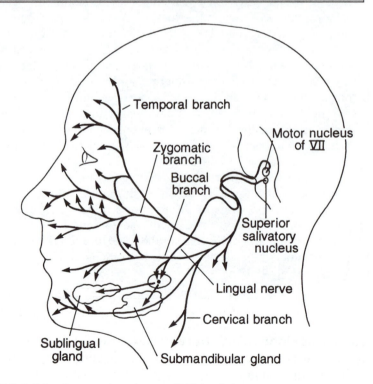

FIGURE 6-15. General course of VII facial nerve.

sensory and motor components. The sensory portion mediates information concerning hearing and balance, while the motor component appears to assist in selectively damping output of hair cells (see Figure 6-16).

IX Glossopharyngeal Nerve. The IX glossopharyngeal nerve serves both sensory and motor functions of the stylopharyngeus muscle and the superior constrictor muscle. The nerve mediates sensation from taste receptors of the posterior one third of the tongue and a portion of the soft palate.

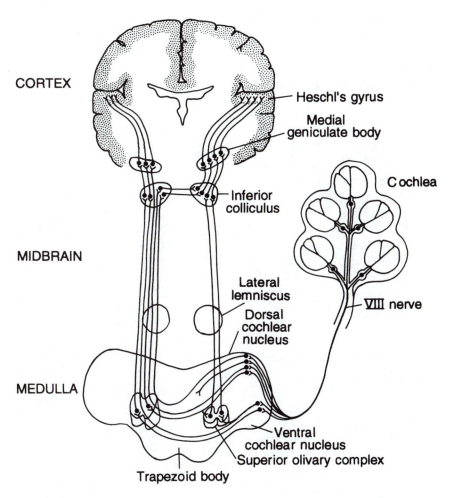

FIGURE 6-16. Course of the VIII vestibulocochlear nerve and auditory pathway.

Lesions of IX Glossopharyngeal Nerve

The IX glossopharyngeal nerve works in concert with the X vagus, making its independent function difficult to determine. Damage to the IX nerve results in paralysis of the stylopharyngeus muscle and may result in loss of general sensation (anesthesia) for the posterior one third of the tongue and pharynx, although the vagus may support these functions as well. The cooperative innervation with the vagus results in little effect on the pharyngeal constrictors, although reduced sensation of the auricle and middle ear may indicate IX damage. Damage to the IX nerve may also cause reduced or absent gag reflex, although absence of the reflex does not guarantee that a lesion exists.

X Vagus Nerve. The motor component of the vagus provides motor innervation of many smooth muscles but, more important, for

Lesions of X Vagus Nerve

The X vagus is the most extensive of the cranial nerves, presenting an important constellation of clinical manifestations. Damage to the pharyngeal branch results in deficit in swallowing, potential loss of the gag reflex through interaction with the IX glossopharyngeal nerve, and hypernasality due to weakness of the velopharyngeal sphincter (all velopharyngeal muscles are innervated by the vagus with the exception of the tensor veli palatine, which is innervated by the trigeminal). Unilateral pharyngeal branch damage results in failure to elevate the soft palate on the involved side (asymmetrical elevation), producing hypernasality. Bilateral lesion produces absent or reduced (but symmetrical) movement of the soft palate producing hypernasality, nasal regurgitation, dysphagia, and paralysis of the pharyngeal musculature.

Lesions of the superior laryngeal nerve may result in loss of sensation of the upper larynx mucous membrane and stretch receptors, as well as paralysis of the cricothyroid muscle. Recurrent laryngeal nerve (RLN) damage produces either unilateral or bilateral flaccid vocal fold paralysis. Besides affecting voice, this condition puts the individual at risk for aspiration pneumonia because of his or her inability to close the airway during swallow.

speech and swallowing, the striated muscles of the larynx used for phonation and protection of the airway are innervated by the recurrent laryngeal nerve and superior laryngeal nerve of the vagus.

The sensory component of the vagus delivers pain, touch, and temperature sense from the skin covering the ear drum, posterior auricle, and external auditory meatus.

XI Accessory Nerve. The XI accessory nerve provides motor innervation directly to the sternocleidomastoid and trapezius muscles and works in conjunction with the vagus to innervate the intrinsic muscles of the larynx, pharynx, and soft palate (see Figure 6-17).

Lesions of XI Accessory Nerve

Lesion of the XI accessory nerve may have an effect on the trapezius and sternocleidomastoid muscles. Unilateral lesion affecting the sternocleidomastoid results in the person's being unable to turn his or her head away from the side of the lesion. (The left sternocleidomastoid rotates the head toward the right side when contracted.) Lesions resulting in paralysis of the trapezius result in restricted ability to elevate the arm or drooping shoulder on the side of the lesion.

XII Hypoglossal. This nerve provides the innervation to motor function of the tongue.

Lesions of XII Hypoglossal Nerve

Lesions that affect the XII hypoglossal have a profound impact on articulation function and speech intelligibility. This nerve provides motor innervation of intrinsic and extrinsic muscles of the tongue. Unilateral lower motor neuron (LMN) lesion results in loss of movement on the side of lesion. Muscular weakness and atrophy on the affected side result in deviation of the tongue toward the side of the lesion. Fasciculations, or abnormal involuntary twitching or movement of muscle fibers, may occur prior to atrophy, arising from damage to the cell body. At rest, the tongue may deviate toward the unaffected side as a result of the tonic pull of the normal styloglossus muscle. Upper motor lesion may result in muscle weakness and impaired volitional movements with accompanying spasticity.

FIGURE 6-17. Spinal accessory nerve origins.

Summary

- Cranial nerves are sensory, motor, or mixed sensorimotor.
- The I olfactory nerve transmits the sense of smell, and the II optic nerve communicates visual information to the brain.
- The III oculomotor, IV trochlear, and VI abducens nerves provide innervation for eye movements.
- The V trigeminal nerve innervates muscles of mastication and the tensor veli palatini and communicates sensation from the face, mouth, teeth, mucosal lining, and tongue to the brain.

- The VII facial nerve innervates muscles of facial expression, and the sensory component transmits taste from the anterior two thirds of the tongue.
- The VIII vestibulocochlear nerve mediates auditory and vestibular sensation.
- The IX glossopharyngeal nerve transmits information from the posterior tongue taste receptors, as well as somatic sense from the tongue, fauces, pharynx, and eustachian tube. The stylopharyngeus and superior pharyngeal constrictor muscles receive motor innervation via this nerve.
- The X vagus nerve is extremely important for autonomic function as well as somatic motor innervation. Somatic sensation of pain, touch, and temperature from the region of the eardrum is mediated by the vagus, as well as pain from pharynx, larynx, esophagus, and many other regions. The recurrent laryngeal nerve and superior laryngeal nerves supply motor innervation for the intrinsic muscles of the larynx.
- The XI accessory nerve innervates the sternocleidomastoid and trapezius muscles, and collaborates with the vagus in activation of palatal, laryngeal, and pharyngeal muscles.
- The XII hypoglossal nerve innervates the muscles of the tongue with the exception of the palatoglossus.

Spinal Cord

The spinal cord comprises tracts and nuclei. The 31 pairs of spinal nerves serve the limbs and trunk. Sensory nerves have cell bodies in dorsal root ganglia and motor neuron bodies lie within the spinal cord. Upper motor neurons have their cell bodies above the segment at which the spinal nerve originates. Lower motor neurons are the final neurons in the efferent chain. Efferent tracts, such as the corticospinal tract, transmit information from the brain to the spinal nerves. Afferent tracts, such as the spinothalamic tract, transmit information concerning the physical state of the limbs and trunk to higher brain centers.

NEUROPHYSIOLOGY

Although extraordinary advances over the past 30 years have vastly expanded our understanding of the workings of the brain, we still have a great deal to learn. We will approach our discussion of nervous system function from the "bottom up," looking first at the simplest responses of the system (communication between neurons) and working our way up to the all-important functions of the cerebral cortex.

The Neuron

Neuron Function

Neurons can be stimulated to send a signal out through the axon, which is how information passes from one neuron to another. When a neuron is stimulated, it can send out a response that either excites the next neuron (*excitatory response*) or inhibits the next neuron (*inhibitory*). Excitation causes an increase in activity, and inhibition causes a reduction in activity. This arrangement lets neurons have very different effects on other neurons.

Synapse

When a neuron is sufficiently stimulated its axon discharges a neurotransmitter into the synaptic cleft, or area between its end bouton and the connecting neuron. The neurotransmitter is a lot like the key to your door. The specific neurotransmitter released into the synaptic cleft is the one to which the adjacent neuron responds. If some other type of neurotransmitter makes its way into that synaptic region, it will have no effect on the adjacent neuron. This "lock-and-key" arrangement lets neurons have specific effects on some neurons while not affecting others.

When a neurotransmitter is released into the synaptic cleft, it stimulates receptor sites on the next neuron. Ion channels in the next neuron's membrane open up and allow ions to enter, and this leads to a discharge, or "firing," of that neuron as well. That firing of a neuron is the *action potential* (see Figure 6-18).

An *action potential (AP)* is a change in electrical potential that occurs when the cell membrane of a neuron is stimulated adequately to permit ions (molecules that are either positively or negatively charged) to pass through the cell wall. When a neuron is stimulated, sodium (Na+) ion "gates" open up and allow sodium ions to flood the intracellular space. This makes the inside of the neuron more positively charged than the area outside the neuron for a brief time. This is termed *depolarization*. For about $\frac{1}{2}$ of one millisecond (0.5 ms), no amount of stimulation of that region of the membrane will cause it to depolarize again; this time is the **absolute refractory period**. The absolute refractory period is the time during which the cell membrane cannot be stimulated to depolarize. During the absolute refractory period, potassium (K+) ions flow into the neuron. The sodium and potassium are actively removed by a protein known as the sodium-potassium pump.

Absolute refractory period:
The time during depolarization when the cell membrane cannot be stimulated to depolarize again.

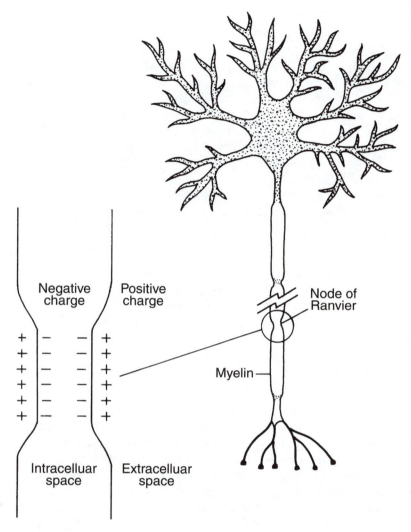

FIGURE 6-18. A quiescent neuron, showing equilibrium of membrane potential.

For an action potential to be generated, the membrane channels have to open up. Portions of the cell membrane may be depolarized, but other parts of the membrane will not be depolarized until a critical threshold has been reached. There have to be sufficient numbers of opened channels for an action potential to be generated. If there are not sufficient numbers, then the membrane returns to the **resting membrane potential (RMP)** which is the state it was in before being stimulated.

Resting membrane potential (RMP): The condition of a neuron at rest, in which it is polarized and ready to discharge.

Myasthenia Gravis

Myasthenia gravis is a neuromuscular disease whose primary effect is on the neuromuscular junction. It appears that an individual's autoimmune system develops an immune response to the neurotransmitter receptor of the neuromuscular junction, building antibodies that block the receptor. Blocked receptors are unable to respond to neurotransmitter substance so that as the disease progresses, greater numbers of receptors become blocked and increasingly fewer ion channels can be activated to depolarize a neuron. As was discussed previously, myasthenia gravis causes a person to have extreme fatigue and weakness, but it is treatable.

This whole cycle from RMP to AP and back to RMP takes about 1 ms in most neurons, and this is a defining time period. This means that a neuron may respond every 1/1,000 of a second, or 1,000 times per second. Even if it is stimulated 2,000 times per second, it will not be able to respond any faster.

Propagation

Propagation: The spreading effect of wave action; in neural responses, the communication of information through the nervous system.

An action potential would do no good at all if it did not pass information to the next neuron or to a muscle fiber. **Propagation** refers to the spreading effect of wave action, much as the wave generated by throwing a rock in a pond spreads out from the stone's point of contact with the water. The depolarization is propagated along the neuron membrane in a wave of depolarization. When the membrane undergoing the local depolarization reaches the critical limit, ions flow rapidly across the membrane. The adjacent membrane contains voltage-sensitive protein channels, which are channels that open when there is a voltage change in their vicinity. The current flow from the first depolarization stimulates regions next to it to depolarize as well. In this manner, the depolarization spreads along the membrane, ultimately reaching the terminal of the axon.

The neuron responds in an all-or-nothing manner. That is, it either depolarizes or it does not. If it fails to depolarize, no action potential is generated and no information is conveyed. If the threshold for depolarization is reached, an action potential will be produced, and information will be transmitted. The neuron acts like a light switch in this sense, and the only variation in information is in the frequency with which the neuron is "turned on," referred to as *spike rate* or *rate of discharge*.

Propagation of the action potential is facilitated by axon diameter and myelin. Axons with larger diameters propagate at a much higher rate than those with smaller fibers, and presence of myelin also speeds propagation. Figure 6-19 shows how myelin is laid down on the axon in "donuts" with nodes of exposed membrane between them. Voltage sensitive ion channels reside in those nodes.

The membrane becomes depolarized at one node, and the effect of that depolarization is felt at the next node, where the membrane depolarizes as well. The propagating action potential is "passed" from node to node, and this jumping is referred to as **saltatory conduction**. Clearly, many precious milliseconds can be saved by skipping from node to node in long fibers.

Saltatory conduction: The process in a neural response in which information in the axon passes from node to node, thereby greatly increasing conduction speed.

When the impulse reaches the terminal point on the axon, a highly specialized process begins. The synaptic vesicles in the terminal end buttons contain a neurotransmitter substance that permits communication between the two neurons. A neurotransmitter is a substance

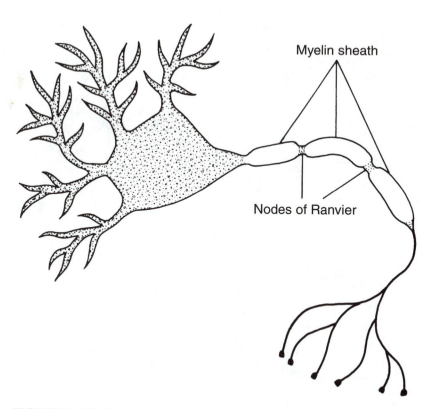

FIGURE 6-19. Myelin sheath and nodes of Ranvier.

released from the terminal end button of an axon that causes either excitation or inhibition of another neuron or excitation of a muscle fiber. When the action potential reaches the terminal point, the vesicles are stimulated to migrate to the membrane wall where they will dump their neurotransmitter through the membrane into the synaptic cleft (see Figure 6-20).

The neurotransmitter travels across the cleft very quickly (100 microseconds [μs]) and is dumped into the cleft to activate receptor proteins on the postsynaptic neuron. Presence of neurotransmitter in the cleft triggers ion channels to open. Neurotransmitters fit specific ion channels, and if a given neurotransmitter does not match a receptor channel protein, the postsynaptic neuron will not fire. That is, the neurotransmitter is a "key" and the receptor is a "lock": If the key does not fit, the gate will not open.

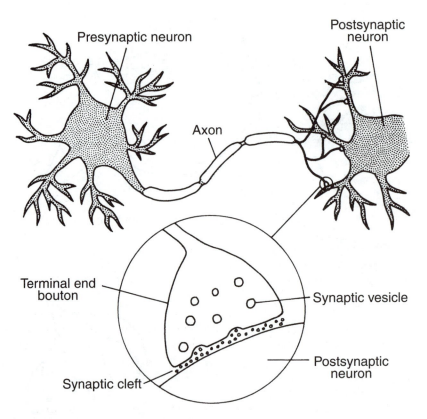

FIGURE 6-20. Expanded view of synapse between two neurons.

The neurotransmitter may have either an excitatory or an inhibitory effect on the neuron. Excitatory effects increase the probability that a neuron will depolarize, whereas inhibition decreases that probability. Excitatory stimulation generates an *excitatory postsynaptic potential (EPSP)*, whereas inhibitory synapses produce *inhibitory postsynaptic potentials (IPSPs)*. Excitation causes depolarization, whereas inhibition causes hyperpolarization, greatly elevating the threshold of firing (making it difficult or impossible for the neuron to fire).

The EPSP actually begins as a *micropotential*, depolarizing the membrane by about only 3 mV. If there is a sufficient number of miniature EPSP depolarizations, the sum of their depolarization will reach the critical threshold and an action potential will be generated, as before. If you imagine a very large teeter-totter with an adult on one end, it would take a large number of children to counteract the effect of that one adult. If there are sufficient numbers of children on the teeter-totter, the adult will rise in the air. If a sufficient number of synapses is activated, there will be an action potential. Likewise, there can be **temporal summation**, in which a smaller number of regions depolarize virtually simultaneously.

Single neurons may take input from thousands of other neurons to produce a single response, a process called **convergence**. In this configuration, a mass of information is distilled into a single response. In contrast, **divergence** occurs when the axon of one neuron makes synapse with many thousands of other neurons. Its single piece of information is transmitted to many other neurons.

Temporal summation: The quality of some neurons wherein the neuron requires virtually simultaneous inputs from other neurons before it can be stimulated to depolarize.

Convergence: The neural process in which outputs of many neurons contribute to the depolarization of a single neuron.

Divergence: The neural process in which one neuron passes information to many other neurons.

Summary

- Communication between neurons of the nervous system occurs at the synapse.
- Neurotransmitter passing through the synaptic cleft either excites or inhibits the postsynaptic neuron.
- If a neuron is excited sufficiently, an action potential will be generated.
- Stimulation of a neuron membrane to depolarize causes exchange of ions between the extracellular and intracellular spaces, and the ion movement results in a large and predictable change in voltage across the membrane.
- The resting membrane potential is the electrical potential measurable prior to excitation.
- The absolute refractory period after excitation is an interval during which the neuron cannot be excited to fire, whereas it

can fire during the relative refractory period, given adequate stimulation.

- Because an action potential always results in the same neural response, the neuron is capable of representing differences in input only through rate of response.
- Myelinated fibers conduct the wave of depolarization more rapidly than demyelinated fibers, primarily due to saltatory conduction.
- Temporal summation is the quality of some neurons wherein the neuron requires virtually simultaneous inputs from other neurons before it can be stimulated to depolarize.
- Single neurons can take input from thousands of other neurons to produce a single response, a process called convergence.
- Divergence occurs when the axon of one neuron makes synapse with many thousands of other neurons.

Muscle Function

Neuromuscular junction: The point of synapse between muscle fiber and motor fiber.

Activation of muscle requires that a nerve make contact with the muscle fiber. The **neuromuscular junction** (point where neuron and muscle connect) looks a lot like a synapse between two neurons. The basic unit of skeletal muscle control is the motor unit, consisting of the motor neuron, its axon, and the muscle fibers it innervates.

Figure 6-21 shows a neuromuscular junction, looking very much like a synapse. In this case, however, there is a terminal endplate on the axon, with a synaptic cleft as before. The neurotransmitter, acetylcholine, is dumped into the active zone, and a *miniature end plate potential (MEPP)* will be generated. If there are sufficient numbers of MEPPs, a muscle action potential will be generated. This is directly analogous to neuron-to-neuron synapse in that it takes many activated regions to excite a muscle fiber. When the MEPP is generated, the muscle fiber twitches, and the whole muscle contracts.

Muscle Control

When the MEPP is generated, the muscle fiber responds in all-or-none fashion and the muscle twitches. Muscles come in all sizes, from the massive to the minute. In addition, muscles must perform vastly different functions, ranging from gross, slow movement to quick, precise action. How do we manage this?

The answer to this question lies largely in allocation of resources. For fine movement, only a limited number of muscle fibers need to be recruited for movement, because you are not trying to move as

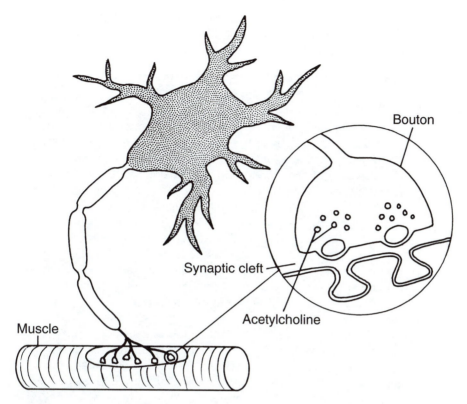

FIGURE 6-21. Neuromuscular Junction between neuron and muscle fiber.

much mass. In contrast, heavy lifting requires recruitment of many muscle fibers.

Summary

- Neuromuscular junctions operate similarly to neuron-to-neuron synapses, except the result is muscle movement.
- Muscle innervation patterns help differentiate fine and gross motor control.

Higher Functioning

We have been discussing responses that occur at the lowest levels of the nervous system and often do not even reach consciousness.

Although it is essential for your brain to know what your tongue muscles are doing, it is obvious that there is more to speech than movement of muscles.

The Great Debate

A lively debate concerning localization of function within the brain has been going on for well over 100 years. On the one hand, *localizationists* (or "materialists" as they were called in the 1860s) held that given sufficiently sensitive tools, specific functions could be localized to specific brain regions. The opposing view, held by "spiritualists," was that it was degrading to think that the human body (much less the brain) could be so mechanically dissected, and that functions such as language or mathematics could not be isolated to a single brain region. Perhaps the first localizationist was Joseph Gall, who also proposed that a properly knowledgeable individual could identify specific cognitive traits of an individual by reading the bumps on that person's head (phrenology) (Kandel, 1991).

Phrenology did not retain many followers, but one admirer of Gall, Paul Broca, was the first to identify the region responsible for expressive language within the dominant hemisphere of the brain (Kandel, 1991). Others provided counter evidence, including people with acquired language deficits that clearly arose from damage to another region distal from the area identified by Broca. Such notables as Sigmund Freud refuted the notion of localization of function, saying that although some specific locations for basic processes might be found, that still did not explain complex cognitive function.

Wernicke entered the battle, clearly identifying a language center within the temporal lobe distinct from that identified by Broca. Indeed, as the twentieth century dawned, localization of function was demonstrated through ablation studies of the occipital and temporal lobes of dogs, eliminating visual and auditory recognition, respectively. Researchers found that they could stimulate specific locales of a dog's cerebrum and cause single, replicable movements of the limbs.

Although such notable researchers as Karl Lashley countered the growing body of evidence, research that examined brain-damaged soldiers during the first and second world wars revealed a great deal of "regional" consistency of symptoms, and these findings led us into the study and treatment of acquired language disorders.

(continues)

Although it is clear that regions of the cerebral cortex, such as the motor strip, are highly specialized for specific functions, other regions of the cortex are less well defined. To further confound things, the developing brain is plastic. The brains of infants who receive trauma are more likely to overcome damage to function than are the brains of adults who receive the same trauma. This and other evidence led to *theories of equipotentiality*, which state that the brain functions as a whole. One could strike a balance with the notion of *regional equipotentiality*. There seems to be a functional unity by regions, but the degree of functional loss to an individual who has received trauma also is related to the total volume of damaged tissue.

In this text, we take a regional approach to function of the cerebral cortex. Our discussion focuses on functional regions and association pathways of the brain and interconnections among regions. The cortex appears to be organized around regions of primary activity for a given area, including the *primary receptive area* for somatic sense, primary motor area, primary auditory cortex, and primary region of visual reception. Adjacent to these are higher-order areas of processing. That is, there are secondary, tertiary, and even quaternary areas of higher-order processing adjacent to the primary receptive areas for sensation. (There also are higher-order areas of processing for motor function, as we will see.) Beyond the higher-order areas of processing are *association areas* where the most complex form of cognitive processing occurs. We receive information from our senses at primary reception areas (Heschl's gyrus for audition; calcarine sulcas for vision; somatosensory cortex of the parietal lobe for body sense) and we extract the information received and put it together with other information associated with the modality at higher-order areas of processing. These higher-order association areas are typically adjacent or close to the primary receptive area. This information is then passed to one of the three association areas for the highest level of cognitive processing.

Afferent Inputs

The motor strip receives input from the thalamus, sensory cortex, and premotor area. There is also heavy sensory input to this motor region, underscoring the notion that control of movement is strongly influenced by information about the ongoing state and position of the musculature. Some muscle stretch sensors (muscle spindles) send information to the motor strip, and spinal reflexes are modified and controlled, at least in part, by activity from this region.

The premotor region is involved in preparation for movement, anticipation of movement, and organization of skilled movement. It receives somatic sensory information from the parietal lobe, as well as sensory information from the thalamus, and projects its output to the motor strip. Afferent parietal information to the supplementary motor area also supports its involvement in active planning and rehearsal of the motor act, as well as decision making about movement. Broca's area (regions of the frontal lobe) uses parietal lobe information to perform a high-level planning function for movement of the speech articulators for speech function.

Association Regions

Association areas are considered to provide the highest order of information processing of the cerebral cortex. It appears that higher-order integration areas extract detailed information from the signal input to the primary areas, whereas association areas permit that information to flow among the various processing sites, effectively connecting modalities. These regions are involved in intellect, cognitive functions, memory, and language.

There are three major association areas: the temporal-occipital-parietal association cortex, the limbic association cortex, and the prefrontal association cortex. The *temporal-occipital-parietal (TOP)* region is of the utmost importance to speech-language pathologists and speech-language pathology assistants because it includes the areas associated with language. This region includes portions of the temporal, parietal, and occipital lobes. It receives input from auditory, visual, and somatosensory regions, permitting the integration of this information into language function.

The *limbic association area* includes regions of the parahippocampal gyrus and temporal pole (temporal lobe), cingulate gyri (parietal and frontal lobes), and orbital surfaces (inferior frontal lobe). The limbic system is involved with motivation, emotion, and memory, making it an ideal association area. Clearly, memory function is served by reception of information from diverse sensory inputs.

The *prefrontal association area* is involved with integration of information in preparation for the motor act, as well as higher-level cognitive processes. The premotor regions, consisting of the premotor gyrus and supplemental motor area, appear to be vital to initiation of motor activity, whereas the prefrontal region anterior to these regions is involved in the motor plan. The premotor region receives input from the primary sensory reception areas, or low-order processing regions, while the prefrontal regions derive their input from the higher-order regions. Premotor and prefrontal regions project to the motor strip, permitting both low-order and abstract sensory perceptions to influence the motor act. Broca's area, the frontal operculum, and the insula also are involved in motor programming. These regions share qualities with both the prefrontal association region and the premotor gyrus because damage to them results in deficits of both motor planning and higher-level language, including word retrieval problems.

In addition to this, the *orbitofrontal region* (the region on the underbelly of the cerebrum that overlays the orbit region) is involved in limbic system function, as well as motor planning memory associated with delayed execution.

Summary

- The complexity of higher functions of the brain is reflected in the inability to assign precise locations for specific functions.
- General regions, such as Wernicke's area, can be ascribed broad function, and this view facilitates examination of brain function and dysfunction.
- A broad view of brain function classifies regions of the cerebrum as primary, higher-order, and association regions.
- Primary sensory and motor regions include the primary reception area for somatic sense, primary motor area, primary auditory cortex, and primary region of visual reception.
- Adjacent to these are higher-order areas of processing, apparently responsible for extracting features of the stimulus.
- Association areas are the regions of highest cognitive processing, integrating sensory information with memory.
- The prefrontal area appears to be involved in higher function related to motor output (such as inhibition of motor function and the ability to change motor responses), whereas the temporal-occipital-parietal association area is involved in language function.
- The limbic association area integrates information relating to affect, motivation, and emotion.

Hemispheric Specialization

Despite the gross similarities between the two cerebral hemispheres, the brain is functionally asymmetrical, and the basic processing differences between the two cerebral hemispheres is of extreme importance to speech-language pathology assistants.

If you write with your right hand, you probably have functional dominance for language and speech in the left hemisphere. Motor pathways decussate as they descend, and auditory pathways decussate in ascension, the result being that your right hand and right ear are dominated by activities of the left hemisphere.

The two hemispheres continually work in concert, being connected via the corpus callosum. Virtually all right-handed individuals have coordination of language function in the left hemisphere, while 30% of left-handers either have their language function in the right hemisphere or have it shared by the two hemispheres. The "dominant hemisphere" for language is the left hemisphere for 90% of the population.

The left hemisphere is specialized for analysis. It takes brief, concise information, analyzes it, categorizes it, and moves on to the next task. It is specialized for processing rapidly changing information (e.g., formant transitions, stop consonant bursts) and information that requires dissection and careful, detailed examination.

In contrast, the right hemisphere is specialized to see the big picture. When presented with a visual image of a group of people sitting in desks, watching a person in front, the right hemisphere will interpret that as a meeting of some sort, and use other cues (chalkboard versus altar) to define the situation as a classroom or church setting. If the left hemisphere were confronted with the same information, it would dutifully list out each of the components (person in chair, person at front, desk, chalkboard) but would not identify the situation as a classroom.

The right hemisphere processes emotion much more readily than the left, and that makes sense given the information we use to encode emotion. Intonation contours of speech are long and change relatively slowly, and the right hemisphere processes that very well. Therefore, if you were listening to a person who was depressed and who was speaking slowly with a monotone voice, your right hemisphere would note that something was wrong. The left hemisphere would miss this information entirely, and a person with a lesion of the right hemisphere might be labeled "insensitive" or "apragmatic" because of this deficit. The right hemisphere takes the details of the face (eyes wide open or squinting, mouth in smile or frown, forehead furrowed or eyebrows lifted) and interprets these details as a cohesive unit. The left hemisphere would simply note and list out the elements of the face without interpreting their meaning as a group. The right hemisphere can recognize faces, but the left hemisphere is weak in that area because recognition requires putting the various parts of the face together into a "whole" identity.

The right hemisphere also has the significant responsibility of providing alternative definitions. When the left hemisphere is presented with the statement, "One swallow doesn't make a summer," it interprets the sentence literally, without regard to metaphor. It is the right hemisphere's responsibility to provide alternative meanings to words, so the meaning fits the context. A person with right-hemisphere damage may not be able to interpret the saying above as meaning, "one sign of something doesn't mean that thing is present," or the even more abstract warning, "wait until you are sure of something before you act."

How have we come to these conclusions? A large body of work is developing based on studies of people with specific left- or right-hemisphere lesions, and the problems they have help us to understand how the two hemispheres operate. For many years, we assumed the right hemisphere was the linguistic lightweight of the cerebral cortex, but we have come to respect it for its ability to help us gain meaning from context and for its depth of word meaning. The left hemisphere performs very well on tasks of demanding precise knowledge and application of syntax, morphology, and phonology, but falls on its face (figuratively) when confronted with the need to make sense of context.

Summary

- The hemispheres of the brain display clear functional differences.
- The left hemisphere in most individuals is dominant for language and speech, processes brief duration stimuli, and performs detailed analysis.
- The right hemisphere, in contrast, appears to process information in a more holistic fashion, processing spatial and tonal information.
- Face recognition appears to be a right-hemisphere function.

Motor Control of Speech

The production of speech is an extraordinarily complex process. The idea, or cognitive input, for speech arises from the anterior frontal lobe and appears to be encoded linguistically at Broca's area, which is a segment of the premotor region. The phonological code seems to develop deep to Broca's area in the insula, and the ability to inhibit or initiate speech is regulated by the basal ganglia and supplementary motor area. When the "idea" has been encoded into phonetic elements, the motor plan is developed in the premotor region, and that plan is conveyed to the motor strip for execution.

The premotor region and motor strip receive significant input about body condition from the thalamus, and the plan for execution is examined and modified by the cerebellum so that adequate force can be applied by the muscles to complete the motor act.

Clearly, the execution of speech involves extensive interaction of the areas of the brain in rapid coordination. Humans are amazingly

Lesions and the Indirect Efferent System

To appreciate the effects of lesions to the indirect motor system, it might help to do a quick exercise. Do this: Reach across the desktop to pick up a pencil. As you do this, pay attention to what your muscles are doing. Even as you reach for the pencil, your elbow rotates to accommodate the needs of your arm and hand to make contact with the object. As you get close to the target, your fingers start to close and the rate of movement of your arm slows down. For all of this to happen, your brain must know how fast your muscles are changing length as well as where the target is located in space relative to your hand and body. Contraction of extensors obviously is important, but your brain must also contract flexors to help control extensor contraction lest the movement be ballistic.

Damage to the cerebellum reduces activation of the fusimotor system. Because this system maintains muscle tone through mild, constant muscle contraction, muscles in a person with lesions in the cerebellum lose tone and become flaccid. In contrast, loss of the moderating control by the cerebrum through lesion causes hypertonia in antigravity musculature and extensors because the stretch reflexes are unrestrained.

Lesions and conditions of the basal ganglia have various effects, among them the rigidity of Parkinson's disease. In this condition, intrafusal systems for both extensors and flexors are unrestrained, resulting in simultaneous contraction of antagonists and rigidity. Other basal ganglia lesions result in general hypertonicity.

A Story with a Happy Ending

Here is a story of aneurysm and hemorrhage that has a happy ending. While at a public event one Saturday a dear friend (S) developed a debilitating headache. When her headache didn't improve after an hour of nursing it in the cab of her truck, her husband began the long drive home. Her husband wisely decided that a stop by the local hospital was in order, and the emergency physician suggested Magnetic Resonance Imaging (MRI) to help determine the source of the pain. As the MRI was activated, S became unconscious.

As we later learned, S had a history of aneurysms in her family and had been examined frequently to ensure that there were no surprises in her future. Despite these precautions, an aneurysm had developed at the base of her brain and hemorrhaged as the MRI was activated. A Life-Flight helicopter took her to a metropolitan center that specialized in management of hemorrhage, and friends and family watched anxiously as S slowly became aware of her surroundings. To everyone's great joy and relief her recovery was remarkably complete so that she was able to return to her life and work unencumbered. The quick action of the emergency room medical team and the stroke unit at the receiving hospital gave S the chance to be called the "miracle woman" by all who know her.

versatile in overcoming obstacles to speech production, which is good news for the speech-language pathology assistant. Try this: Say "Sammy is a friend of mine." Now place your pencil between your molars on one side of your mouth, bite down lightly, and say it again a few times. Were you able to produce intelligible speech? Although the pencil interfered with some dental or labial productions, on the whole you were probably not only intelligible, but accurate. If the program for the individual articulators were "written in stone," you would not have been able to tolerate this aberration (use of a "bite block"), and your speech would have been unintelligible. Through this sort of examination, we realize that we probably develop an internal standard of what we want our speech to sound like, and then we do whatever is necessary to match that standard. Thus, your role as a speech-language pathology assistant could well include helping your client develop that internal standard and take stops to improve his or her communication.

Impact of Aphasia

The life of an individual with aphasia caused by a stroke is significantly changed by the cerebrovascular event. With the brain lesion comes an instant change in how the individual can interact with his or her environment, with how readily linguistic information can be used to process information and to communicate, and with how easily cognitive processes can be performed.

The individual with left-hemisphere stroke of the frontal lobe faces dysfluency while being very aware of the jumble of verbal output. If the lesion is in the posterior regions, speech will be more fluent but may be "empty" of content, and the person may have difficulty with comprehension, not realizing that his or her speech is not doing what was intended.

It is extremely important that a speech-language pathology assistant, enlist the help of a client's family or close friends very early in the process. These significant others will be most able to extend the therapy into every aspect of the person's life, and they will become the individual's most valuable communication partners. Including a partner early in treatment affords the opportunity to move the client back into the world of communication.

CHAPTER SUMMARY

The nervous system is a complex, hierarchical structure. Voluntary movement, sensory awareness, and cognitive function are the domain of the cerebral cortex. The communication links of the nervous system are spinal nerves, cranial nerves, and tracts of the brainstem and spinal cord. Several organizational schemes characterize the nervous system. It can be divided functionally into the autonomic and somatic nervous systems. The nervous system can also be divided anatomically into the central and peripheral nervous systems. Neurons communicate through synapses by means of neurotransmitter substances. Effects on the receiving neurons are excitatory or inhibitory. Glial cells provide the fatty sheath for myelinated axons, as well as support structure for neurons.

The cerebral cortex is protected from physical insult by cerebrospinal fluid and the meningeal linings—the dura, pia, and arachnoid maters. The cerebrum is divided into two hemispheres connected by the corpus callosum. The gyri and sulci of the hemisphere provide important landmarks for lobes and other regions of the cerebrum. The temporal lobe is the site of auditory reception. The frontal lobe is responsible for most voluntary motor activation and is the site of the important speech region known as Broca's area. The parietal lobe is the region of somatic sensory reception. The occipital lobe is the site of visual input to the cerebrum. The insular lobe lies deep in the lateral sulcus and is revealed by deflecting the temporal lobe. The operculum overlies the insula. The functionally defined limbic lobe includes the cingulate gyrus, uncus, parahippocampal gyrus, and other deep structures.

The basal ganglia are subcortical structures involved in control of movement, and the hippocampal formation of the inferior temporal lobe is deeply implicated in memory function. The thalamus of the diencephalon is the final relay for somatic sensation directed toward the cerebrum and other diencephalic structures. The hypothalamus controls many bodily functions and desires. The regions of the cerebral cortex are interconnected by means of a complex network of projection fibers, connecting the cortex with other structures; association fibers, which connect regions of the same hemisphere; and commissural fibers, which provide communication between corresponding regions of the two hemispheres.

The anterior cerebral arteries serve the medial surfaces of the brain, and the middle cerebral artery serves the lateral cortex, including the temporal lobe, motor strip, Wernicke's area, and much of the parietal lobe. The vertebral arteries branch to form the anterior and posterior spinal arteries, with ascending components serving the ventral brainstem. The basilar artery gives rise to the superior and anterior inferior cerebellar arteries to serve the cerebellum, while the posterior inferior cerebellar artery arises from the vertebral artery. The basilar artery divides to become the posterior cerebral arteries, serving the inferior temporal and occipital lobes, upper midbrain, and diencephalon. The Circle of Willis is a series of communicating arteries that provide redundant pathways for blood flow to regions of the cerebral cortex, equalizing pressure and flow-rate of blood.

The cerebellum coordinates motor and sensory information, communicating with the brainstem, cerebrum, and spinal cord. It communicates with the rest of the nervous system via the superior, middle, and inferior cerebral peduncles. Position in space, adjustment against gravity, and fine motor adjustments are mediated by the cerebellum. The superior cerebellar peduncle enters the pons and serves the dentate nucleus, red nucleus, and thalamus.

The brainstem is divided into medulla, pons, and midbrain. It is more highly organized than the spinal cord and mediates higher-level body functions such as vestibular responses. The pyramidal decussation of the medulla is the point at which the motor commands originating in one hemisphere of the cerebral cortex cross to serve the opposite side of the body. The reticular formation is a phylogenetically old set of nuclei essential for life function. The pons and midbrain set the stage for communication with the higher levels of the brain, including the cerebellum and cerebrum. This communication link permits not only complex motor acts, but also consciousness, awareness, and volitional acts.

Cranial nerves mediate articulatory, phonatory, and auditory functions. Cranial nerves are sensory, motor, or mixed sensorimotor, and are categorized based on function as general or specialized and as serving visceral or somatic organs or structures. The V trigeminal innervates muscles of mastication and the tensor veli palatini, and it communicates sensation from the face, mouth, teeth, mucosal lining, and tongue. The VII facial nerve innervates muscles of facial expression, and the sensory component serves taste of the anterior two thirds of the tongue. The VIII vestibulocochlear nerve mediates auditory and vestibular sensation. The IX glossopharyngeal nerve serves the posterior tongue taste receptors, as well as somatic sense from the tongue, fauces, pharynx, and eustachian tube. The stylopharyngeus and superior pharyngeal constrictor muscles receive motor innervation via this nerve. The X vagus serves autonomic and somatic functions, mediating pain, touch, and temperature from the eardrum and pain from the pharynx, larynx, and esophagus. The recurrent laryngeal nerve and superior laryngeal nerves supply motor innervation for the intrinsic muscles of the larynx. The XI accessory nerve innervates the sternocleidomastoid and trapezius muscles, and it collaborates with the vagus nerve in activation of palatal, laryngeal, and pharyngeal muscles. The XII hypoglossal nerve innervates the muscles of the tongue with the exception of the palatoglossus.

Communication between neurons of the nervous system occurs at the synapse, and neurotransmitter passing through the synaptic cleft either excites or inhibits the postsynaptic neuron. When a neuron is sufficiently stimulated, an action potential is generated, which causes membrane depolarization and exchange of ions between the extracellular and intracellular spaces. Ion movement results in a change in voltage across the membrane. Resting membrane potential is the relatively stable state of the neuron at rest, whereas the absolute refractory period after excitation is an interval during which the neuron cannot be excited to fire. Neurons are capable of representing differences in input only through rate of response. Myelinated fibers conduct the wave of depolarization more rapidly than demyelinated fibers, primarily due to saltatory conduction.

Higher function of the brain defies a strict localization approach to functional organization. Brain function is classified into regions of primary, higher-order, and association regions. Primary sensory and motor regions include the primary reception area for somatic sense, primary motor area, primary auditory cortex, and primary region of visual reception. Higher-order areas of processing are apparently responsible for extracting features of the stimulus. Association areas are the regions of highest cognitive processing, integrating sensory information with memory. The prefrontal area appears to be involved in higher function related to motor output, and the temporal-occipital-parietal association is involved in spoken and written language function. The limbic association area integrates information relating to affect, motivation, and emotion.

The hemispheres of the brain display clear functional differences. Language and speech, brief duration stimuli, and detailed information are processed in the left hemisphere in most individuals. The right hemisphere appears to process information in a more holistic fashion, preferring spatial and tonal information.

Movement is initiated at the motor strip, but there is a great deal of planning that occurs prior to that point. The premotor regions, including Broca's area, are involved in planning for the motor act, and project that plan to the motor strip. The prefrontal association area also provides input to the motor strip concerning higher cognitive elements of the speech act, and the lowest levels of information (information about muscle stretch and tension) are also fed to the motor strip.

Study Questions

1. The _____ governs voluntary actions.

2. The _____ is responsible for coordinating movement.

3. _____ are groups of cell bodies in the PNS with functional unity.

4. The _____ system includes the cerebrum, cerebellum, subcortical structures, brainstem, and spinal cord.

5. The _____ system consists of the 12 pairs of cranial nerves and 31 pairs of spinal nerves, as well as the sensory receptors.

6. The _____ system governs involuntary activities of involuntary muscles.

7. The _____ system governs voluntary activities.

8. Information directed toward the brain is termed _____ and information directed from the brain is termed _____.

9. On the following figure identify the indicated parts of the neuron.

   A. _____

   B. _____

C. _____

D. _____

E. _____

F. _____

G. _____

H. _____

I. _____

10. On the following figure identify the indicated parts of the cerebrum.

A. _____ lobe

B. _____ lobe

C. _____ lobe

D. _____ lobe

E. _____ gyrus

F. _____ gyrus

G. _____ sulcus

H. _____ sulcus

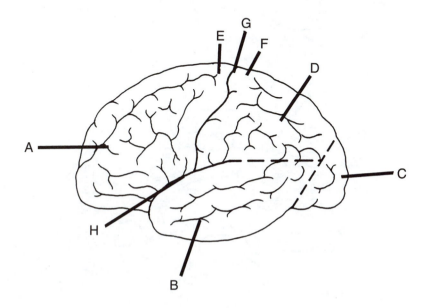

11. On the following figure identify the parts of the surface of the cerebrum.

A. _____ gyrus

B. _____

C. _____ gyrus

D. _____ area

E. _____ area

F. _____ gyrus

G. _____ gyrus

H. _____ sulcus

12. On the following figure identify the indicated arteries and structures.

A. _____ artery

B. _____ artery

C. _____ artery

D. _____ artery

E. _____ artery

F. _____ artery

G. _____ artery

H. _____ artery

I. _____

13. _____ is a change in electrical potential that occurs when a cell membrane is stimulated adequately to permit ion exchange between intracellular and extracellular spaces.

14. The _____ period is the time during which the cell membrane cannot be stimulated to depolarize.

15. The _____ is a period during which the membrane can be stimulated to excitation again, but only with greater than typical stimulation.

16. The _____ of the axon myelin promote saltatory conduction.

17. The substance known as _____ is discharged into the synaptic cleft, stimulating the postsynaptic neuron.

18. Higher cognitive processing occurs generally in _____ areas.

19. The _____ area is involved in language function.

20. The _____ area of the cerebrum appears to be involved in higher function related to motor output (such as inhibition of motor function and the ability to change motor responses), whereas the temporal-occipital-parietal association area is involved in language function.

21. The _____ area integrates information relating to affect, motivation, and emotion.

22. The _____ hemisphere in most individuals is dominant for language and speech, processes brief duration stimuli, and performs detailed analysis.

23. The _____ hemisphere appears to process information in a more holistic fashion, preferring spatial and tonal information.

REFERENCES

Albom, M. (1997). *Tuesdays with Morrie.* New York: Broadway Books.

Bateman, H. E., & Mason, R. M. (1984). *Applied anatomy and physiology of the speech and hearing mechanism.* Springfield, IL: Charles C. Thomas.

Bear, M. F., Connors, B. W., & Paradiso, M. A. (1996). *Neuroscience: Exploring the brain.* Baltimore: Williams & Wilkins.

Bhatnagar, S. C., & Andy, O. J. (2002). *Neuroscience for the study of communicative disorders* (2nd ed.). Baltimore: Williams & Wilkins.

Bly, L. (1994). *Motor skills acquisition in the first year.* Tucson, AZ: Therapy Skill Builders.

Bowman, J. P. (1971). *The muscle spindle and neural control of the tongue.* Springfield, IL: Charles C. Thomas.

Carpenter, M. B. (1991). *Core text of neuroanatomy* (4th ed.). Baltimore: Williams & Wilkins.

Chusid, J. G. (1985). *Correlative neuroanatomy and functional neurology* (17th ed.). Los Altos, CA: Lange Medical Publications.

Cotman, C. W., & McGaugh, J. L. (1980). *Behavioral neuroscience.* New York: Academic.

Darley, F. L., Aronson, A. E., & Brown, J. R. (1975). *Motor speech disorders.* Philadelphia: Saunders.

Edvinsson, L., & Krause, D. N. (2002). *Cerebral blood flow and metabolism.* Philadelphia: Williams & Wilkins.

Filskov, S. B., & Boll, T. J. (1981). *Handbook of clinical neuropsychology.* New York: Wiley.

Fiorentino, M. R. (1973). *Reflex testing methods for evaluating CNS development.* Springfield, IL: Charles C. Thomas.

Flege, J. E. (1988). Anticipatory and carry-over nasal coarticulation in the speech of children and adults. *Journal of Speech and Hearing Research, 31,* 525–536.

Ganong, W. F. (2003). *Review of medical physiology* (21st ed.). New York: McGraw-Hill/Appleton & Lange.

Gelfand, S. A. (2001). *Essentials of audiology* (2nd ed.). New York: Thieme Medical.

Kandel, E. R. (1991). Brain and Behavior. In E. R. Kandel, J. R. Schwartz, & T. M. Jessell (Eds.), *Principles of neural science* (3rd ed.) pp. 9–48. Norwalk, CT: Appleton & Lange.

Kandel, E. R., Schwartz, J. H., & Jessell, T. M. (2000). *Principles of neural science* (4th ed.). New York: McGraw Hill.

Kuehn, D. P., Lemme, M. L., & Baumgartner, J. M. (1991). *Neural bases of speech, hearing, and language.* Boston: Little, Brown.

MacKay, L. E., Chapman, P. E., & Morgan, A. S. (1997). *Maximizing brain injury recovery.* Gaithersburg, MD: Aspen.

McMinn, R. M. H., Hutchings, R. T., & Logan, B. M. (1994). *Color atlas of head and neck anatomy*. London: Mosby-Wolfe.

Moore, K. L. (1988). *The developing human*. Philadelphia: Saunders.

Netsell, R. (1986). A neurobiologic view of speech production and the dysarthrias. San Diego: College-Hill.

Netter, F. H. (1983a). *The CIBA collection of medical illustrations*. (Vol. 1.) Nervous System. Part I. Anatomy and physiology. West Caldwell, NJ: CIBA Pharmaceutical Company.

Netter, F. H. (1983b). *The CIBA collection of medical illustrations*. (Vol. 1.) Nervous system. Part II. Neurologic and neuromuscular disorders. West Caldwell, NJ: CIBA Pharmaceutical Company.

Netter, F. H. (1997). *Atlas of human anatomy*. Los Angeles: Icon Learning Systems.

Noback, C. R., Demarest, R. J., & Strominger, N. L. (1991). *The nervous system: Introduction and review*. Philadelphia: Williams & Wilkins.

Nolte, J. (2002). *The human brain* (5th ed.). St. Louis, MO: Mosby.

Poritsky, R. (1992). *Neuroanatomy: A functional atlas of parts and pathways*. St. Louis: Mosby Year Book.

Rohen, J. W., & Yokochi, C. (1993). *Color atlas of anatomy*. New York: Igaku-Shoin.

Spirduso, W. W. (1995). *Physical dimensions of aging*. Champaign, IL: Human Kinetics.

Twietmeyer, A., & McCracken, T. D., (1992). *Coloring guide to regional human anatomy* (2nd ed.). Philadelphia: Lea & Febiger.

Winans, S. S., Gilman, S., Manter, J. T., & Gatz, A. J. (2002). *Manter and Gatz's essentials of clinical neuroanatomy and neurophysiology* (10th ed.). Philadelphia: Davis.

Wood, P. J., & Criss, W. R. (1975). *Normal and abnormal development of the human nervous system*. Hagerstown, MD: Harper & Row.

Yost, W. A. (2000). *Fundamentals of hearing: An introduction* (4th ed). New York: Academic.

Zemlin, W. R. (1998). *Speech and hearing science. Anatomy and physiology* (4th ed.). Needham Heights, MA: Allyn & Bacon.

APPENDIX

Study Question Answers

CHAPTER 1

1. <u>ANATOMY</u> is the study of the structure of an organism.

2. <u>PHYSIOLOGY</u> is the study of the function of a living organism and its parts.

3. <u>CLINICAL</u>, or <u>APPLIED</u>, anatomy is anatomical study for diagnosis and treatment of disease.

4. <u>SYSTEMIC ANATOMY</u> is involved in the description of individual parts of the body without reference to disease, viewing the body as a composite of systems that function together.

5. Skin and mucous membrane are made up of <u>EPITHELIAL</u> tissue.

6. CARTILAGE is a particularly important connective tissue because it is both strong and elastic.

7. MUSCLE is contractile tissue.

8. LIGAMENTS bind organs together or hold bones to bone or cartilage.

9. FASCIA is a sheetlike membrane surrounding organs.

10. TENDONS attach muscle to bone or to cartilage.

11. The relatively immobile point of attachment of a muscle is the ORIGIN.

12. The relatively mobile point of attachment of a muscle is the INSERTION.

13. Identify the systems from their definitions:

    A. MUSCULAR SYSTEM This system includes smooth, striated, and cardiac muscles of the body.

    B. SKELETAL SYSTEM This system includes the bones and cartilages that form the structure of the body.

    C. RESPIRATORY SYSTEM This system includes the passageways and tissues involved in gas exchange with the environment, including the oral, nasal, and pharyngeal cavities, the trachea and bronchial passageway, and the lungs.

    D. DIGESTIVE SYSTEM This system includes the esophagus, liver, intestines, and associated glands.

    E. NERVOUS SYSTEM This system includes the nerve tissue and structures of the central and peripheral nervous systems.

14. Identify the systems of speech from their definitions:

    A. RESPIRATORY SYSTEM This system includes the passageways and tissues involved in gas exchange with the environment, including the oral, nasal, and pharyngeal cavities, the trachea and bronchial passageway, and the lungs.

    B. PHONATORY SYSTEM This system is involved in production of voiced sound and uses components of the respiratory system (the laryngeal structures).

    C. ARTICULATORY SYSTEM This system is the combination of structures used to alter the sounds of speech, including parts of the anatomically defined digestive and respiratory systems (the tongue, lips, teeth, soft palate, etc.).

    D. RESONATORY SYSTEM This system includes the nasal cavity and soft palate and portions of the anatomically defined respiratory and digestive systems.

15. On the figure, identify the descriptive terms indicated.

    A. TRANSVERSE plane

    B. SAGITTAL plane

    C. CORONAL, or FRONTAL, plane

    D. ANTERIOR, or VENTRAL, aspect

    E. POSTERIOR, or DORSAL, aspect

    F. ABDUCT (movement away from midline)

    G. ADDUCT (movement toward midline)

    H. DISTAL (located away from midline)

    I. MEDIAL (located near midline)

    J. LATERAL (related to the side)

    K. SUPERIOR (above)

    L. INFERIOR (below)

16. Pathology is the study of diseased tissue. By extension, a speech-language pathologist is one who studies the "pathology" of our field, communication disorders.

CHAPTER 2

1. PRESSURE is defined as force distributed over area.

2. NEGATIVE pressure causes air to enter the container until the pressure is equalized.

3. How many of each of the following vertebrae are there?

   7 cervical vertebrae

   12 thoracic vertebrae

   5 lumbar vertebrae

   5 sacral vertebrae (fused)

4. On the following figure, identify the indicated landmarks.

   A. SPINOUS process

   B. TRANSVERSE process

   C. CORPUS

   D. SUPERIOR ARTICULAR facet

      E. INFERIOR COSTAL facet

      F. SUPERIOR COSTAL facet

      G. VERTEBRAL foramen

5. The SPINAL CORD passes through the vertebral foramen.

6. On the following figure, identify the indicated landmarks.

      A. ILIUM

      B. ISCHIUM

      C. PUBIC BONE

      D. SACRUM

      E. ILIAC CREST

      F. PUBIC SYMPHYSIS

      G. COCCYX

      H. CLAVICLE

      I. SCAPULA

      J. MANUBRIUM STERNI

      K. XIPHOID or ENSIFORM PROCESS

      L. CORPUS STERNI

      M. STERNAL NOTCH

7. On the following figure, identify the indicated landmarks.

      A. TRACHEA

      B. MAINSTEM BRONCHUS

      C. SECONDARY BRONCHUS

      D. TERTIARY BRONCHUS

8. On the following figure, identify the indicated muscles and structures.

      A. EXTERNAL OBLIQUE ABDOMINIS

      B. INTERNAL OBLIQUE ABDOMINIS

      C. RECTUS ABDOMINIS

      D. TRANSVERSUS ABDOMINIS

      E. LINEA ALBA

      F. INGUINAL LIGAMENT

      G. LINEA SEMILUNARIS

9. On the following figure, identify the indicated muscles.

   A. <u>Serratus Posterior Superior</u>

   B. <u>Levator Costarum Brevis</u>

   C. <u>Levator Costarum Longis</u>

10. Identify the muscles indicated in the following figure.

    A. <u>Scalenus Anterior</u>

    B. <u>Scalenus Medius</u>

    C. <u>Scalenus Posterior</u>

11. Identify the muscles and portions of muscles indicated in the following figure.

    A. <u>Sternocleidomastoid</u>

    B. <u>Clavicular</u> head

    C. <u>Sternal</u> head

    D. <u>Pectoralis Major</u>

    E. <u>Pectoralis Minor</u>

12. Contraction of the diaphragm increases the <u>Vertical</u> dimension of the thorax.

13. Contraction of the accessory muscles of inspiration increase the <u>Transverse</u> dimension of the thorax.

14. Contraction of the muscles of expiration <u>Decrease</u> the volume of the thorax.

15. Passive expiration involves the forces of <u>Torque, Elasticity,</u> and <u>Gravity</u>.

16. Identify the described volumes and capacities.

    A. <u>Tidal Volume</u>

    B. <u>Inspiratory Reserve</u> volume

    C. <u>Expiratory Reserve</u> volume

    D. <u>Residual</u> volume

    E. <u>Vital</u> capacity

    F. <u>Functional Residual</u> capacity

    G. <u>Total Lung</u> capacity

17. DEAD AIR SPACE is the volume of air that cannot undergo gas exchange.

18. INTRAORAL pressure is the air pressure in the oral cavity.

19. SUBGLOTTAL pressure is the air pressure below the vocal folds.

20. ALVEOLAR, or PULMONIC, pressure is the pressure in the alveolus.

21. INTRAPLEURAL, or PLEURAL, pressure is the pressure between the visceral and parietal pleural membranes.

22. When the diaphragm contracts, pressure in the alveolus DECREASES.

23. When air pressure in the lungs is lower than that of the atmosphere, air will ENTER the lungs.

24. When the body is reclining, the resting lung volume DECREASES.

25. Use of the muscles of inspiration to impede the outward flow of air during speech is termed CHECKING ACTION.

26. In advanced emphysema the diaphragm is pulled down and stretched relatively flat by the flaring of the rib cage. In normal inspiration contraction of the diaphragm causes the central tendon to pull down, causing air to enter the lungs (Boyle's law dictates that a drop in alveolar pressure causes airflow into the lungs). When the diaphragm of an individual with advanced emphysema contracts, it pulls the ribs closer together because they were distended by the "barrel chest." As a result, the alveoli are compressed, causing an increase in alveolar pressure and causing air to leave the lungs. Thus, the inspiratory gesture of the diaphragm causes expiration. The single inspiratory avenue left to the individual is to elevate the sternum and clavicle using clavicular breathing.

CHAPTER 3

1. Identify the structures indicated on the figure.

   A. EPIGLOTTIS cartilage

   B. THYROID cartilage

   C. CRICOID cartilage

   D. ARYTENOID cartilage

   E. CORNICULATE cartilage

   F. HYOID bone

2. Identify the landmarks indicated on the figure.

   A. SUPERIOR CORNU

   B. INFERIOR CORNU

   C. OBLIQUE LINE

   D. THYROID NOTCH

   E. ANGLE OF THYROID

   F. LAMINA

3. Identify the landmarks indicated on the figure.

   A. MUSCULAR process

   B. VOCAL process

4. Identify the muscles indicated in the following figure.

   A. TRANSVERSE ARYTENOID

   B. OBLIQUE ARYTENOID

   C. POSTERIOR CRICOARYTENOID

5. Identify the muscles indicated in the following figure.

   A. MYLOHYOID

   B. DIGASTRICUS ANTERIOR

   C. DIGASTRICUS POSTERIOR

   D. STYLOHYOID

6. Identify the muscles indicated in the following figure.

   A. GENIOHYOID

   B. DIGASTRICUS ANTERIOR

   C. DIGASTRICUS POSTERIOR

   D. MYLOHYOID

7. This is a view of the laryngeal opening from above. Identify the indicated structures.

   A. ARYEPIGLOTTIC FOLD

   B. TRUE VOCAL FOLDS

   C. VALLECULAE

   D. EPIGLOTTIS

8. Identify the two muscles in the following figure.

   A. THYROVOCALIS

   B. THYROMUSCULARIS

9. The CRICOTHYROID muscle is the primary muscle responsible for change of vocal fundamental frequency.

10. The space between the vocal folds is the GLOTTIS.

11. The BERNOULLI effect states that given a constant volume flow of air or fluid, at a point of constriction there will be a decrease in air pressure perpendicular to the flow and an increase in velocity of the flow.

12. Removal of the larynx would leave the airway unprotected from intrusion of foreign matter during swallowing. To avoid this danger, the airway is sealed off surgically, and a stoma is surgically opened up through the trachea to permit unhampered respiration.

13. ABDOMINAL FIXATION is the process of capturing air in the thorax to provide the muscles with a structure upon which to push or pull.

14. In GLOTTAL attack, the vocal folds are adducted before initiation of expiratory flow.

15. In BREATHY attack, the vocal folds are adducted after the initiation of expiratory flow.

16. In SIMULTANEOUS attack, the vocal folds are adducted simultaneous with initiation of expiratory flow.

17. During modal phonation, the vocal folds open from INFERIOR to SUPERIOR. The folds close from INFERIOR to SUPERIOR.

18. The minimum subglottal driving pressure for speech is 3 cm to 5 cm H_2O.

19. In the mode of vibration known as GLOTTAL FRY, the vocal folds vibrate at a much lower rate than in modal phonation, and the folds exhibit a syncopated vibratory pattern.

20. In the mode of vibration known as FALSETTO, the vocal folds lengthen and become extremely thin and reedlike.

21. Presence of vocal nodules or other space-occupying laryngeal pathology may result in BREATHY phonation.

22. To increase vocal intensity, one must INCREASE subglottal pressure and INCREASE medial compression.

23. To increase vocal fundamental frequency, one must INCREASE vocal fold tension by LENGTHENING the vocal folds.

24. OPTIMAL PITCH is the pitch of phonation that is optimal or most appropriate for an individual.

25. HABITUAL PITCH is the vocal pitch habitually used during speech.

26. As vocal intensity increases, the closed phase of the vibratory cycle INCREASES.

27. The vocal folds vibrate as a function of the transglottal pressure drop: The subglottal pressure is higher than the supraglottal (oral) pressure, so air flows through the glottis and the vocal folds vibrate. When the fistula was unoccluded, the transglottal pressure drop increased markedly, making control of the vocal folds difficult and causing the aperiodicity we saw. We have seen the same phenomenon in individuals with neurological diseases such as multiple sclerosis. In that case, we saw increased aperiodicity as a function of open vowel position, but the principle still holds.

CHAPTER 4

1. The SOURCE-FILTER theory of vowel production states that the voicing source is routed through the vocal tract where it is shaped into the sounds of speech by the articulators.

2. On the following figure, identify the indicated bones and landmarks.

    A. MAXILLA (bone)

    B. MANDIBLE (bone)

    C. ZYGOMATIC bone

    D. NASAL bone

    E. FRONTAL bone

    F. FRONTAL process

    G. ALVEOLAR process

    H. SYMPHYSIS MENTE

3. On the following figure, identify the indicated bones and land-marks.

   A. SPHENOID bone

   B. OCCIPITAL bone

   C. TEMPORAL bone

   D. CRISTA GALLI

   E. CRIBRIFORM PLATE

   F. FORAMEN MAGNUM

4. On the following figure, identify the indicated bones and land-marks.

   A. ZYGOMATIC bone

   B. TEMPORAL bone

   C. MAXILLAE (bone)

   D. MANDIBLE (bone)

   E. NASAL bone

   F. FRONTAL bone

   G. PARIETAL bone

   H. OCCIPITAL bone

   I. RAMUS

   J. ANGLE

   K. ZYGOMATIC process

   L. CONDYLAR process

   M. CORONOID process

   N. CORPUS

   O. MASTOID process

   P. STYLOID process

   Q. EXTERNAL AUDITORY MEATUS

5. On the following figure, identify the indicated structures.

   A. PALATINE process

   B. MAXILLAE (bone)

   C. PALATINE bone

   D. PREMAXILLA

  E. INCISIVE foramen

  F. INTERMAXILLARY suture

  G. STYLOID process

  H. MEDIAL PTERYGOID plate

  I. LATERAL PTERYGOID plate

  J. MASTOID process

  K. FORAMEN MAGNUM

  L. PTERYGOID HAMULUS

6. On the following figure, identify the indicated muscles.

  A. LEVATOR VELI PALATINI

  B. TENSOR VELI PALATINI

  C. PALATOGLOSSUS

  D. PALATOPHARYNGEUS

7. On the following figure, identify the indicated muscles.

  A. BUCCINATOR

  B. ORBICULARIS ORIS SUPERIORIS

  C. ORBICULARIS ORIS INFERIORIS

  D. DEPRESSOR ANGULI ORIS

  E. DEPRESSOR LABII INFERIORIS

  F. ZYGOMATIC MAJOR

  G. ZYGOMATIC MINOR

  H. LEVATOR LABII SUPERIORIS ALAEQUE NASI

  I. LEVATOR ANGULI ORIS

  J. LEVATOR LABII SUPERIORIS

  K. RISORIUS

  L. PLATYSMA

8. On the following figure, identify the indicated muscles.

  A. MASSETER

  B. TEMPORALIS

  C. LATERAL PTERYGOID

  D. MEDIAL PTERYGOID

9. On the following figure, identify the indicated muscles.

    A. GENIOGLOSSUS

    B. HYOGLOSSUS

    C. DIGASTRICUS POSTERIOR

    D. STYLOGLOSSUS

    E. STYLOHYOID

    F. PALATOGLOSSUS

    G. INFERIOR LONGITUDINAL

    H. SUPERIOR LONGITUDINAL

10. On the following figure, identify structures the indicated muscles.

    A. VOMER (bone)

    B. PALATINE process

    C. HORIZONTAL plate

    D. PERPENDICULAR plate

    E. CARTILAGINOUS SEPTUM

    F. NASAL bone

11. MASTICATION refers to the processes involved in food preparation, such as chewing food, moving the food onto the molars, and so forth.

12. DEGLUTITION refers to swallowing.

13. In the ORAL PREPARATORY stage of swallowing, food is prepared for swallowing.

14. In the ORAL stage of swallowing, mastication ceases, the tongue drops down and pulls posteriorly, and the anterior tongue elevates to the hard palate and squeezes the bolus back toward the faucial pillars.

15. In the PHARYNGEAL stage of swallowing, the bolus contacts the anterior faucial pillars, the soft palate elevates, respiration stops, the vocal folds tightly adduct, the larynx elevates and moves forward, and the cricopharyngeus relaxes as food enters the pharynx.

16. During the ESOPHAGEAL stage of swallowing, the bolus is transported through the esophagus.

17. Identify the muscle that best fits the statement (In some cases more than one muscle fills the bill.)

    A. SUPERIOR LONGITUDINAL INTRINSIC elevates tongue tip.

    B. INFERIOR LONGITUDINAL INTRINSIC depresses tongue tip.

    C. GENIOGLOSSUS, POSTERIOR PORTION protrudes tongue.

    D. GENIOGLOSSUS, ANTERIOR PORTION; STYLOGLOSSUS retracts tongue.

    E. PALATOGLOSSUS elevates posterior tongue.

    F. TRANSVERSE INTRINSIC narrows tongue.

    G. VERTICAL INTRINSIC; GENIOGLOSSUS flattens tongue.

    H. PALATOGLOSSUS; PALATOPHARYNGEUS depresses soft palate.

    I. TENSOR VELI PALATINI tenses soft palate.

    J. CRICOPHARYNGEUS constricts esophageal opening.

    K. SUPERIOR PHARYNGEAL CONSTRICTOR constricts upper pharynx.

    L. LEVATOR VELI PALATINI elevates velum.

18. Motor control in the body develops from HEAD to TAIL and from PROXIMAL to DISTAL.

19. Elevation of the posterior tongue requires active contraction of the palatoglossus, perhaps the styloglossus, and the vertical intrinsic muscle. In addition, the tongue is pulling against the soft palate to achieve elevation because the palatoglossus is a velar depressor as well. When the palatoglossus contracts to elevate the tongue, the tensor and levator veli palatine must contract to keep the soft palate elevated.

CHAPTER 5

1. The PINNA of the outer ear is important for localization of sound in space.

2. Resistance to flow of energy is called IMPEDANCE.

3. The area ratio between the tympanic membrane and the oval window provides a 25-dB gain, and the level advantage gives a 2-dB gain.

4. The cochlea performs both SPECTRAL analysis and TEMPORAL analysis.

5. Compression in the fluid of the scala vestibuli is translated directly to the basilar membrane, and the disturbance at the basilar membrane causes the initiation of T<small>RAVELING</small> wave.

6. High-frequency sounds are resolved at the base of the cochlea, with progressively lower sounds processed at progressively higher positions on the cochlea. This array is called T<small>ONOTOPIC</small>.

7. The frequency analysis ability of the basilar membrane is determined by graded W<small>IDTH</small>, S<small>TIFFNESSS</small>, and T<small>HICKNESS</small>.

8. At the apex, the basilar membrane is T<small>HICKER</small> than at the base.

9. At the apex, the basilar membrane is W<small>IDER</small> than at the base.

10. F—The cilia of the outer hair cells are embedded in the tectorial membrane.

11. T—The cilia of the inner hair cells are embedded in the tectorial membrane.

12. H<small>IGH</small>-T<small>HRESHOLD</small> neurons require a higher intensity and encompass the higher end of our auditory range of signal intensity, whereas L<small>OW</small>-T<small>HRESHOLD</small> neurons respond at very low signal levels and display random firing even when there is no stimulus.

13. F<small>REQUENCY</small> S<small>PECIFICITY</small> refers to the ability of the cochlea to differentiate spectral components of a signal.

14. The C<small>HARACTERISTIC</small> frequency of a neuron is the frequency to which it responds best.

15. Tuning curves are composites of the responses of a single fiber at each frequency of presentation. The sharper the tuning curve is, the greater is the F<small>REQUENCY</small> S<small>PECIFICITY</small> of the basilar membrane.

16. Rate of firing of neurons increases as the I<small>NTENSITY</small> increases.

17. Stimulation of the C<small>ROSSED</small>-O<small>LIVOCOCHLEAR</small> bundle and the U<small>NCROSSED</small>-O<small>LIVOCOCHLEAR</small> bundle reduces the firing rate of neurons innervated by them.

18. The E<small>XTERNAL</small> A<small>UDITORY</small> meatus is a conduit for sound reaching the tympanic membrane.

19. The I<small>NTERNAL</small> A<small>UDITORY</small> meatus is a conduit for the VIII nerve fibers coursing to the brainstem.

20. The tympanic membrane (or eardrum) is made up of T<small>HREE</small> layers of tissue.

21. The outer layer of the tympanic membrane is continuous with the E<small>PITHELIUM OF</small> E<small>XTERNAL</small> A<small>UDITORY</small> M<small>EATUS</small>.

22. The INTERMEDIATE layer of the tympanic membrane is made up primarily of radiating fibers.

23. The UMBO is a landmark produced by the most distal part of the manubrium malli.

24. The MALLEUS is the bone of the middle ear directly attached to the tympanic membrane.

25. The STAPES is the bone of the middle ear directly communicating with the oval window.

26. The MANUBRIUM of the malleus attaches to the tympanic membrane.

27. The FOOTPLATE of the stapes articulates with the oval window.

28. The STAPEDIUS muscle pulls the stapes posteriorly.

29. The TENSOR TYMPANI muscle pulls the malleus anteromedially.

30. The entryway to the cochlea and vestibular system is via the space known as the VESTIBULE.

31. The OSSEOUS LABYRINTH is the system of cavities within bone that houses the membranous labyrinth.

32. The scala VESTIBULI and scala TYMPANI are incomplete spaces in the osseous labyrinth.

33. The ROUND window provides communication between the scala tympani and the middle ear.

34. The OVAL window permits communication between the scala vestibuli and the middle ear space.

35. The MEMBRANOUS LABYRINTH is a fluid-filled sac attached to the walls of the osseous labyrinth and is filled with endolymph.

36. REISSNER'S membrane separates the scala vestibuli and the scala media; the BASILAR membrane separates the scala media from the scala tympani.

37. The TUNNEL OF CORTI separates the outer and inner hair cells.

38. The hair cells are innervated by the VIII VESTIBULOCOCHLEAR nerve.

39. As with any other body structure, the ossicles are subject to trauma. A frequent cause of disarticulation of the ossicles is head trauma that involves the temporal bone (this may also cause a perilymph fistula, which is a tear in the basilar or Reissner's membrane that allows perilymph and endolymph to mingle). Another cause of disarticulation is noise or high-pressure trauma: The high-pressure forces associated with explosions can easily cause disarticulation.

40. The fruit bat cochlea is, naturally enough, smaller than that of the human. In addition, the cochlea of the bat is extremely sensitive to ultra-high frequencies (above human range of hearing), because high-frequency sounds are more efficient for echolocation. Elephants, on the other hand, have larger cochleas than humans. They process sounds that are lower than those we can hear!

CHAPTER 6

1. The CEREBRUM governs voluntary actions.

2. The CEREBELLUM is responsible for coordinating movement.

3. GANGLIA are groups of cell bodies in the PNS with functional unity.

4. The CENTRAL NERVOUS SYSTEM includes the cerebrum, cerebellum, subcortical structures, brainstem, and spinal cord.

5. The PERIPHERAL NERVOUS SYSTEM consists of the 12 pairs of cranial nerves and 31 pairs of spinal nerves, as well as the sensory receptors.

6. The AUTONOMIC NERVOUS SYSTEM governs involuntary activities of involuntary muscles.

7. The SOMATIC NERVOUS SYSTEM governs voluntary activities.

8. Information directed toward the brain is termed AFFERENT and information directed from the brain is termed EFFERENT.

9. On the following figure, identify the indicated parts of the neuron.

    A. AXON

    B. DENDRITE

    C. TELODENDRIA

    D. TERMINAL END BOUTON

    E. SYNAPTIC CLEFT

    F. SYNAPTIC VESICLES

    G. POSTSYNAPTIC NEURON

    H. MYELIN SHEATH

    I. SOMA

10. On the following figure, identify the indicated parts of the cerebrum.

    A. <u>Frontal</u> lobe

    B. <u>Temporal</u> lobe

    C. <u>Occipital</u> lobe

    D. <u>Parietal</u> lobe

    E. <u>Precentral</u> gyrus

    F. <u>Postcentral</u> gyrus

    G. <u>Central</u> sulcus

    H. <u>Lateral</u> sulcus

11. On the following figure, identify the parts of the surface of the cerebrum.

    A. <u>Cingulate Gyrus</u>

    B. <u>Corpus Callosum</u>

    C. <u>Superior Temporal Gyrus</u>

    D. <u>Wernicke's Area</u>

    E. <u>Broca's Area</u>

    F. <u>Precentral Gyrus</u>

    G. <u>Heschl's Gyrus</u>

    H. <u>Central Sulcus</u>

12. On the following figure, identify the indicated arteries and structures.

    A. <u>Anterior Cerebral Artery</u>

    B. <u>Middle Cerebral Artery</u>

    C. <u>Posterior Cerebral Artery</u>

    D. <u>Anterior Communicating Artery</u>

    E. <u>Superior Cerebellar Artery</u>

    F. <u>Internal Carotid Artery</u>

    G. <u>Basilar Artery</u>

    H. <u>Vertebral Artery</u>

    I. <u>Circle of Willis</u>

13. Action Potential is a change in electrical potential that occurs when a cell membrane is stimulated adequately to permit ion exchange between intracellular and extracellular spaces.

14. The Absolutely Refractory period is the time during which the cell membrane cannot be stimulated to depolarize.

15. The Relatively Refractory Period is a period during which the membrane can be stimulated to excitation again, but only with greater than typical stimulation.

16. The Nodes of Ranvier of the axon myelin promote saltatory conduction.

17. The substance known as Neurotransmitter is discharged into the synaptic cleft, stimulating the postsynaptic neuron.

18. Higher cognitive processing occurs generally in Association areas.

19. The Temporo-Occipital-Parietal Association area is involved in language function.

20. The Frontal Association area of the cerebrum appears to be involved in higher function related to motor output (such as inhibition of motor function and the ability to change motor responses), whereas the temporal-occipital-parietal association area is involved in language function.

21. The Limbic Association area integrates information relating to affect, motivation, and emotion.

22. The Left hemisphere in most individuals is dominant for language and speech, processes brief duration stimuli, and performs detailed analysis.

23. The Right hemisphere appears to process information in a more holistic fashion, preferring spatial and tonal information.

GLOSSARY

Abdomen	The region represented externally as the front (anterior) abdominal wall.
Abduction	The process of moving two structures farther apart.
Absolute refractory period	The time during depolarization when the cell membrane cannot be stimulated to depolarize again.
Abduction	The process of moving two structures closer together.
Adipose tissue	Areolar tissue that is richly impregnated with fat cells.
Aditus	The entrance of the larynx.
Agonists (prime movers)	Muscles that move a structure.
Alveolar pressure (P_{al})	Pressure in the alveolus. Also referred to as pulmonic pressure.
Alveoli	Air sacs in the lungs.
Anastomoses	Points of communication among arteries.
Anatomical position	The body is erect and the palms and arms face forward.
Anatomy	The study of structure of an organism.
Antagonists	Muscles that oppose a prime mover or agonist.
Anterior	In front of.

Anterior commissure of glottis	The anterior-most region of the glottis.
Aphonia	Loss of voicing.
Aplasia	Lack of development.
Aponeurosis	Sheetlike tendon.
Appendicular skeleton	The portion of the skeleton that includes only the lower and upper limbs.
Applied anatomy	The subdiscipline of anatomy concerned with diagnosis, treatment, and surgical intervention. Also referred to as *clinical anatomy*.
Approximation	When referring to vocal folds, making contact.
Areolar tissue	Supportive connective tissue. Also referred to as *loose connective tissue*.
Arm	The region from the shoulder to the elbow.
Articulate	Join.
Articulation	The process of bringing the mobile and immobile articulators into contact for the purpose of shaping the sounds of speech.
Atmospheric pressure (P_{atm})	Pressure generated as a result of the weight of atmospheric gasses.
Atresia	Absence.
Auditory physiology	The study of auditory function.
Autonomic nervous system	The division of the central nervous system that is responsible for involuntary functions.
Average fundamental frequency	The average frequency of vibration taken over a given time period of phonation.
Axial skeleton	The portion of the skeleton that is the head and trunk, with the spinal column being the axis.
Axes	The real or imaginary line running through the center of a body or structure.
Axon	The terminal point of a neuron, through which information passes.
Baseplate membrane	Thin, membranous subsurface of epithelial tissue that serves structural, functional, and developmental purposes depending on its location. Also referred to as *basement membrane*.
Beating ciliated epithelia	Cells with hairlike protrusions that actively beat to remove contaminants from the epithelial surface.

Bernoulli effect (principle)	Given a constant volume flow of air or liquid, at a point of constriction there will be a decrease in air pressure perpendicular to the flow and an increase in velocity of flow.
Bifurcates	Divides into two parts.
Blood	Connective tissue that contains plasma and blood cells.
Bolus	A mass of masticated food ready to be swallowed.
Bone	Dense, inelastic connective tissue.
Boyle's law	Given a gas of constant temperature, increasing the volume of the chamber in which the gas is contained will cause a corresponding decrease in pressure.
Breaths per minute (bpm)	The number of complete inhalations and exhalations performed in one minute.
Breathy phonation	The mode of phonation produced with extra airflow through the partially adducted vocal folds. Also referred to as *pressed phonation*.
Breathy vocal attack	Phonation by expiration before adduction of the vocal folds.
Broca's area	The region of the third frontal convolution of the dominant hemisphere responsible for speech motor planning.
Buccoversion	Tilted toward the cheek.
Capacity	Functional unit that is a combination of respiratory volumes, used to express physiological limits.
Cardiac muscle	Muscle of the heart, composed of cells that interconnect like a net.
Cartilage	Connective tissue that is elastic.
Caudal	Toward the tail.
Central nervous system (CNS)	The division of the nervous system that contains the brain and spinal cord.
Cephalo-caudal	Development occurs from head to tail.
Cerebrovascular system	The vascular supply of the central and peripheral nervous systems.
Checking action	Using the muscles of inspiration to impede the outflow of air during expiration.
Class I occlusal relationship	The normal occlusal relationship characterized by the maxillary and mandibular molar relationship in which the maxillary first molar is retracted one-half tooth relative to the mandibular first molar. Also referred to as *neutroclusion*.

Class II malocclusion	The occlusal relationship characterized by the maxillary and mandibular molar relationship in which the maxillary first molar is retracted at least one tooth relative to the mandibular first molar.
Class III malocclusion	The occlusal relationship characterized by the maxillary and mandibular molar relationship in which the maxillary first molar is advanced at least one tooth relative to the mandibular first molar.
Clinical eruption	Eruption of dentition through the gum.
Compact bone	Sheetlike bone.
Comparative anatomy	The study of anatomical structures across species.
Compressive strength	The ability of a material to resist crushing.
Connective tissue	Tissue that supports and connects other tissue.
Convergence	The neural process in which outputs of many neurons contribute to the depolarization of a single neuron.
Cornu	Horn.
Corpus	Body.
Cough	Forceful expiration of air following tight adduction of the vocal folds, for the purpose of expelling foreign matter from the airway.
Cranium	The part of the skull that houses the brain.
Cubic centimeter (cc)	A milliliter, or one thousandth of a liter.
Dead air space	The space, representing the conductive passageway of the respiratory system, that contains a volume of air that never undergoes gas exchange (approximately 150 cc in adults).
Deciduous teeth	The primary set of teeth. Also referred to as *shedding teeth*.
Deep	Closer to the central axis of the body.
Dendrite	The component of a neuron that generally receives input from another neuron or sensor.
Descriptive anatomy	The description of individual parts of the body without reference to disease. Also referred to as *systemic* or *systematic anatomy*.
Developmental anatomy	The study of development of the organism's anatomy from conception to adulthood.
Diarthrodial joints	Highly mobile joints lubricated with synovial fluid. Also referred to as *synovial joints*.

Direct motor system	The motor system under voluntary control. Also referred to as *pyramidal motor system.*
Distal	Away from midline.
Distoversion	Tilted away from the midline of the dental arch.
Divergence	The neural process in which one neuron passes information to many other neurons.
Dorsal	The back surface of a body.
Dorsal trunk	The region commonly referred to as "the back."
Dorsiflexion	Hyperextension.
Dysphagia	Disorder of swallowing.
Elasticity	Having the ability and tendency to return to original position.
Electromyography	The study of forces exerted by muscles.
Electrophysiology	Measurement and study of the electrical activity of cells.
Epithelial tissue	Tissue that provides a protective lining for the surface of the body and internal surfaces of cavities.
Eversion	Turning the foot outward.
Expiration	The process of eliminating air from the lungs for respiration.
Expiratory reserve volume (ERV)	The volume of air that can be expired following passive, tidal expiration (approximately 1,000 cc for adults).
Extension	The act of pulling two ends farther apart; the opposite of flexion.
External	Outside a cavity or body.
Extrinsic laryngeal muscles	Muscles with one attachment in the larynx and one attachment outside the larynx.
Falsetto	Phonation high in frequency, which is produced by significant increase in laryngeal tension that results in thinned vocal fold margins.
Fascia	Sheetlike membrane of connective tissue that surrounds organs.
Fibrocartilage	Smooth cartilage with a glassy, blue cast.
Fibrous tissue	Tissue that binds structures together.
Fissure	Significant infolding or complete separation of two structures of the cerebral or cerebellar cortex.
Flexion	Bending at a joint, usually toward the ventral surface.

Force physiology	The study of forces exerted by muscles.
Fossa	Indentation or cavity.
Frontal section	Section that divides the body into front and back portions.
Functional residual capacity (FRC)	The volume of air in the thorax after a passive exhalation (approximately 2,100 cc for adults).
Functional unity	Groups of tissues working for a single functional purpose.
Fundamental frequency	The lowest component of a harmonic series. In phonation, the lowest frequency of the voiced source.
Glandular epithelium	Epithelium that secretes fluids.
Glia (glial cells)	Nervous system tissue that provides support and nutrients in the nervous system.
Glottal attack	Phonatory onset that occurs with the adduction of the vocal folds before expiration.
Glottal fry	A low-frequency mode of vibration characterized by syncopated rhythm and generated by low subglottal air pressure.
Glottis	The space between the vocal folds.
Gross anatomy	The study of structures visible without the aid of microscopy.
Gustation	Sense of taste.
Gyri	Outfolding of tissue on the cerebral or cerebellar cortex.
Habitual pitch	The frequency of vibration of the vocal folds habitually used by an individual during speech.
Hyaline cartilage	Smooth, glassy, blue cartilage for surfaces of bones that come together in joints.
Hyperextension	Extension that continues to the point where the dorsal surfaces approach each other.
Hypertonus	Abnormal increase in muscle tone.
Indirect (extrapyramidal) motor system	The motor system that provides background support for the direct motor system.
Inferior	Below, closer to the ground.
Infraversion	Inadequate eruption relative to the other teeth in the arch.
Innervation	Process of communication of muscles from and to the brain.
Insertion	The point of attachment of a muscle that is mobile when a muscle contracts.
Inspiration	The process of bringing air into the lungs for respiration.

Inspiratory capacity	The maximum inspiratory volume possible after tidal expiration (approximately 3,000 cc in adults).
Inspiratory reserve volume (IRV)	The volume of air that can be inhaled after a tidal inspiration (approximately 2,475 cc for adults).
Internal	Within a cavity or body.
Intonation	The changes in pitch in continuous speech.
Intraoral pressure (P_m)	Pressure in the oral cavity.
Intraosseous eruption	Eruption of dentition through bone.
Intrapleural pressure (P_{pl})	Pressure between the visceral and parietal pleurae.
Intrinsic laryngeal muscles	Muscles with both origin and insertion in the larynx.
Inversion	Turning the sole of the foot inward.
Labioversion	Tilted toward the lip.
Laryngeal stridor	Harsh sound produced upon inhalation or exhalation.
Lateral	To the side.
Lesion	Damage to tissue.
Ligament	Band of connective tissue responsible for binding structures together.
Linguaversion	Tilted toward the tongue.
Loudness	The perceptual correlate of intensity.
Lower extremity	The region that includes the thigh, calf, ankle, and foot.
Lymphoid tissue	Specialized connective tissue in tonsils and adenoids.
Manometer	Device that measures pressure.
Matrix	Intercellular material of connective tissue.
Medial	Toward midline. Also referred to as *mesial*.
Mediastinal	Referring to the mediastinum of the thorax.
Mesioversion	Tilted toward the midline of the dental arch.
Micrognathia	Small mandible relative to the maxillae.
Microscopic anatomy	The study of structures not visible to the unaided eye.
Microtia	Small ear.
Midsagittal section	Section that cuts the body into left and right halves.
Milliliter (mL)	One thousandth of a liter.

Modal register	The mode of vibration used for daily speaking.
Monoloud	Of unvarying vocal loudness.
Monopitch	Speech with little or no perceived variation in pitch.
Morphology	Form.
Motor (efferent/excitatory) innervation	Innervation that causes muscles to contract or glands to secrete.
Motor nerve	Nerve that activates muscle or glands.
Motor unit	Tissue consisting of one motor nerve fiber and the muscle fibers to which it attaches.
Muscular tissue	Tissue that is capable of contraction.
Nares	Nostrils.
Nasal regurgitation	Loss of masticated food through the nasal cavity.
Necrotic tissue	Dead tissue.
Neural tissue	Tissue that is specialized to transmit information.
Neuraxis	The axis of the nervous system, including spinal cord, brainstem, and cerebrum.
Neuromuscular junction	The point of synapse between muscle fiber and motor fiber.
Neurons (nerve cells)	Tissue specialized for communication.
Neutroclusion	The normal occlusal relationship characterized by the maxillary and mandibular molar relationship in which the maxillary first molar is retracted one-half tooth relative to the mandibular first molar.
Occlusion	Closing.
Olfaction	Sense of smell.
Optimal pitch	The most efficient frequency of vibration of the vocal folds.
Origin	The point of attachment of a muscle that is immobile when a muscle contracts.
Oscillation	Repeated vibration of a body at the same frequency.
Overjet	Condition of normal dentition in which the upper incisors overlap and hide the lower incisors.
Palmar grasp reflex	Reaction of stimulation of the palm that causes the fingers to grasp.
Palmar	Referring to the palm of hand.
Palpation	Feeling a structure using one's hands.

Paralysis	Loss of voluntary motor function due to lesion in the nervous system.
Parasternal	Near the sternum.
Parasympathetic nervous system	The component of the autonomic nervous system responsible for body system responses.
Paresis	Weakness arising from lesion in the nervous system.
Pathological anatomy	The area of study concerned with diseased tissue.
Pelvis	The area of the hip bones.
Pericardium	The membranous sac enclosing the heart.
Perimysium	Special fascia surrounding muscle.
Periosteum	Fibrous membrane covering of a bone.
Peripheral	Away from the center of the body.
Peripheral nervous system (PNS)	The division of the nervous system that contains cranial and spinal nerves.
Persistent closed bite	The posterior dentition fails to occlude properly as a result of supraversion of the anterior teeth.
Persistent open bite	Anterior dentition fails to occlude properly as a result of supraversion of the posterior teeth.
Pharyngeal recesses	Valleculae and pyriform sinuses.
Physiology	The study of an organism's function.
Pitch	The perceptual correlate of frequency of vibration.
Pitch range	The range of phonation possible, calculated as the highest frequency of vibration minus the lowest frequency of vibration.
Plane	A flat or relatively smooth surface.
Plantar flexion	Extension of the toes.
Plantar grasp reflex	Reaction to stimulation of the sole of the foot that causes the toe of the feet to "grasp."
Plasma	Fluid component of blood.
Posterior	Toward the back; behind.
Posterior commissure of glottis	The posterior-most region of the glottis.
Process	An anatomical structure protruding from a surface.
Pronation	Rotation of the hand so the palmar surface is directed inferiorly.
Prone	Lying on the belly.

Propagation	The spreading effect of wave action; in neural responses, the communication of information through the nervous system.
Prosody	Combination of changes in fundamental frequency and vocal intensity that provides linguistically relevant information (e.g., vocal pitch, intonation, loudness, duration, and rhythm).
Proximal	Near a body or structure.
Proximo-distal	Development occurs from medial to distal structures.
Quiet tidal volume	Tidal volume at rest.
Residual volume (RV)	The volume of air in the lungs after a maximum exhalation; the volume of air that cannot be expelled (approximately 1,100 cc in adults).
Respiration	Exchange of gas between an organism and its environment.
Respiratory physiology	The study of all processes involved in breathing.
Resting membrane potential (RMP)	The condition of a neuron at rest, in which it is polarized and ready to discharge.
Rostral	Toward the head.
Sagittal plane	Plane created by a sagittal section.
Sagittal section	Section that divides the body into left and right parts.
Saltatory conduction	The process in a neural response in which information in the axon passes from node to node, thereby greatly increasing conduction speed.
Sensory (afferent) innervation	Innervation that provides the central nervous system with information about the state of the body or tissues.
Sign	Measurable or objective component of illness or condition.
Simultaneous vocal attack	Phonation initiated through simultaneous adduction and expiration of vocal folds.
Skeletal ligaments	Connective tissue that binds bone to bone.
Smooth muscle	Muscular tissue not under voluntary control, especially of the digestive tract and blood vessels.
Soma	The cell body of a neuron.
Somatic nervous system	The subdivision of the nervous system responsible for voluntary motor function and nonvisceral sensation.
Spatial summation	The quality of some neurons wherein they require multiple synaptic inputs from a broad array of neurons in order to be stimulated to depolarize.

Spectral analysis	Analysis of a signal that identifies frequency components of that signal.
Spirometer	Device that measures volume of air expelled or inspired.
Spongy bone	Porous bone.
Stenosis	Narrowing.
Stress	The emphasis on a word produced in continuous speech, relative to the emphasis of the entire utterance.
Striated muscle	Skeletal muscle, voluntary muscle.
Subglottal pressure (P_s)	Pressure beneath the level of the vocal folds.
Successional teeth	Teeth in the mature dental arch that replace corresponding teeth of the deciduous arch.
Sulci	Minor infolding of tissue on the cerebral or cerebellar cortex.
Superficial	Confined to the surface.
Superior	Above; farther from the ground.
Supination	Rotation of the hand so the palmar surface is directed superiorly.
Supine	Lying on the back.
Supraglottal	The region above the vocal folds.
Suprasegmental	Information in the speech signal that spans two or more phonemes; generally called prosodic elements.
Supraversion	Excessive eruption relative to the majority of teeth in the arch.
Surface anatomy	The study of the form and structure of the surface of the body, especially with reference to the organs beneath the surface.
Sympathetic nervous system	The component of the autonomic nervous system responsible for body system responses that prepare the body to cope with stressful situations.
Synergists	Muscles used to stabilize structures.
Temporal summation	The quality of some neurons wherein the neuron requires virtually simultaneous inputs from other neurons before it can be stimulated to depolarize.
Tendons	Connective tissue bands that are part of the muscle and attach muscle to bone or cartilage.
Tensile strength	The ability of a material to resist being pulled apart.
Thorax	The chest region.
Tidal volume	The volume of air exchanged during one cycle of respiration.

Torquing	Twisting of a shaft while one end does not move.
Torsiversion	Twisted on the long axis.
Total lung capacity (TLC)	The total volume of the respiratory system that can undergo gas exchange, equaling the sum of tidal volume, inspiratory reserve volume, expiratory reserve volume, and residual volume (approximately 5,100 cc in adults).
Transverse section	Section that divides the body into upper and lower halves.
Upper extremity	The region consisting of the arm, forearm, wrist, and hand.
Valleculae	Pair of small indentations between the tongue and epiglottis.
Ventral	The front surface of a body.
Ventricular	Referring to cavities or passageways to structures.
Visceral ligaments	Connective tissue that binds organs together or holds structures in place.
Vital capacity (VC)	The combination of inspiratory reserve volume, expiratory reserve volume, and tidal volume, representing the capacity of air available for speech (approximately 4,000 cc in adults).
Vocal folds (vocal cords)	The vibrating component of the larynx used to produce sound.
Vocal tract	The oral cavity, the pharynx, and the nasal cavity.
Volume	In respiration, the displacement of air that represents specifically partitioned components of the respiratory system, measured in cubic centimeters or cubic inches.
Whispered speech	Speech produced without vocal fold vibration by causing air to pass along the edges of the tensed vocal folds, thus producing a friction sound source.
White fibrous tissue	Connective tissue that is strong, dense, and highly organized.
Yellow (elastic) cartilage	Cartilage that has greater elasticity than other forms of cartilage.
Yellow elastic tissue	Connective tissue in cartilage.

INDEX

Installing Anatesse

1. Insert CD-ROM in CD-ROM drive on your computer.
2. Before program can be installed, you will be queried to read and agree to the Thomson Delmar Learning licensing agreement. You will not be able to continue with the installation until you click the AGREE button.
3. Installation should continue automatically and a SKULL icon will appear on the desktop.
4. If this does not happen, double-click on SETUP.EXE in the CD and follow the instructions in the installer. When done, you should have an icon for Anatesse showing on your desktop.
5. If the installer finished properly but you don't have a SKULL icon, you can run Anatesse from the Start button or create an icon.

Running Anatesse for the First Time

1. Anatesse is a study guide that always gives you a grade report at the end of each lesson. Your instructor will decide whether that report is to be recorded for actual grading. If so, you should keep a floppy disk to hold your grades and turn in the disk when your instructor requests it.
2. On the first use of Anatesse, insert an empty disk in the computer's slot, then start the program. You will be asked for a name or ID; your instructor should specify a form of identification, such as last name or student number. Then you will need to enter a password. This should consist of letters and/or numbers, with no spaces or punctuation. Capitalization does not matter: if you set up your password as SNAP and later enter snap or sNaP, it will still work. Once the floppy has been registered, you can continue on to the actual lessons.
3. After the first use, simply insert the same floppy disk before starting the program; you will be asked for your password.
4. When this initial stage is over, you will see a Select Lesson list; from there you will proceed to work whichever lesson is assigned or is next.
5. If you have to leave a lesson before finishing, a Bookmark will be created on your floppy disk. The next time you start up the Select Lesson menu will indicate a Bookmark for that lesson and you will be able to start where you left off by clicking the "Start from Bookmark" button instead of the regular Start.
6. You can see your own grades by starting Anatesse and hitting the Read Grades button. (A separate Help text is available inside that action.)
7. Anatesse looks best at a screen resolution of 800×600. At larger resolutions the frame expands to fill the screen, but some images will look rough. If you prefer a frame that stays the same size, switch the desktop shortcut from ANATESSE.EXE to ANATESSE2.EXE.

License Agreement for Delmar Learning, a division of Thomson Learning, Inc.

Educational Software/Data

You the customer, and Delmar Learning, a division of Thomson Learning, Inc. incur certain benefits, rights, and obligations to each other when you open this package and use the software/data it contains. BE SURE YOU READ THE LICENSE AGREEMENT CAREFULLY, SINCE BY USING THE SOFTWARE/DATA YOU INDICATE YOU HAVE READ, UNDERSTOOD, AND ACCEPTED THE TERMS OF THIS AGREEMENT.

Your rights:

1. You enjoy a non-exclusive license to use the software/data on a single microcomputer in consideration for payment of the required license fee (which may be included in the purchase price of an accompanying print component), or receipt of this software/data, and your acceptance of the terms and conditions of this agreement.
2. You acknowledge that you do not own the aforesaid software/data. You also acknowledge that the software/data is furnished "as is," and contains copyrighted and/or proprietary and confidential information of Delmar Learning, a division of Thomson Learning, Inc. or its licensors.

There are limitations on your rights:

1. You may not copy or print the software/data for any reason whatsoever, except to install it on a hard drive on a single microcomputer and to make one archival copy, unless copying or printing is expressly permitted in writing or statements recorded on the diskette(s).
2. You may not revise, translate, convert, disassemble or otherwise reverse engineer the software/data except that you may add to or rearrange any data recorded on the media as part of the normal use of the software/data.
3. You may not sell, license, lease, rent, loan or otherwise distribute or network the software/data except that you may give the software/data to a student or and instructor for use at school or temporarily at home.

Should you fail to abide by the Copyright Law of the United States as it applies to this software/data your license to use it will become invalid. You agree to erase or otherwise destroy the software/data immediately after receiving note of termination of this agreement for violation of its provisions from Delmar Learning.

Delmar Learning, a division of Thomson Learning, Inc. gives you a LIMITED WARRANTY covering the enclosed software/data. The LIMITED WARRANTY follows this License.

This license is the entire agreement between you and Delmar Learning, a division of Thomson Learning, Inc. interpreted and enforced under New York law.

LIMITED WARRANTY

Delmar Learning, a division of Thomson Learning, Inc. warrants to the original licensee/purchaser of this copy of microcomputer software/data and the media on which it is recorded that the media will be free from defects in material and workmanship for ninety (90) days from the date of original purchase. All implied warranties are limited in duration to this ninety (90) day period. THEREAFTER, ANY IMPLIED WARRANTIES, INCLUDING IMPLIED WARRANTIES OF MERCHANTABILITY AND FITNESS FOR A PARTICULAR PURPOSE, ARE EXCLUDED. THIS WARRANTY IS IN LIEU OF ALL OTHER WARRANTIES, WHETHER ORAL OR WRITTEN, EXPRESS OR IMPLIED.

If you believe the media is defective please return it during the ninety day period to the address shown below. Defective media will be replaced without charge provided that it has not been subjected to misuse or damage.

This warranty does not extend to the software or information recorded on the media. The software and information are provided "AS IS." Any statements made about the utility of the software or information are not to be considered as express or implied warranties.

Limitation of liability: Our liability to you for any losses shall be limited to direct damages, and shall not exceed the amount you paid for the software. In no event will we be liable to you for any indirect, special, incidental, or consequential damages (including loss of profits) even if we have been advised of the possibility of such damages.

Some states do not allow the exclusion or limitation of incidental or consequential damages, or limitations on the duration of implied warranties, so the above limitation or exclusion may not apply to you. This warranty gives you specific legal rights, and you may also have other rights which vary from state to state. Address all correspondence to: Delmar Learning, a division of Thomson Learning, Inc., 5 Maxwell Drive, P.O. Box 8007, Clifton Park, NY 12065-8007. Attention: Technology Department